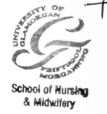

Illustrated Manual of
ORTHOPAEDIC MEDICINE

ILLUSTRATED MANUAL
OF
ORTHOPAEDIC MEDICINE

James Cyriax M.D., M.R.C.P.

Honorary Consultant in Orthopaedic Medicine
St Thomas's Hospital, London
Visiting Professor in Orthopaedic Medicine
University of Rochester Medical Centre, New York

Patricia Cyriax M.C.S.P.

Butterworths
London   Boston   Durban   Singapore   Sydney   Toronto   Wellington

First published 1983
Reprinted 1984
Reprinted 1985

© OM Publications 1983, 206 Albany Street, London NW1

British Library Cataloguing in Publication Data

Cyriax, James
    Illustrated manual of orthopaedic medicine.
    1. Orthopedia
    I. Title   II. Cyriax, Patricia
    617'.3   RD731

    ISBN 0-407-00262-6

Library of Congress Cataloging in Publication Data

Cyriax, James Henry.
    Illustrated manual of orthopaedic medicine.
    Includes index.
    1. Orthopedia.
    I. Cyriax, Patricia.   II. Title.
    [DNLM: 1. Orthopedics.   WE 168 C997i]
    RD731.C897   1983   617'.3   83-3763

    ISBN 0-407-00262-6

Typeset by Scribe Design Ltd, Gillingham, Kent
Origination by Peak Litho Ltd, Tonbridge, Kent
Printed by Cambus Litho Ltd, Scotland
Bound by Hunter & Foulis Ltd, Scotland

This book is dedicated to S.J.N.

PREFACE

*The role and
development of
orthopaedic medicine*

Few conditions are as common as soft-tissue lesions; not many ailments respond so readily to treatment. Yet all too often their care is regarded as a matter of indifference or, little better, as the province of a narrow and complex specialty beyond ordinary reach.

Both views are misconceived; orthopaedic medicine is a straightforward and practical discipline for the profession at large. With the publication of this book, the work has at last been distilled into terms suitable for ready adoption by the ordinary practitioner, whether family doctor, physiotherapist or sports therapist.

This represents an important step forward; orthopaedic medicine may have been born in 1929, but only now is it coming of age. Since the early years tremendous strides have been realised in diagnostic theory but, perhaps for want of a working textbook, the subject has not made its deserved headway towards widespread implementation. To take just two examples, since the mid-1940s it has been possible to abort arthritis of the shoulder, saving the patient anything up to a year's pain; and likewise by a simple injection to deal with many cases of otherwise intractable backache. But in only a tiny proportion of cases do patients needing such treatment actually receive it, and this kind of neglect means that over the years orthopaedic medicine has retained its anomalous status as a discipline that has been overlooked but not superceded. Only its resolute insistence on the virtues of clinical examination, accurate diagnosis and accurate treatment might be termed old-fashioned, but no substitutes can replace these skills.

It is true that all sorts of sophisticated new technologies have developed over the last 50 years—arthrograms, myelograms, ultrasound, blood tests, computerised diagnostic aids and so on. Naturally these are indispensible in the appropriate circumstances, but it so happens that they have no bearing on the ordinary soft-tissue lesion. Thus a patient with, say, a sprained ligament has nothing wrong with his blood or his bones, and an arthrogram may show up an osteoarthrosis that is in reality painless. Procedures boasting the latest equipment, whether diagnostic or therapeutic, are no advance when meted out indiscriminately. The most modern exercise machines or heat delivery systems cannot be regarded as up to date if the patient does not need these treatments; what matters is to establish what is wrong with the patient and then to treat him for that condition.

This was the challenge facing me in 1929. I then found, starting as an orthopaedic house surgeon, that patients were divisible into two categories—those whose defects showed up on the X-ray and those whose X-rays were normal. At that time it was the custom to pass the latter on for physiotherapy, consisting of various kinds of heat therapy, general diffuse massage, and exercises. It was a question of divided responsibility. No diagnosis was made or attempted in either the Orthopaedic or Physiotherapy Departments, and the treatments were not given because they were indicated or even specified but simply because they were available. Fifty years later one still hears of patients diagnosed as 'painful shoulder' and batched for heat therapy or exercise classes.

To be effective, treatment must be an appropriate countermeasure for the condition diagnosed, and this is as much the concern of the doctor as the physiotherapist. The doctor cannot wash his hands of the patient merely by referral elsewhere with some vague label; for he can rest assured that no one else will make good any shortcomings in his initial diagnosis. Whenever a patient is sent for physiotherapy, it must be with the diagnostic certainty not only that physiotherapy is the appropriate recourse but also that the physiotherapist knows the work, that is, how to treat the right tissue in the right way. In such an informed context, the relationship between physician and physiotherapist becomes complementary; he can inject where she cannot; she can take much time-consuming work off his hands by massage or manipulation. Between the two of them, nearly all patients can be dealt with on the spot; generally the last thing needed is to call in a specialist, least of all a specialist outside the field of soft-tissue lesions.

To summarize the basic principles of orthopaedic medicine is now the matter of a few minutes, but from 1929 it took nearly two decades to establish the theoretical groundwork; the findings first saw publication in 1947 in book form as *Rheumatism and Soft-Tissue Lesions*. Over the years this work grew until it now stands as the *Textbook of Orthopaedic Medicine* Volumes 1 and 2, together spanning some 900 closely-argued pages. These titles are the repository of the sum total of my investigations into soft-tissue lesions and are, I believe, the standard reference work.

But as interest in orthopaedic medicine blossomed, so a need arose for a renewed publishing programme. One fundamental requirement was an introductory textbook with a broader appeal for the working practitioner, uniting the entire discipline in a single volume. This was the genesis of the *Illustrated Manual of Orthopaedic Medicine*. Nearly all the processes—whether examination, injection, massage or manipulation—lend themselves readily to step-by-step photography; hence the major role in this new book accorded to the illustrations, which constitute virtually a complete presentation of orthopaedic medicine in their own right. Indeed, it seemed only logical to press on to make a 'film of the book' and accordingly a companion series of 10 half-hour videotapes has now been completed.

The trail for this substantial undertaking was blazed by the *Textbook of Orthopaedic Medicine*; with the arrival of the *Illustrated Manual* the profession has at last a practical guide. Although it is true that exclusive reliance on this work alone will mean the rare and difficult cases remain obscure, as a rule the material has been not so much simplified as clarified. This book sets out to equip the reader to face the great bulk of his patients with confidence. Everyone sees these cases; with a little effort nearly everyone can diagnose and treat them with gratifying success.

James Cyriax
London 1982

Note on the drawings
Where injections are depicted only the exterior portion of the needle is portrayed, with a small marker indicating the spot at which the skin is punctured. The point or points of delivery of the solution is designated by red dots.

In site drawings which feature multiple arrows, the size of the arrow is directly related to the frequency with which the lesion occurs at any given location.

ACKNOWLEDGEMENTS

No project of this kind can be undertaken without the help of many friends and colleagues.

In particular I am grateful to my wife both for her assistance on the text and for the production of the anatomical drawings.

The live-action photography was most ably contributed by Pablo Keller. My thanks are also due to Robert de Coninck, founder of the Belgian Scientific Society of Orthopaedic Medicine, for his advice and suggestions on the manuscript; any errors that remain are, of course, mine alone.

Finally I should mention this undertaking was initiated at the insistence of, and supervised by, OM Publications under whose direction the illustrations and photographs were executed, the text prepared for publication and the book designed. They in their turn wish, through me, to acknowledge a considerable debt to the long-suffering editorial staff at Butterworths who have taken this venture through to fruition.

J.H.C.

CONTENTS

PART ONE

GENERAL PRINCIPLES

CHAPTER ONE

PRINCIPLES OF
DIAGNOSIS

Orthopaedic medicine is concerned with the diagnosis and treatment of soft-tissue lesions. These disorders affect a substantial proportion of all patients in general and family medicine; cases are additionally found in the departments of orthopaedic surgery, rheumatology, neurology, casualty and, in particular, physiotherapy and sports clinics. Sooner or later nearly everyone suffers some such complaint.

In broad terms these disorders embrace conditions commonly called arthritis, rheumatism, fibrositis, backache, lumbago, sacroiliac strain, sciatica, frozen shoulder, tennis elbow, strained wrist, 'gammy' knee, sprained ankle, aches, sprains, inflammation and sports injuries generally.

However, this broad nomenclature encompasses what is, in reality, a multitude of distinct and readily distinguishable conditions. Once accurately diagnosed they permit the formulation of rapid and effective treatment—lacking which the pain and disability may persist for weeks, months or years. Soft-tissue lesions are thus a common cause of avoidable pain.

The scope of orthopaedic medicine.

Diagnostic problems

The X-ray

The soft moving tissues share one thing in common—they are all radiotranslucent.

The tissues in question are the joint capsule, the ligaments, the fasciae, muscles, tendons, bursae and discs; at the spine the dura mater and dural sheaths to the emergent nerve roots are included. Any of these structures can cause pain; none of them, inflamed or otherwise, is visible on the radiograph.

If the pain does arise from a soft tissue, the X-ray can show only one of two things.

First, it may reveal the bones are normal, in which case the X-ray plays a negative role.

Second, the X-ray may disclose some symptomless abnormality, which is then mistakenly regarded as the source of pain. In this case the radiograph is positively misleading. For example, many patients with a stiff neck have cervical osteoarthrosis or cervical spondylosis. But enquiry may reveal that the patient's pain started only last month,

whereas the osteophytes have been in existence for a decade or more. After the pain has vanished a couple of months later, it turns out that the osteophytes remain unchanged. In fact, cervical osteoarthrosis is all but universal to those over 40 and is of itself symptomless. The cause of pain lies elsewhere.

To the physician confronted by a soft-tissue lesion the radiograph is at best of doubtful assistance. This poses a serious diagnostic problem. The patient complains, say, of a painful arm but there are no objective signs. In fact, the lesion might lie at any one of a number of sites in the joint capsule, supraspinatus, infraspinatus, subscapularis, subdeltoid bursa, biceps or neck.

Palpation

The difficulty is compounded because a lesion of any of these tissues can make the whole shoulder and arm ache, giving rise to apparently indistinguishable symptoms. Before effective treatment can be administered, the one defective tissue must be singled out. If not, any therapy will be directed not at the disordered structure but at an adjacent or even relatively distant healthy structure. All pain has a source; the job of the diagnostician is to find it.

Palpation is often assumed to provide the answer. But nearly all pain is felt at other than its point of origin. The symptoms may be referred by as little as a centimetre or as much as a metre, but in either case the margin of error is too great. Effective treatment must be delivered not just to the right tissue, but to the right part of the right tissue—to the lesion itself. It is no good treating the infraspinatus if the supraspinatus is at fault, nor is it any improvement if the supraspinatus is treated at the distal site when the lesion lies proximally.

Palpation will regularly deceive. The soft tissues—with one exception—refer pain on a segmental basis. Thus the great majority of shoulder structures refer pain in identical fashion to the dermatome corresponding to their embryological derivation: C5. But the C5 dermatome does not include the point of the shoulder or the scapular area; it extends down the arm. So the painful area outlined by the patient may not even contain the lesion. Any tenderness that is found may itself be referred; in any case, many spots are normally sensitive. The lesion may be buried beyond the reach of the physician's fingers and furthermore he will be unable to distinguish symptoms of psychogenic origin.

The least reliable way to diagnose in soft-tissue lesions is to palpate or prod immediately in the area delineated by the patient. Neither the discovery of trigger or myalgic spots nor any description of the nature of the pain—throbbing, burning, stabbing or otherwise—do much, if anything, to indicate their origin and cause. In common with the X-ray, palpation does a great deal to mislead.

The diagnostic approach

Like other medical disciplines, orthopaedic medicine relies for its diagnosis on assessment of function. With the soft tissues this is relatively easy: a joint moves within certain known limits, certain muscles are responsible for certain movements. It is merely necessary to devise a system to detect abnormalities and relate any defect to a specific tissue.

Clinical examination is the key. A healthy structure will function painlessly; a faulty structure will not. Thus each tissue from which pain could arise is put through its paces in turn and as each structure has a known and separate function this presents few obstacles. The tissue that cannot operate without bringing on the pain is the culprit.

The mechanism of diagnosis is tension, applied manually. The physician subjects each tissue about the incriminated joint to tension in turn. This process is known as 'selective tension'.

Inert and contractile structures

A basic distinction is drawn between contractile structures—the muscle and its attachments—and those which are inert. These latter lack the capacity to contract and relax.

The inert structures are the joint capsule, the ligaments, fasciae, bursae, the dura mater and the dural sheaths to the nerve roots. From this distinction the possibility of the clinically pure movement is derived. Tension can be applied manually by the examiner to assess the contractile and inert structures separately.

Passive movements

If the patient relaxes her limb and the physician moves it for her (*Figure 1.1*) the inert structures will be stretched; but no material strain is brought to bear on the contractile tissues. So if a passive movement hurts, an inert structure is at fault. The inert structures are stretched at the extreme of range of the joint and it is then that any pain would be apparent.

Fig 1.1 *A passive movement. Passive internal rotation stretches one aspect of the shoulder capsule. As the patient is relaxed, the contractile structures are not subjected to strain.*

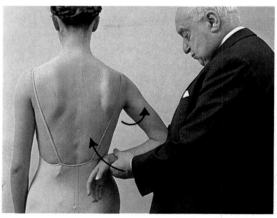

1.1

Resisted movements

If the physician holds the joint still while the patient exerts her muscles to their utmost against his resistance, no material strain falls on the inert structures. Instead it devolves upon the particular muscle or muscle group responsible for the attempted movement. For example, if the patient tries to adduct her arm while the movement is thwarted by the doctor (*Figure 1.2*), then tension is put on the pectoralis major, both teres muscles and the latissimus dorsi. Thus if a resisted movement brings on or accentuates the pain the relevant contractile structure is incriminated. The joint is best held at mid-range.

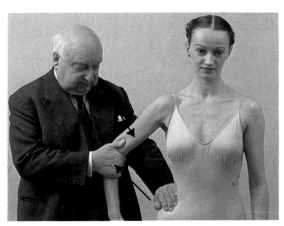

1.2

Any suspected joint can thus be appraised by subjecting the tissues about it to a routine of passive and resisted movements. A distinctive pattern of pain and limitation emerges, based on applied anatomy, which allows for identification of the tissue (and often the part of the tissue) at fault. The state of the structure under examination is thus divulged not by palpation but in the conventionally accepted way—by seeing how well it functions. Palpation may or may not follow but will, in any case, be confined to the tissue at fault, and even then is only performed if the structure lies within reach of the fingers.

Finally, each lesion has a distinctive history, and the taking of a thorough chronological history together with the clinical examination will seldom fail to identify the condition. The history is an integral part of the examination.

Structure of this chapter

The inferences to be drawn from this and the preceding pages are set out in tabular form below to which progressive addition is made in the course of the chapter. The theoretical discussion in the following pages takes the basic principles first, commencing with resisted movements and ending with history and referred pain; it goes over in greater depth the ground already covered in outline.

However, in the consulting room these principles are implemented in the reverse order: the clinical examination starts with the taking of a history and finishes by testing the movements against resistance. In the chart below it is this layout, corresponding to the actual routine of clinical work, that is adopted. The table is built up in succeeding variants; as new theoretical findings derived from the text are incorporated they are highlighted.

Examination: an example

The physician confronted by, say, a patient with a shoulder pain will, after first clarifying the history, see if moving the patient's neck brings on the pain. If not, there is nothing wrong with structures responsible for movement of the neck. Similarly, he then ascertains whether movement at the shoulder elicits the pain. If so, the shoulder is then subjected to a routine of 12 passive and resisted movements. A common finding would be painful resisted abduction pointing to a defect of the supraspinatus. A painful arc, if present, will reveal the exact site of the lesion in the supraspinatus. Painful resisted lateral rotation incriminates the infraspinatus. No individual glenohumeral ligaments at the shoulder malfunction, but inflammation of the

Fig 1.2 *A resisted movement. The doctor forcibly resists the patient's adduction. Resisted movements provide clear information on the state of each muscle group.*

CLINICAL EXAMINATION: SUMMARY I

The moving soft tissues are radiotranslucent. Palpate only after examination, along structure already identified as at fault.		
A. History/Referred Pain	**B. Assessment by Function**	
1. Take a history.	2. Examine incriminated joint by selective tension employing:	
	PASSIVE MOVEMENTS for inert structures: *joint capsule, ligaments, bursae, fascia, displacements, dura mater, nerve roots.*	RESISTED MOVEMENTS for contractile structures: *muscles, tendons and attachment to bone.*

joint capsule will limit passive abduction as well as passive medial and passive lateral rotation.

Although the history at the shoulder is generally insignificant, if immobility of spontaneous origin comes on over 3 days rather than over a more protracted period, acute subdeltoid bursitis is the probable cause.

Only finally will the physician palpate. The patient is first positioned so the defective structure by now identified is rendered accessible to the examiner's fingers. If assessment of function has revealed only that the lesion is situated in an extensive structure

(e.g. the subdeltoid bursa) but not the exact part, the physician palpates for tenderness along that structure to pinpoint the lesion's precise location. Otherwise (i.e. if the disorder is known to lie in a small tissue) palpation is simply used to locate the tissue itself prior to treatment. Sensitivity of neighbouring structures is ignored. For example, even when the supraspinatus is inflamed the bone of the tuberosity lying anterior to it is still more tender. Throughout this book any recommendation to palpate refers to the search for tenderness conducted in a tissue already singled out by assessment of function.

Resisted movements

If one resisted movement proves painful, the overwhelming likelihood is that the other resisted movements will be painless. Furthermore, the fact that a resisted movement increases the pain means that a particular contractile structure is the source of pain. The passive movements should therefore be painless and of full range. The physician thus seeks congruous positive and negative findings; in the absence of a double lesion all the symptoms should be referrable to a single source. Simple although resisted movements are, various considerations should be borne in mind:

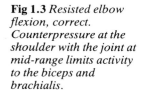

Fig 1.3 *Resisted elbow flexion, correct. Counterpressure at the shoulder with the joint at mid-range limits activity to the biceps and brachialis.*

Fig 1.4 *Resisted adduction, incorrect.*

(1) The joint should be held at mid-range (*Figure 1.3*) so that no inert structures are stretched.
(2) No movement should take place at the joint.
(3) Muscles other than those being tested must not be included (*Figure 1.4*). For instance, where resisted movements at the shoulder

are tested, the examiner must make sure that the trunk muscles are not activated.
(4) The patient must be encouraged to rally all her reserves of strength.
(5) The examiner should pay considerable attention to where he stands and how he manages his hands. This is particularly so because he is examining not just for increased pain but also for weakness.

Weakness
When strong muscles are tested, minor weakness cannot be detected unless the hands are well placed for resistance and counterpressure; the examiner's body must be properly positioned. For example, when the power of resisted abduction at the shoulder is tested, if the examiner stands facing the patient's side then he is toppled over backwards. But if he is stationed in front of or behind the patient, one hand at her elbow and the other on the far flank at her waist, a true assessment is arrived at.

Findings on resisted movements
(1) *Strong and painless:* nothing is the matter with the contractile structures.
(2) *Strong and painful:* this common finding designates a minor lesion of some part of a muscle or tendon, both almost invariably susceptible to treatment.
(3) *Weak and painless:* this can suggest a complete rupture of the relevant muscle or tendon, but much more often implicates a disorder of the nervous system. Impaired conduction along a nerve leads to muscle weakness; thus if a lesion at the cervical spine compresses the C5 nerve root then abduction will be weak.
(4) *Weak and painful:* serious trouble is present, for example a fracture or secondary deposits.

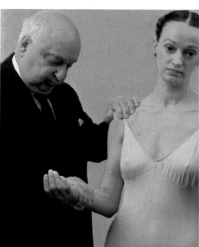
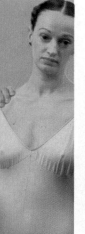

1.3   1.4

CLINICAL EXAMINATION: SUMMARY II

The moving soft tissues are radiotranslucent. Palpate only after examination, along structure already identified as at fault.		
A. History/Referred Pain	**B. Assessment by Function**	
1. Take a history.	2. Examine incriminated joint by selective tension employing:	
	PASSIVE MOVEMENTS for inert structures: *joint capsule, ligaments, bursae, fascia, displacements, dura mater, nerve roots.*	**RESISTED MOVEMENTS for** contractile structures: *muscles, tendons and attachment to bone.*
		Examine for: a) pain b) weakness. *Principal findings* a) pain: lesion of appropriate contractile structure. b) painless weakness: interference with conduction of appropriate nerve. c) strong and painless: normal.

(5) *Painful on repetition:* if a movement is strong and painless but is found to hurt after a number of repetitions, intermittent claudication is the probability.

(6) *All the resisted movements hurt:* this could be a gross lesion lying proximally, but is more likely to stem from neurosis.

In practice the resisted movements are performed after the passive movements which take precedence as joint signs.

Passive movements

With the exception of partial rupture in a muscle, a lesion of a contractile structure will not produce limitation on passive movement. Thus if there is limitation of passive movement an inert structure must be at fault and 5° restriction of passive range carries quite a different significance from full range. The exact situation must be determined, and in cases of doubt the examiner may have to push fairly hard to arrive at a true picture; where a painful arc is present it may take some persuasion to get beyond it to establish that pain does in fact cease at full range.

If the movements show the lesion to lie in an inert structure, the primary question is whether the lesion involves the entire capsule or some other inert structure, that is, whether the lesion is capsular or non-capsular. If the latter, there are various possible explanations, by far the commonest of which are internal derangement and ligamentous sprain, although occasionally the cause of non-capsular limitation on passive movement may be extra-articular.

These classifications are considered below.

Findings on passive movements

Capsular lesions

If an entire joint capsule is inflamed, all or most passive movements of that joint will strain a different part of the capsule so that all or most of the passive movements will prove painful and limited.

This constitutes one of the most important concepts in orthopaedic medicine, namely that a lesion of the entire capsule will give rise to limitation in the capsular pattern. Thus arthritis is designated by the capsular pattern which:

(1) varies from joint to joint.
(2) is denoted by limitation not in a fixed degree but in a fixed proportion.

Thus at the wrist the capsular pattern is equal limitation of flexion and extension with little limitation of deviations. At the shoulder the pattern is so much limitation of abduction, more limitation than that of lateral rotation and less limitation than that of medial rotation.

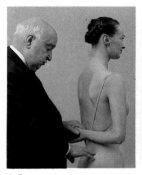
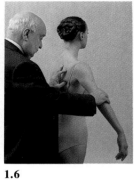
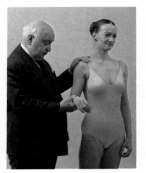

1.5　　　　**1.6**　　　　**1.7**

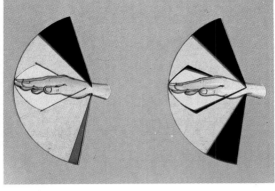

1.8, 1.9

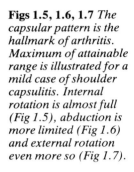

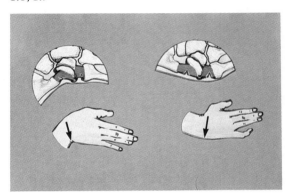

1.10, 1.11

Figs 1.5, 1.6, 1.7 *The capsular pattern is the hallmark of arthritis. Maximum of attainable range is illustrated for a mild case of shoulder capsulitis. Internal rotation is almost full (Fig 1.5), abduction is more limited (Fig 1.6) and external rotation even more so (Fig 1.7).*

Figs 1.8, 1.9 *The non-capsular and capsular patterns. A carpal capitate subluxation limits extension and hurts on flexion (Fig 1.8), whereas arthritis limits both equally (Fig 1.9).*

Figs 1.10, 1.11 *A strained ligament causes pain on one passive movement only (right). Passive ulnar deviation does not stretch the ulnar collateral ligament (left).*

In a severe case the limitations would amount to, for example, 80°, 110° and 30° respectively. In a less pronounced case they would adhere to similar proportions, coming to, for example, 30°, 60° and 5° respectively (*Figures 1.5; 1.6; 1.7*).

The pattern is the same whatever the cause of arthritis. The reason for the existence of the capsular pattern appears to be merely that different aspects of the joint capsule resent stretching more than others.

In the early cases it is muscle spasm springing into play to prevent capsular stretching beyond a certain point that protects the joint. The restriction of mobility will, however, still be in the capsular pattern. The spasm is secondary to the capsular lesion at the joint and is itself painless.

For the traditional notion of arthritis recognised by limitation of movement in every direction should be substituted the concept of limitation conforming to the capsular pattern for that particular joint. The arthritis can continue for many months without giving rise to any radiological evidence of disease.

The capsular pattern for every joint is listed in Appendix III.

Internal derangement
If limitation of passive movement is discovered in proportions not conforming to the capsular pattern, arthritis is absent and lesions capable of restricting range, but not involving the entire joint, have to be considered. The principal possibilities are ligamentous strain (discussed below) and internal derangement. Thus a carpal capitate subluxation at the wrist would give rise to painful but full passive flexion, painful limited extension and painless full deviations (*Figure 1.8*). By contrast a capsular lesion would be distinguished by equal limitation of flexion and extension (*Figure 1.9*).

Similarly at the neck, in the capsular pattern five of the six possible movements are limited, whereas with an intra-articular cervical displacement the limitation is generally present only on two, three or four movements.

Ligamentous sprains
A sprained ligament will generally give rise to pain on one passive movement. Thus at the wrist if passive radial deviation is painful, a lesion of the ulnar collateral ligament (*Figure 1.10*) is suggested and if the ulnar collateral ligament is involved the other three passive movements—flexion, extension and ulnar deviation—will be painless (*Figure 1.11*).

End-feel
At the extreme of each passive movement the joint will transmit some specific sensation to the examiner's hands. For example, on extension of the elbow the normal end-feel of the joint is hard: bone is felt to engage bone. Were, therefore, the end-feel of elbow extension not hard, the joint would be abnormal.

The significance of the end-feel is thus the degree to which it corresponds to or differs from what the end-feel would be if the joint were normal. Different types of end-feel imply different disorders. The categories include:

(1) Bone to bone: this is the standard end-feel for elbow extension but not, for example, for elbow flexion (see (4) below).

(2) A springy block points to internal derangement.

(3) The abrupt stop imposed by muscle spasm coming actively into play may indicate severe arthritis, a displacement for example at the knee, cancer or a fracture. Knowledge of the joint in question narrows down the possibilities.

(4) Soft tissue approximation: a normal end-feel when the joint cannot be pushed further because of engagement against another part of the body, for example, on elbow flexion.

(5) Empty feel: this happens when the movement causes considerable pain before the extreme of range is reached, yet the sensation imparted to the examiner's hand is 'empty', that is, lacking in organic resistance with further range clearly possible were it not for the patient's pain. Acute bursitis, extra-articular abscess or neoplasm should be strongly considered.

End-feel is an important diagnostic indicator.

Extra-articular limitation
Limitation of passive movement at a joint may occasionally exculpate the joint. Thus if the amount of limitation of movement at one joint is dictated by the position in which another joint is held, the restricting tissue must lie outside any joint. The relationship shows that the lesion lies in a structure that spans at least two joints; this excludes any articular disorders. A prime example is straight-leg raising. Limitation of hip flexion is found when the knee is in extension but not when it is flexed.

Occasionally, disproportionate limitation is encountered with gross restriction in one direction combined with full painless range in all other directions. Again this suggests that the joint itself is normal but that an extra-articular contracture will not permit that movement. Examples are found at the gastrocnemius muscle (where a partial rupture grossly limits dorsiflexion of the ankle joint), if there is a haematoma in the popliteal space (which will limit knee flexion) and in acute subdeltoid bursitis.

CLINICAL EXAMINATION: SUMMARY III

The moving soft tissues are radiotranslucent. Palpate only after examination, along structure already identified as at fault.		
A. History/Referred Pain	**B. Assessment by Function**	
1. Take a history.	2. Examine incriminated joint by selective tension employing:	
	PASSIVE MOVEMENTS for inert structures: *joint capsule, ligaments, bursae, fascia, displacements, dura mater, nerve roots.* Examine for: a) pain b) limitation c) end-feel. *Principal Findings* a) capsular pattern: capsular lesion. Pain and limitation in a fixed proportion on some/all movements of a joint. b) non-capsular pattern of i) ligamentous sprain *or* ii) internal derangement One/some movements of a joint painful/limited, but not in the capsular pattern. c) extra-articular limitation.	RESISTED MOVEMENTS for contractile structures: *muscles, tendons and attachment to bone.* Examine for: a) pain b) weakness. *Principal findings* a) pain: lesion of appropriate contractile structure. b) painless weakness: interference with conduction of appropriate nerve. c) strong and painless: normal.

Clinical examination

The physical examination cannot be conducted in a vacuum simply by assessing the patient's response to passive and resisted movements. First, the physician must start by taking a history. Second, he must appreciate the workings of referred pain. These are two essentials of the examination without which accurate diagnosis will not be realised.

History

The examination begins with the physician talking to the patient; a clear chronological history is a prerequisite. The patient is asked about the events leading up to the onset of the symptoms, what they were then, what brought them on and is then told to recount week by week or year by year what has happened since. All the time the physician compares the patient's account with his own knowledge of the likelihoods of the various conditions and, in particular, with his mental map of the dermatomes. By the time the physical examination gets under way the physician should have a clear idea of the probable cause of the trouble. Any diagnosis subsequently arrived at must be compatible with the known chronological facts. It will be seen that:

(1) Many, if not most, soft-tissue lesions have a distinctive history.
(2) The treatment for many disorders varies according to the stage reached in each one's history.

The following examples illustrate the above two points:

(1) Traumatic arthritis at the shoulder is confined to those over 45 and causes little or no pain in the first days following trauma. During the first few weeks the entire condition may be aborted by capsular stretching; in the second stage, stretching aggravates and injection is the treatment of choice.
(2) A disc lesion that gives pain on movement down the arm recovers spontaneously in four months and no treatment avails after the first couple of weeks.
(3) Pain from a tennis elbow will generally not make its mark for about two weeks following the causative trauma.
(4) If the patient continually wakes at 2 am with acute pins and needles in his arms and complains of numbness persisting the following morning, the thoracic outlet syndrome is strongly suggested.
(5) The patient falls and his knee locks; a meniscus should be considered. But if the

patient falls and his knee locks momentarily, a small loose body is more probable.
(6) A sharp pain in the heel on the first few steps after sitting is suggestive of plantar fasciitis.
(7) A patient afflicted by a lumbar disc lesion of rapid onset for the first time may benefit from manipulation. But if he suffers regular recurrences following manipulative reduction, sclerosants may be indicated. If he is over 60, no benefit will accrue from traction. If pain from a lumbar disc lesion has been down the leg for six months or more, manipulation will not succeed.

Diagnosis and treatment depend on history. Questions include the patient's age and occupation followed by detailed enquiries to cover the onset and subsequent evolution of the condition. The physician should spare no pains to establish what by way of trauma, if any, provoked the symptoms, where they were first felt, where they have spread to since and the general progression of the disorder. Throughout, he will bear in mind the workings of referred pain.

Referred pain

Pain perceived elsewhere than at its true site is termed 'referred'. Nearly all pain is referred; the diagnostician's task is to ascertain from where.

The site where symptoms are referred to is determined by the sensory cortex which attributes the sensory impulses it receives to the appropriate areas of the body (*Figure 1.12*). With stimuli to the skin, the sensory

Fig 1.12 *Referred pain. The symptoms are attributed by the sensory cortex to the corresponding dermatome. C5 shown.*

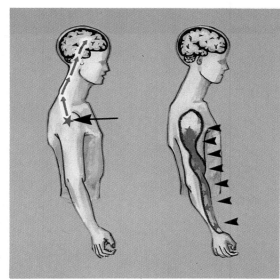

1.12

cortex achieves a high degree of accuracy. Over the years a stimulus reaching certain cells in the sensorium comes to bear the meaning that damage is being inflicted on a certain area of skin.

When a painful stimulus arising from a deep seated structure (e.g. a soft tissue) is received by the same cells, the sensory cortex interprets this new impulse on the basis of past experience. The pain is referred to the area of skin connected with those particular cortical cells.

This area of skin is the dermatome, and the dermatome to which any given pain is allocated corresponds to the segment from which the structure was embryologically derived. Thus a pain in a tissue of C5 segmental origin will be referred by the sensory cortex to the C5 dermatome, and from a C6 structure to the C6 dermatome. So when dealing with a lesion suspected of arising from, for example, a C5 structure, it is vital to know the boundaries of the C5 dermatome (*Figure 1.13*). Pain felt outside that area cannot emanate from a C5 structure, and knowledge of the C5 dermatome will show that a pain at the back of the elbow cannot originate from a structure of C5 derivation, whereas pain at the anterior aspect might. It might, of course, also come from any other segments whose dermatomes overlie that area.

It is with symptoms in the upper and lower limbs that the role of referred pain is particularly important. The dermatomes do no more than represent the original relationship of the limb buds to the trunk at the earliest stage of development of the embryo. The 40 segments in a month old fetus are distributed horizontally (*Figure 1.14*). At this stage the dermatomes are superimposed directly over the segments from which they are derived. But the growth of the four limbs draws the dermatomes out down the arms and legs (*Figure 1.15*). At the trunk, however, the original arrangement of circular dermatomic bands remains relatively intact.

This means that the upper limb is covered by the C5, C6, C7, C8, T1 and T2 dermatomes. Pain within the appropriate area of the arm could arise from structures of matching embryological derivation. The L2, L3, L4, L5, S1, S2 and S3 dermatomes all extend down the leg. Thus when examining the patient for the cause of pain in the limbs it will be borne in mind that the symptoms may originate not just locally but proximally (*Figure 1.16*).

In practice this is simpler than it sounds. For example, the front of the knee falls within (*inter alia*) the L3 dermatome (*Figure 1.17*).

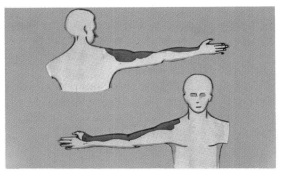

1.13

Fig 1.13 *The C5 dermatome. Nearly all shoulder pain is felt within this area.*

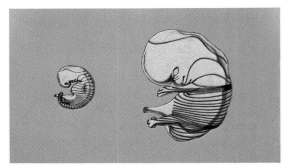

1.14, 1.15

Figs 1.14, 1.15 *Embryological derivation. During growth, the limb projections deform the original shape of the segments.*

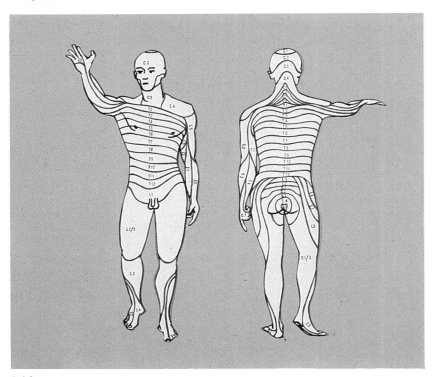

1.16

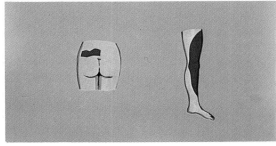

1.17

Fig 1.16 *The dermatomes. The diagrams give an adequate overall impression of the segmentation of the skin; they do not allow for the areas of overlap.*

Fig 1.17 *The L3 dermatome.*

Thus in addition to pain of local origin, symptoms at the knee may be emitted by any L3 structure. The primary possibilities will be osteoarthrosis of the hip and a disc lesion pressing on the L3 nerve root.

So if a patient complains of anterior pain at the knee, as before the first thing to do is to take a history. It should emerge whether the pain is connected with:

(1) Trauma to the knee.
(2) A rheumatoid–type disorder occurring spontaneously at the knee.
(3) Pain from the groin to the front of the knee, coming from the hip.
(4) A history typical of backache coupled with pain down the leg.

Turning to the physical examination, the various possibilities may be swiftly confirmed or eliminated. If spinal movements are painless, the pain does not come from the spine. If hip movements are painless, the pain does not stem from the hip. If the knee movements bring on the pain, the pain does come from the knee—which is then examined in detail by the appropriate routine of passive and resisted movements.

These principles are duplicated at the upper limb. Most shoulder structures are of C5 derivation. The biceps also has an element of C6. Additionally the arm is served by the various nerve roots emerging from the cervical spine. A cervical disc lesion may compress a nerve root at C3 (rare), C4, C5, C6, C7 (common), C8, T1 (rare) or T2 (rare). Pain would be felt in the corresponding dermatomes, each of which occupies a fairly well defined but frequently overlapping section of the arm, elbow, wrist or hand. Likewise, after a careful history, examination of the upper limb may have to start off at the neck, proceed to the shoulder and only ultimately will the structures about, for example, the elbow, be identified as containing the causative lesion. This is a simple enough procedure and, in fact, knowledge of referred pain can simplify diagnosis.

Pain is referred in compliance with certain rules, which can be deployed by the physician to define:

(1) from which tissues the pain could arise;
(2) from which tissues the pain could not arise.

CLINICAL EXAMINATION: SUMMARY IV

The moving soft tissues are radiotranslucent. Palpate only after examination, along structure already identified as at fault.			
A. History/Referred Pain	**B. Assessment by Function**		
1. Take a history. Consider:	2. Examine incriminated joint by selective tension employing:		
a) the probable lesion and the stage it has reached; treatment is governed by both factors. *b) referred pain.*	PRELIMINARY EXAMINATION Where necessary begin by rough outline examination consisting of active movements to establish which joint is at fault. Then proceed to examination in detail of the incriminated joint by a routine of passive and resisted movements.	PASSIVE MOVEMENTS for inert structures: *joint capsule, ligaments, bursae, fascia, displacements, dura mater, nerve roots.* Examine for: a) pain b) limitation c) end-feel. *Principal Findings* a) capsular pattern: capsular lesion. Pain and limitation in a fixed proportion on some/all movements of a joint. b) non-capsular pattern of i) ligamentous sprain *or* ii) internal derangement One/some movements of a joint painful/limited, but not in the capsular pattern. c) extra-articular limitation.	RESISTED MOVEMENTS for contractile structures: *muscles, tendons and attachment to bone.* Examine for: a) pain b) weakness. *Principal findings* a) pain: lesion of appropriate contractile structure. b) painless weakness: interference with conduction of appropriate nerve. c) strong and painless: normal.

Rules governing the reference of pain

(1) Pain is referred segmentally
Thus a C5 tissue refers pain to the C5 dermatome. It should be remembered that—subject to (2) below—the pain can occupy all or any part of the dermatome. For example, with acute traumatic arthritis at the shoulder, the pain may run all the way down the arm to the wrist. But initially the pain resides locally and only spreads by degrees to the elbow and finally to the wrist. As the disorder wears off, the symptoms recede proximally. Throughout, the pain has been confined to the C5 dermatome.

It follows that the physician will be particularly on the alert if the patient describes symptoms straddling more than one dermatome at once, or those that migrate from one dermatome to another.

Four possibilities arise:

(a) The patient is describing a pain devoid of organic basis.
(b) The lesion itself is shifting. This often happens with displacements at the spine.
(c) The lesion is spreading. Consider, for example, metastases.
(d) The pain stems from a tissue that does not refer pain on a segmental basis (*see below*).

Exception to the rule of segmental reference
The dura mater refers pain extrasegmentally —an exception of the greatest importance dealt with on page 14.

(2) Pain is referred distally
The source of symptoms must thus be sought locally or proximally. The structures about the knee and elbow stand almost alone in setting up pain felt to radiate equally in both directions, but in both cases the patient seldom fails to realise where his symptoms originate.

(3) Referred pain never crosses the midline
Thus a T5 left rib will not cause discomfort on the right of the body. A pain felt centrally must originate from a central structure and cannot be accounted for by a unilateral structure; similarly, the source of bilateral pain must be sought centrally. A pain alternating from one side of the body to the other must have a central source that can shift from one side to another (e.g. a displacement at the spine).

(4) The extent of reference is controlled by
(a) The size of the dermatome and the position in that dermatome of the tissue at fault. Clearly, a large dermatome permits greater reference than a small one. Furthermore, a lesion in the proximal part of the dermatome tends to refer pain further than a lesion in the distal part. At the extremities of each limb the capacity for accurate localisation increases. At the wrist, hand, ankle and foot useful results may be obtained from palpation after assessment by function.
(b) The strength of the stimulus. The more intense the pain the greater the number of cortical cells touched off. The spread to adjacent cells in the sensory cortex is regarded by the patient as an enlargement of the painful area.
(c) The depth of the tissue at fault. The deeper a soft tissue lies the larger the reference to be expected. However, bone sets up a pain that hardly radiates at all.

Symptoms referred from the nervous system
There are four aspects to be analysed: the spinal cord, the dural sleeve of a nerve root, a nerve trunk and a small nerve. The symptoms from each vary in important respects and thus may be differentiated.

(1) Compression of the spinal cord
Pain does not result. Pins and needles are apt to be bilateral and to disregard the segmentation of the body. Serious trouble is present.

(2) Compression of the dural sleeve to a nerve root
At the point of emergence from the dura, the nerve roots are invested with a dural sleeve. Pressure on the dural sleeve (*Figure 1.18*) will produce all or any of the following:

Figs 1.18, 1.19, 1.20
Pressure on the dural sheath at the cervical spine. Compression of the C7 root (Fig 1.18) can produce both pain down the arm (Fig 1.19) and pins and needles in the appropriate fingers (Fig 1.20).

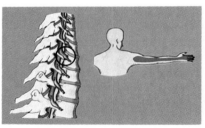 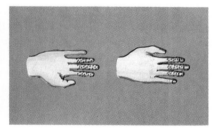

1.18   1.19   1.20

(a) Pain in all or any part of the relevant dermatome. Thus pressure on the C7 root will give pain down the arm (*Figure 1.19*); pressure on the L4 root engenders pain down the leg extending to the big toe.
(b) Pins and needles—a compression phenomenon—generally felt at the distal end of the dermatome and often conspicuously occupying an area not supplied by any one nerve trunk (*Figure 1.20*). The paraesthesia has neither edge nor

aspect, being felt, for example, within the fingers.

(c) Numbness which, as it comes on, tends to displace the pins and needles. Major pressure on a nerve root causes analgesia; minor pressure evokes pins and needles.

Weakness results not from interference with the dural sleeve but from compression of the nerve root within—the parenchyma. Weakness will be discernible on resisted movements.

(3) Compression of a nerve trunk
The results are:

(a) No pain (although pressure on the surrounding dural cladding at the transverse process will hurt).
(b) Weakness. Impaired conduction along a nerve leads to muscle weakness manifested on resisted movements.
(c) Pins and needles (*Figures 1.21; 1.22*) rather than numbness, generally brought on as a release phenomenon. Thus pressure on, for example, the sciatic nerve while sitting causes no symptoms; the pins and needles come when the subject relieves the pressure by standing up. The paraesthesia is concentrated in the distal part of the cutaneous area supplied by that peripheral nerve; the lesion always lies proximal to the upper edge of the paraesthetic area.

(4) Compression of a small nerve
The results are:

(a) No pain.
(b) Normally no weakness because the efferent fibres have left the body of the nerve proximally.
(c) Numbness rather than pins and needles, occupying the cutaneous area supplied by that nerve (*Figure 1.23*). The edge is well defined and towards the centre of the area full anaesthesia is often demonstrable.

Figs 1.21, 1.22, 1.23
Pins and needles. Contrasting symptoms are caused by pressure on the median nerve above and below its point of division.

Fig 1.24 *The dura mater. Pressure on this structure is responsible for much backache. The pain is referred extrasegmentally.*

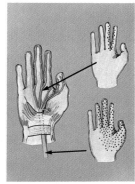

1.21, 1.22, 1.23

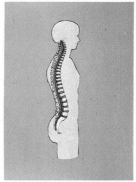

1.24

Examination of the nervous system
Pins and needles from any source are findings that are thrown up in the course of the history. Pain from compression of the dural sleeve to a nerve root may be aggravated by spinal movements.

In addition, because the nerve roots at the lumbar spine are mobile, any impingement restricting a nerve root's mobility can be tested for by indirect traction to the nerve. Thus pain may be elicited by straight-leg raising or prone-lying knee flexion.

Interference with motor conduction is evident as weakness on resisted movements. Interference with sensory conduction will show itself as cutaneous analgesia.

An example
Apparently similar symptoms may readily be traced back to source. Thus a trigger finger would compress the two digital nerves at their point of division engendering numbness of the two adjacent sides of the two relevant fingers. This could not come from the median nerve because the pins and needles would then be felt in the thumb, index, long and the radial side of the ring finger. If, however, a cervical nerve root is pinched, the pins and needles occupy fingers that no single nerve in the arm runs to; the thumb and index finger, for example, are served only by the C6 root.

Exception to the rule of segmental reference
For reasons that remain obscure, the dura mater does not obey the rules of segmental reference. The dura mater descends from the foramen magnum of the skull to the caudal edge of the first or second sacral vertebra (*Figure 1.24*) and keeps the spinal cord buffered in cerebrospinal fluid. From it protrude 30 pairs of nerve roots covered by the dural sheath.

Whereas pressure on the nerve roots engenders segmentally referred pain, compression or stretching of the dura mater itself gives rise to extrasegmentally referred pain. The dura mater is, throughout its extent, adjacent to the intervertebral discs and is thus vulnerable to posterior pressure exerted via the posterior longitudinal ligament.

Pain from pressure on the dura mater at cervical levels (*Figure 1.25*) may be felt anywhere from the head to mid-thorax, often pervading many dermatomes simultaneously. It is a frequent cause of scapular pain (but not of brachial symptoms which may, however, be accounted for by pressure on a nerve root). The symptoms are usually central or unilateral.

Pressure on the dura mater at thoracic levels (*Figure 1.26*) may radiate pain to the base of

CLINICAL EXAMINATION: SUMMARY V

The moving soft tissues are radiotranslucent. Palpate only after examination, along structure already identified as at fault.

A. History/Referred Pain	B. Assessment by Function		
1. Take a history. Consider:	2. Examine incriminated joint by selective tension employing:		
a) the probable lesion and the stage it has reached; treatment is governed by both factors. *b) referred pain.* Consider: i) dermatome occupied/segmental derivation, particularly with pain in upper or lower limb. ii) rules of reference, i.e. referred pain – is referred segmentally – is referred distally – never crosses the mid-line. iii) site of interference (if any) with nervous system – spinal cord: no pain, pins and needles – nerve root sheath: pain, pins and needles, numbness – nerve trunk: no pain; weakness, pins and needles – small nerve: no pain, no weakness; numbness iv) extrasegmentally referred pain from dura mater if spinal lesion.	PRELIMINARY EXAMINATION Where necessary begin by rough outline examination consisting of active movements to establish which joint is at fault. Then proceed to examination in detail of the incriminated joint by a routine of passive and resisted movements.	PASSIVE MOVEMENTS for inert structures: *joint capsule, ligaments, bursae, fascia, displacements, dura mater, nerve roots.* Examine for: a) pain b) limitation c) end-feel. *Principal Findings* a) capsular pattern: capsular lesion. Pain and limitation in a fixed proportion on some/all movements of a joint. b) non-capsular pattern of i) ligamentous sprain *or* ii) internal derangement One/some movements of a joint painful/limited, but not in the capsular pattern. c) extra-articular limitation.	RESISTED MOVEMENTS for contractile structures: *muscles, tendons and attachment to bone.* Examine for: a) pain b) weakness. *Principal findings* a) pain: lesion of appropriate contractile structure. b) painless weakness: interference with conduction of appropriate nerve. c) strong and painless: normal.

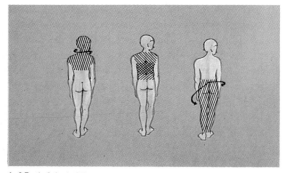

1.25, 1.26, 1.27

the neck or to the posterior or anterior aspect of the trunk. It will often spread over many dermatomes simultaneously. The symptoms are usually central or unilateral.

Pressure on the dura mater at lumbar levels (*Figure 1.27*) may cause pain reaching the lower thorax posteriorly, the lower abdomen, the upper buttocks, sacrum and coccyx. The symptoms may extend bilaterally or unilaterally down the legs as far as the ankle but not beyond to the foot. Once again, many dermatomes may be occupied simultaneously.

The mere fact that the patient describes a reference of pain otherwise impossible should focus attention on the dura mater. It is a mobile, inert structure and consequently is specifically examined by passive movements.

Diagnosis at the spine

Diagnosis at the joints of the spine adheres to exactly the same general principles but is governed by the sensitivity of the dura mater.

Examination of the spine for backache conducted in the light of this information regularly produces the following findings:

(1) Painless resisted movements, exculpating the contractile structures.
(2) Painful passive movements incriminating the inert structures (e.g. the dura mater).
(3) Painful passive movements in the non-capsular pattern characteristic of internal derangement.
(4) Frequently signs of:
  (a) Interference with dural mobility.
  (b) Interference with mobility of the dural

Figs 1.25, 1.26, 1.27 *Extrasegmental reference. The areas in which pain may be felt as a result of interference with the dura at cervical (left), thoracic (centre) and lumbar levels (right).*

Figs 1.28, 1.29 *A central displacement impinges on the dura mater (left) whereas a lateral protrusion can compress the nerve root sheath.*

sleeve to a nerve root, sometimes with signs of impaired nerve root conduction.

(5) A history consistent only with an intra-articular displacement.

Clinical evidence thus points firmly to the conclusion that the great majority of spinal pain has a single unified cause: minor and remediable displacements of disc material compressing the dura mater or nerve roots (*Figures 1.28; 1.29*). This deduction may be confirmed by abolition of the symptoms following:

(1) Manipulative reduction of the displacement (see page 142).
(2) Reduction of the displacement by traction.
(3) An injection of epidural local anaesthetic rendering insensitive the superficial aspect of the dura mater and nerve roots.

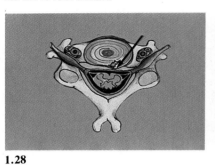

1.28

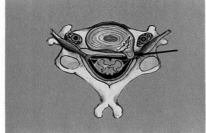

1.29

Diagnostic skills

Diagnosis is a skill and clearly the physician learns from experience. Nevertheless, satisfactory results are soon achieved. It is as well to remember that the object of the physical examination is to find the movement that elicits the pain of which the patient complains, rather than some other nebulous symptom of which he was previously unaware. Nor is it sufficient for a movement to prove painful; it must actually increase the patient's pain. During examination the patient is of course questioned in a neutral manner, being asked whether a movement has any influence on (rather than aggravating) his symptoms.

The examination for any given joint should always be performed in its entirety and it should always be performed in the same order—first the history, then the passive movements and finally the resisted movements. Only by sticking to a standard sequence will the physician be sure of leaving nothing out and only by leaving nothing out are true findings feasible. The physician arrives at a diagnosis not from the evidence furnished by one painful movement but by careful detection of a consistent pattern.

Corroboration or disproof of the diagnosis may often be obtained by induction of local anaesthesia—a 1:200 solution of procaine is recommended. Following its infiltration, the patient is asked to repeat whichever movement was found to be most painful on examination. If the pain has gone, the anaesthetic was injected into the correct site. No other mode of endorsement is comparably effective.

Slight pains often make for problems. It is sometimes wise to ask the patient to return a week later, by which time he may be either better or worse; if the latter, a more conclusive examination is now on the cards.

Very severe pain may render clinical examination impossible on account of an excess of physical signs. Justifiable fear of pain may prevent the patient from moving; every movement may provoke intense exacerbation. In these cases history must be awarded its full weight, and gross signs are viewed in the light of the fact that only a limited number of disorders engender agonising pain.

Double lesions are a source of confusion, with the signs pointing, for example, to a lesion of both the infraspinatus and supraspinatus, or to a lesion of both the shoulder and cervical spine. In such cases it is best to tackle one lesion at a time, beginning with the more tractable, common or painful. After one condition has cleared up the second suspected lesion will be easier to identify.

Psychogenic pain is no rarity. Detection is seldom difficult as the patient is ignorant of the principles of referred pain and of the way the supposed lesion should behave. A host of contradictions with no coherent picture swiftly become apparent during the history and physical appraisal. The more thorough and systematic the questioning and examination the more inconsistencies come to light.

The examiner should be on his guard against dismissing the symptoms of hypersensitive patients as psychogenic.

CHAPTER TWO

PRINCIPLES OF
TREATMENT

Once an exact diagnosis has been made it is possible to prescribe treatment. Treatment is:

(1) Administered to the specific site of the lesion diagnosed.
(2) Of a kind to exert a beneficial effect on the lesion.

It follows that for soft-tissue lesions the non-specific remedies such as heat, cold, water, exercises, ointment, bandages, diffuse massage and analgesics are, with insignificant exceptions, palliative rather than curative.

The object of scientific treatment is recovery and accordingly the criterion is not whether the patient has received a course of therapy but whether the treatment has yielded any amelioration. Thus the patient is continually reassessed to see if range has improved and pain diminished. If not, either the diagnosis or the treatment has been misconceived.

The requisite therapeutic skills are readily acquired and can be easily learned and applied. Virtually no special equipment is needed.

Disadvantages of conventional treatment.

Joints other than the spine

Disorders

The salient disorders are discussed here; the appropriate treatments are dealt with in the immediately ensuing section.

Muscles

Strain in a muscle causes a few fibres to part. The resultant scar tissue mats the fibres together not just longitudinally but also transversely and these microscopic adhesions generate pain when the muscle broadens on contraction (*Figures 2.1, 2.2* and *2.3*). They can be broken up by deep massage (*Figure 2.4*).

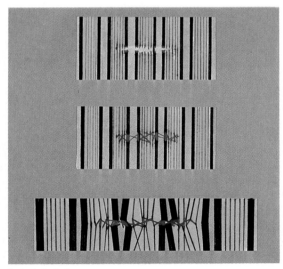

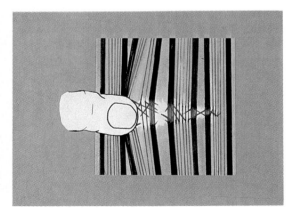

Figs 2.1, 2.2, 2.3 *Minor muscular tears. The formation of intramuscular scarring (top and centre) can painfully limit full broadening (bottom).*

Fig 2.4 *Deep massage. The muscle fibres are teased apart.*

2.1, 2.2, 2.3

2.4

Aborting muscular adhesions

If the tear lies clear of the tendon and in the belly of the muscle, active exercises and an induction of local anaesthesia may also play their part in speeding recovery immediately after injury. The infiltration of local anaesthesia allows for normal movement of the uninjured part of the muscle, and off-weight exercises encourage the formation of a supple scar that quickly becomes painless.

The nearer towards the tendon the scar lies, the less likely these techniques are to succeed. The tactic is effective only during the first few days (at most) following injury and is strongly recommended, notably for sports injuries where the patient tends to seek immediate professional advice. Resisted exercises are best avoided until recovery is well established.

The outstanding conditions to which this approach applies are lesions of the gastrocnemius, hamstrings and quadriceps. The pectoralis major, latissimus dorsi and trapezius also benefit.

Tendons

Strain on a tendon tears a few fibres and each muscle contraction thereafter is apt to renew the rupture in the healing breach. The result is an inflamed scar. Either the inflammation or the scar itself can be disposed of, the former by an injection of steroid suspension and the latter by deep massage. The injection is faster and less painful. But with massage the incidence of recurrence is lower as the scar itself is effectively abolished.

The joint capsule

The joint capsule may become inflamed whether through traumatic or rheumatoid arthritis. In rheumatoid-type cases without irretrievable damage to the joint and where the condition is in a reasonably chronic phase, an intra-articular injection of steroid suspension can be relied on to bring immediate relief lasting many months.

Traumatic arthritis of the shoulder, elbow, radioulnar joint and foot also respond well to steroid therapy. With traumatic arthritis of the shoulder or capsular contracture at the hip, manipulative stretching may also be helpful.

Rheumatoid arthritis strongly contra-indicates manipulation.

Displacements

An intra-articular displacement will momentarily strain the capsule or ligaments about a joint. The loose body takes up intra-articular space and either distorts the capsule or enlarges the distance spanned by the ligaments. The displacement itself is insensitive being constructed of cartilage, a tissue devoid of nerves.

The treatment is manipulative reduction to return the displacement to a more favourable site. Loose bodies are found with varying degrees of frequency at most joints except the shoulder.

Ligaments

A ligament may be strained giving rise to painful stretching on further use. As healing proceeds, scar tissue may bond the ligament to adjacent bone (*Figures 2.5; 2.6*).

The treatment differs according to the site but consists of massage or an injection of steroid suspension. The infiltration clears up the inflammation. The massage physically moves the ligament in imitation of its normal behaviour, preventing the formation of adhesions which, if allowed to bind, must be manipulatively ruptured (*Figure 2.7*).

Figs 2.5, 2.6, 2.7
Ligamentous sprain. Following injury (top) macroscopic adhesions bind the ligament down (centre); if untreated, they must be manipulatively ruptured (bottom).

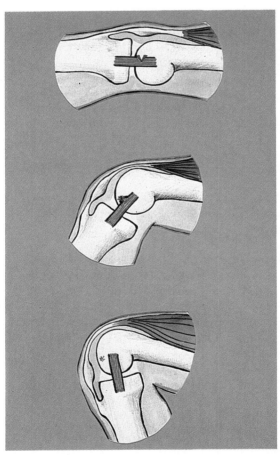

2.5, 2.6, 2.7

Tenosynovitis

At the wrist and ankle this is a primary lesion of the gliding surfaces of the external aspect of the tendon. The sheath becomes roughened and inflamed from over-use and can be dealt with by an injection of steroid suspension or massage.

TREATMENT AT THE PERIPHERAL JOINTS: SUMMARY

Disorder	Strained muscle	Strained tendon	Capsular inflammation	Intra-articular displacement	Ligamentous sprain	Tenosynovitis
Treatment	Deep massage.	Deep massage *or* injection of steroid suspension as appropriate.	*Traumatic:* injection of steroid suspension *or* manipulative stretching as appropriate. *Rheumatoid:* injection of steroid suspension.	Manipulative reduction.	Deep massage and/or injection of steroid suspension as appropriate.	Injection of steroid suspension *or* massage.

Table 2

Treatments

Both deep massage and steroid injections are purely local in effect and assist only when administered to the precise site of the lesion. No vestige of benefit is reaped by treating healthy tissues nearby.

Deep massage

Deep massage, otherwise known as 'transverse friction', bears no relationship to conventional effleurage. Reduced to its simplest, the physiotherapist's digit is placed on the exact site of the lesion (*Figure 2.8*) and rubbed hard *across* the grain of the muscle, tendon, tendon sheath or ligament. The sessions are painful and last for about 20 minutes. Six to 12 treatments may be necessary at intervals of seldom less than every other day, otherwise the lesion will still be too tender from the previous day's encounter to tolerate adequate treatment. The key is that the therapeutic movement is confined to a very small spot (*Figures 2.9; 2.10*).

In muscular lesions, the effect of deep massage is to break down the adhesions formed by the scar tissue between individual muscle fibres. On the tendon, the scar is eroded by the abrasive action. During the period of healing, the ligament is moved in imitation of its normal behaviour, thus preventing the formation of adhesions. In tenosynovitis it appears that the manual rolling of the tendon sheath to and fro against the tendon serves to smooth off the roughened surfaces.

The approach varies slightly for each condition, but the principles remain constant. First the lesion must be brought within reach of the physiotherapist's finger. This entails positioning the patient carefully according to the dictates of applied anatomy. For instance in supraspinatus tendinitis the patient's arm

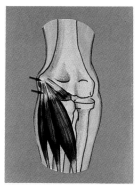

2.8

Fig 2.8 *Tendinitis, golfer's elbow. There are two sites; treatment to either must be given with scrupulous accuracy.*

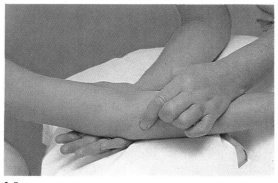

2.9

Figs 2.9, 2.10 *Massage, golfer's elbow. Note the movement is of little more than 1cm. It is the lesion itself that receives the friction.*

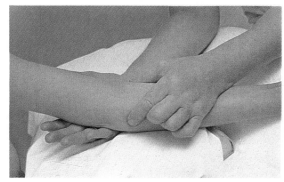

2.10

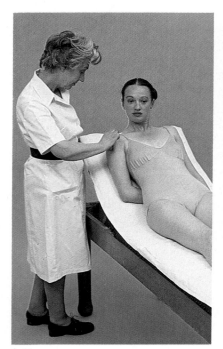

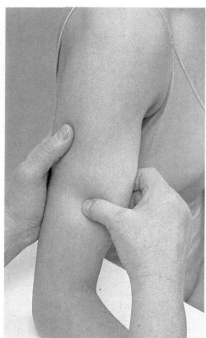

2.11

2.12

Fig 2.12 *Deep massage, the biceps belly. The patient must be taught to stay relaxed. It is the substance, not the surface, of the muscle that needs treatment.*

Fig 2.13 *Deep massage, extensor carpi radialis. The wrist is flexed over the pillow to tauten the tendon.*

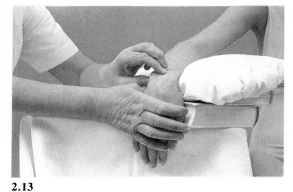

2.13

Fig 2.11 *Deep massage, supraspinatus. In this position the tendon is bent through a right angle and lies exposed in the sagittal plane.*

must be placed behind her back (*Figure 2.11*). This brings the tendon out from under the acromion which would otherwise shield the entire structure.

Second, the tissue to receive the massage should be appropriately tensioned. If a muscle is to be treated, it must be relaxed so the massage can penetrate deeply to tease the fibres apart (*Figure 2.12*). A tendon without a sheath is simply put into the most accessible position. By contrast, with tenosynovitis the tendon must be tautened to form an immobile basis against which to rub the tendon sheath (*Figure 2.13*). For a ligament, the joint may have to be moved as far as possible in one direction, and the massage administered in that position, then taken in the other direction and the massage repeated there.

Third, the physiotherapist's fingertip(s) apply the treatment. The technique is to move the whole hand, with the patient's skin and the physiotherapist's finger operating as one. The friction must be *across* the fibres of the affected structure with sufficient amplitude of sweep to ensure that the frictional element (and not the pressure) is paramount. In general the digit, hand and forearm should comprise a straight line kept parallel to the movement imparted, the distal interphalangeal joint being slightly flexed. In practice, however, there are many variations.

Two fingers may be needed for a large lesion, or more often one finger reinforces the other. The thumb is often used to supply counterpressure so that the digit can bear strongly on the lesion. For certain disorders the

massage is transmitted by alternate pronation and supination of the hand, thus rotating the digit. In others, the physiotherapist's finger stays stationary while the limb is moved underneath it. Occasionally, the lesion—typically in the belly of a muscle—must be squeezed between thumb and finger.

Finally, both physiotherapist and patient must assume a position allowing sufficient leverage and comfort for the treatment to be kept up for 20 minutes at a time. The standard approach is shown for each lesion. But, provided the massage itself is correctly administered, the physiotherapist may devise some variant of her own or change position during a session to relieve fatigued muscles.

DEEP MASSAGE: SUMMARY

1. Administer to precise site of lesion.

2. The digit is rubbed *across* structure undergoing treatment.

3. Frictional element not pressure is paramount.

4. Position the patient to:
   a) render lesion accessible.

   b) put tissue under treatment into appropriate tension, eg muscles relaxed.

5. Generally six to twelve sessions required, twenty minutes each on alternate days.

NB Precise procedure varies from joint to joint.

Steroid therapy

Fibrous tissue appears capable of supporting an inflammation, originally traumatic, as the result of a habit continuing long after the cause has ceased to operate. But if this cycle of chronic inflammation is broken for only two weeks the scar becomes painless and usually remains so. This may be achieved by infiltration of steroid suspension at the exact site of the lesion.

Often the injections demand the utmost exactitude (see below) but none call for more than routine asepsis. The treatment is thus eminently suited to outpatient/family medicine.

Steroid suspension

Injections of anti-inflammatory agents work, but only where they are put. A suspension of insoluble steroid material is used, and being insoluble, the powder stays where it is injected and is slowly destroyed there so its active action is confined to the cells with which it lies in contact. In consequence, no systemic effect is evoked. The lack of solubility also has the advantage of an intense anti-inflammatory effect being exerted at the point of application. But it also implies that great precision in diagnosis and injection techniques must be maintained in order to get the suspension to the correct spot. At tendinous sites (*cf.* capsular injections) delivery must be accurate to within a millimetre or so (*Figures 2.14; 2.15*).

(b) in many cases feel the bubbles forming under his fingers as the injection proceeds?
(5) Where should the needle be inserted; in what direction and how deeply?
(6) How long a needle is required and what size of syringe?
(7) How much suspension is required to infiltrate the whole affected area?

The data relevant to each lesion is detailed in the ensuing chapters.

Injection into a joint can be contrasted with injection into a tendon or ligament. The intra-articular injection is, on the whole, simpler but whatever the site of injection the patient is instructed not to exert the limb for the week following infiltration. This gives the anti-inflammatory effect of the hormone the most favourable environment in which to act. No matter how well the patient may appear to himself to be, too early violent exercise could lead to relapse.

Intra-articular injections

The infiltration is made as soon as the needle has passed through the capsule of the joint and the point lies intra-articularly. The suspension (10mg/ml) then distributes itself throughout the inside of the joint. Traction applied by an assistant is useful at the small joints of the fingers or toes where only 0.5–1ml of steroid is required; at the larger joints the dosage ranges up to 5ml.

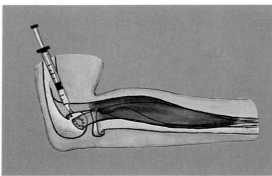

2.14

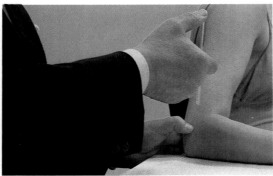

2.15

Figs 2.14, 2.15 *Injection, steroid suspension. Delivery must be absolutely precise if the steroid is to abate the localised inflammation.*

The following factors should be considered before undertaking an injection of steroid suspension:

(1) In what tissue does the lesion lie?
(2) In what part of that tissue in a horizontal plane?
(3) In what part of that tissue in a vertical plane?
(4) How should the doctor best place his finger on the relevant structure so that he can:
    (a) identify the tissue at fault?

Little local reaction is provoked, though the benefit is not evident until 24 hours have elapsed.

Although the rheumatoid-type arthritises have been shown to respond very favourably to intra-articular injections, it is the symptoms and not the cause that are abolished. Thus if the relief is to be maintained, the injections must be repeated at whatever intervals prove necessary; in practice, they can often be semi-lastingly discontinued. But although the injections are free from systemic effect, there is a ceiling to the number of intra-articular infiltrations that can be absorbed by a weight-bearing joint without courting the risk of a steroid arthropathy.

In acute cases, where many joints are flaring at the same time, the treatment is impracticable.

Tendinous injections
At the tendons a more precise approach is needed. Generally 1ml steroid suspension is enough at a dilution of 10mg/ml. This solution also suffices for capsular injections, but the strength is vital for short tendons where rupture has been reported after using a strength of 40mg/ml. However, such ruptures are probably more attributable to faulty technique.

A tuberculin syringe with a thin needle must be employed and the entire suspension is never pumped into the same spot. Instead, a series of half-withdrawals and reinsertions are made with a dozen droplets or so injected over the three-dimensional area constituting the lesion—if part of the affected area is left out the symptoms will persist. Normally, only one or two injections are required. With these safeguards, athletes or dancers need not fear the rupture that may occasionally result from lax procedure.

The anti-inflammatory effect takes 12 to 48 hours to establish itself and before this has happened a local irritant effect is manifest. Thus injection into, say, a tendon may create such discomfort that the patient is more or less unable to use the part for a day or two. Then the anti-inflammatory effect comes into play and the symptoms are relieved with dramatic speed.

Steroid therapy and deep massage
Steroid injections do not help muscle or musculo-tendinous lesions; for these conditions the remedy is deep massage. But one cannot generalise about the selection of treatment for the tendons and ligaments. Some lesions respond better to massage, others better to steroid infiltration; in such cases the preferences for each structure are set out in the text. There remain some disorders where the physician has a choice of therapy but it must be stressed these are *alternatives*. Both approaches are not to be adopted at a time.

The advantage of steroid infiltration is the rapid success of the injection; six to 12 sessions of painful deep massage may be needed to secure the same result. But unlike massage, steroids provoke quite a strong reaction lasting one or two days. There is also a tendency to a higher rate of recurrence of the lesion because the scar, although the inflammation in it has been inhibited for the time being, has not been removed. This consideration will weigh particularly with athletes, dancers and manual workers. Aside from the guidelines above, deep massage may be indicated in the following cases:

(1) Diagnostic uncertainty, where the exact site of the lesion cannot be satisfactorily defined. Each of the physiotherapist's fingers is about 1cm wide and the amplitude of her sweep at least 2cm. Hence the margin of diagnostic error allowable for adequate treatment by massage is greater than for 1ml of steroid suspension is used.
(2) A large lesion, particularly at the knee, should be tackled by massage first with any residual spots polished off by injection.

STEROID INJECTIONS: SUMMARY

Capsular injections					
Strength	**Equipment**	**Delivery**	**After-effects**	**After care**	**Caution**
10 mg/ml	Syringe with thinnest possible needle.	Relatively simple. Anywhere inside capsule.	Little pain following injection, symptoms rapidly abate.	Avoid or minimise use of limb for a week.	Avoid repeated injections to weight bearing joints.
Non-capsular injections					
As above.	As above.	Relatively difficult. Precisely into exact cubic extent of the lesion, injected in droplets all over affected area.	Pain for 1–2 days following infiltration, thereafter symptoms rapidly abate.	As above.	Follow individual procedures as set out in text.

Manipulation

To 'manipulate' means to move. In orthopaedic medicine manipulation is used in three distinct situations: in the presence of capsular contracture, in the presence of an adhesion and in the presence of a displacement. In each of these classifications, the movement is undertaken with different intent and therefore in a different way.

Manipulative stretching to counter capsular contracture is a slow, steady movement carried out over a number of sessions. Manipulative rupture of adhesions consists of a sharp jerk. Both techniques are of narrow application, the latter employed at the knee and ankle and the former only at the shoulder and hip; they are dealt with at the appropriate stages in the text.

Manipulative reduction

Manipulative reduction of a displacement is an important tactic, regularly called for at the elbow, wrist, hip, knee and ankle as well as at the cervical, thoracic and lumbar spine. Despite its reputation, the treatment is straightforward, logical and safe, and although much is gained from experience, competence and proficient results are rapidly achieved. Manipulation is part of the standard armamentarium of the family physician or physiotherapist.

The basic principles are simple (*Figures 2.16; 2.17; 2.18*) and hardly vary from joint to joint.

First, the manipulator pulls as hard as he can on the affected joint, distracting the joint surfaces and allowing the loose fragment room to move.

Second, the joint is twisted in an endeavour to shift the loose fragment.

Third, the patient is re-examined to see if the displacement now lies in a more favourable position. This is readily ascertained as, if it does, the patient's pain will have eased and/or his range increased. The manipulator therefore asks the patient to repeat the movements found to be limited before the manipulation commenced, observes whether range has improved and asks if his pain has altered.

If a particular manipulation has helped, it is repeated. If not, some variation is resorted to that imposes a different strain on the joint. This may amount to no more than twisting the limb in the other direction. Alternatively, it may be a more elaborate refinement entailing adoption of a different posture by patient and operator to apply a different leverage to magnify the forces brought to bear. The methods for each joint and the standard progressions are displayed in the relevant chapters.

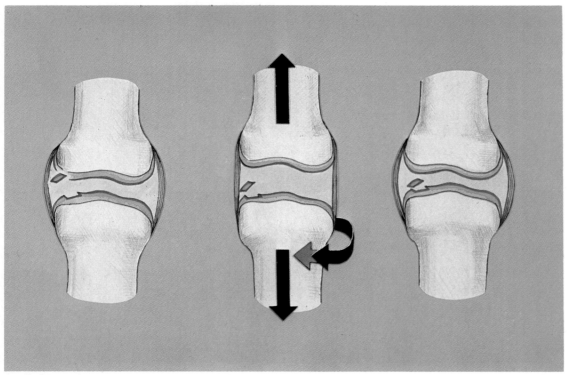

Figs 2.16, 2.17, 2.18
Manipulation. Manipulative reduction during traction may return a displaced intra-articular structure (left) towards its bed (right). Traction is applied and the joint twisted (centre). The patient is re-examined after each manoeuvre. Partial improvement shown.

2.16, 2.17, 2.18

Figs 2.19, 2.20, 2.21
Manipulative reduction, a loose body in the elbow. The doctor leans back to separate the joint surfaces (Fig 2.19) and extends the patient's arm during repeated pronation and supination (Figs 2.20, 2.21).

Two points are worth amplifying. First, manipulation is a vigorous business but not an uncontrolled wrench. It is a strict step-by-step process (*Figures 2.19; 2.20; 2.21*). To start with, manual traction is applied. Then the operator takes the joint to the starting point for the manipulation. For instance, at the elbow the forearm is swung towards extension. At the cervical spine the neck is twisted until the tissue resistance that heralds the end of range. At the knee, the tibia is rotated during increasing extension. Finally, the operator applies his over-pressure. In many cases this may be a movement of tiny amplitude. Thus at the elbow, as the end of range is reached a small jerk secures additional extension and full rotation. At the neck, rotation is accentuated by a sharp twist of a couple of degrees. At the knee, a final thrust is given towards extension and rotation.

Second, re-examination after each manipulation is indispensable. Without it the operator has no idea of what progress has been made. To report on any alteration in his condition, naturally the patient must be conscious; anaesthesia is therefore highly unwise and in any case is not required (except occasionally for a meniscus at the knee), as manipulation is not painful.

The objective of manipulation is the restoration of full painless movement, and treatment is discontinued once the maximum benefit has been exacted. This is soon achieved as manipulation works quickly or not at all; most success will be registered during the first or second sessions, and many patients are quite well after the first. It is rare that a fourth treatment produces enhanced results. Each session may go on for a long as half an hour; elderly patients are manipulated with equal vigour but for a shorter span.

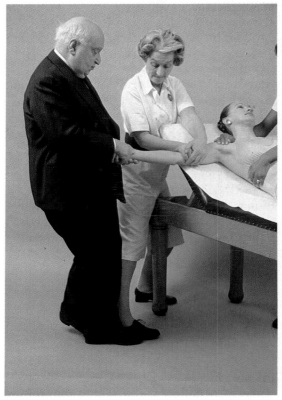

2.19

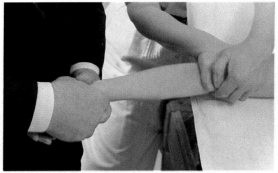

2.20

MANIPULATION: GENERAL SUMMARY

> 1. Purpose: to reduce a displacement.
>
> 2. Technique:
>
>   a) apply manual traction.
>
>   b) take joint to extreme of range.
>
>   c) apply over-pressure.
>
>   d) re-examine patient.
>
> *NB Precise procedure varies from joint to joint.*

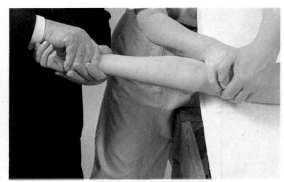

2.21

Treatment at the spine

Disorders at the spine fall neatly into two categories. A number of relatively rare conditions occur such as spondylitis, metastases, myeloma, chordoma, fracture, tuberculosis and Paget's disease. None is within the therapeutic scope of the orthopaedic physician who should, nevertheless, diagnose each case correctly. But a substantial proportion of patients suffer from minor radiotranslucent displacements of disc material. Such a loose body may exert pressure either on the dura mater to give rise to extrasegmental referred pain, or on the dural investment of the nerve roots to produce segmentally referred pain. The disc lesion may consist either of a cartilaginous fragment or part of the *nucleus pulposus*.

Principal treatments

A small cartilaginous displacement at any spinal level can usually be put back by manipulation (*Figures 2.22; 2.23; 2.24*). The principles are the same as for manipulation of the peripheral joints.

Manual traction is applied except at the lumbar spine, where it is ineffective. The joints are rotated and the patient is then re-examined. Twisting the spine turns all the joints along any given extent and the treatment is thus to some degree non-specific. But the strain will be borne by the blocked joint (i.e. the joint with the displacement) as it is there the movement is restricted. For further background information the reader is referred to page 142.

A small lumbar displacement of nuclear material can usually be reduced by a course of sustained traction (*Figure 2.25*). A distracting force of never less than 80lb (35kg) and not more than 180lb (80kg) is used. Sessions are daily for half an hour and are given for two to three weeks.

The pain from a large lumbar disc lesion can ordinarily be abolished or permanently mitigated by desensitisation of the dura mater and its sleeve. Accordingly a solution of 50ml 1:200 procaine is injected into the sacral hiatus (*Figure 2.26*).

Again, the above treatments are easily mastered and often afford immediate relief.

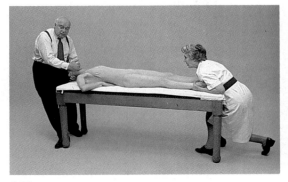

2.22

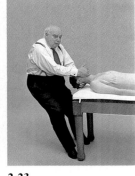

2.23

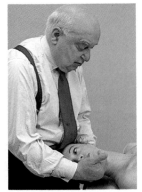

2.24

Figs 2.22, 2.23, 2.24
Manipulation. Nearly all cervical displacements respond to manipulation during traction. The neck is turned towards the extreme of range and then twisted a little further.

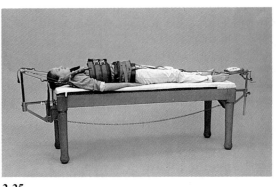

2.25

Fig 2.25 *Lumbar traction. Distraction of the vertebrae can suck a nuclear protrusion back into place. The treatment is useless if the pull is intermittent or too light.*

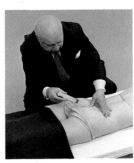

2.26

Fig 2.26 *Epidural injection. The dura mater and nerve roots are bathed in anaesthetic, often resulting in permanent alleviation of pain.*

TREATMENT OF AN INTERVERTEBRAL DISC LESION: SUMMARY

Cervical displacement	Thoracic displacement	Lumbar displacement

Manipulative reduction.	Manipulative reduction.
	
	To forestall relapse: Sclerosants.
		Manipulative reduction if cartilaginous.
		
		Traction if nuclear.
		
		Epidural local anaesthesia if irreducible.
		
		To forestall relapse:
		   1. Posture.
		   2. Corset.
		   3. Sclerosants.
		
		Only a tiny proportion of cases go to operation.

Note that signs or symptoms may strongly contraindicate manipulation or traction.

Orthopaedic medicine

Equipment
The physical resources for the diagnosis and treatment of the soft tissue lesions are minimal. Two couches are needed; both must be firm as manipulation cannot be conducted against a yielding surface. One couch should be about 15 inches high, the other about 30 inches high and a traction attachment and harness will serve to convert the latter into a traction table. The inventory is completed by supplies of procaine and steroid suspension. The doctor works in conjunction with one or more trained physiotherapists.

Application
Such resources are universally available within the existing medical framework. There is no shortage of patients.

Orthopaedic medicine and sports injuries

In this volume sports injuries are not considered as a separate entity; they are incorporated as an integral part of the book. It may generally be assumed that trauma to soft tissue will form one component of a sports injury whether or not accompanied by fracture. By no means are all soft-tissue lesions sports injuries, but most sports injuries are soft-tissue lesions. The issue is not whether the patient was playing sport when he suffered injury but what injury he suffered, and this is established in the same way whether a road accident or athletics was the cause.

Structure of this book
As spinal lesions frequently generate symptoms in the upper or lower limbs, a thorough understanding of the spine is essential before the peripheral joints are fully comprehensible. However, to avoid an accumulation of introductory material, the immediately ensuing chapters are devoted to the upper and lower limbs, while details on the complicating effect of the spine are held back to pages 133 and 222.

One chapter is reserved for each joint. In the appendices will be found:

(1) An illustration of each dermatome.
(2) A list of the capsular patterns.
(3) A summary of the examination and findings at each joint with treatment(s) for each condition.
(4) A consolidated tabulation of the various causes of pins and needles in the upper and lower limbs.

Teaching facilities are discussed in Appendix V.

PART TWO

THE
PERIPHERAL
JOINTS

CHAPTER THREE

THE
SHOULDER

The shoulder is the most rewarding and straightforward joint to deal with in the whole body and the finding of a limited or painful movement regularly means exactly what it should mean on anatomical grounds. Lesions of the joint and soft tissues are easily treated; once relieved, they seldom recur.

The mechanism of shoulder elevation is not always appreciated but has important diagnostic implications.

The 'best' joint in the body.

Referred pain

Nearly all shoulder structures are derived from the C5 segment. Pain will be felt within the C5 dermatome (*Figures 3.1* and *3.2*); it will be recalled this does not include the scapular area. The point of the shoulder is within the C4 dermatome (*Figures 3.3* and *3.4*)—the acromioclavicular joint refers pain to this area.

The pre-eminent cause of unilateral scapular pain is a cervical disc displacement giving rise to extrasegmental reference. With a cervical lesion the neck movements prove painful.

A lateral disc protrusion impinging on the C5, C6, C7 or C8 nerve root produces root pain felt down the arm in the relevant dermatome (see page 164).

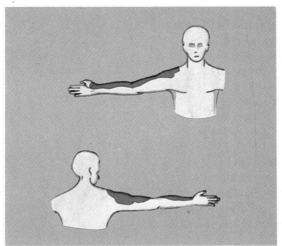

3.1, 3.2

Figs 3.1, 3.2 *The C5 dermatome.*

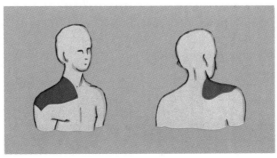

3.3, 3.4

Figs 3.3, 3.4 *The C4 dermatome.*

History

The history will suggest whether a cervical or shoulder lesion is involved. Once it is established the source of the pain lies at the shoulder, the history is relatively unrewarding—the ache is apt to be felt at the same place whatever the disorder. But the patient's age, the site of pain, whether other joints were affected and whether there was any trauma must be established.

Three further enquiries are made if the capsular pattern is found. Does the pain reach below the elbow? Does the arm ache all the time, even when held still? Can the patient sleep on that side at night?

Examination

A brief preliminary examination is required to exculpate the neck; provided the six active cervical movements prove painless, the patient then undergoes a routine of 12 shoulder movements.

Active and passive movements

The first step is active elevation (*Figure 3.5*). The patient is asked to raise her arm as far as she is able and it may later transpire that any limitation is devoid of organic basis; in genuine cases, either the joint range is restricted or the muscle is weak.

The patient's arm is now elevated passively as far as it will go (*Figure 3.6*). The possibilities are full range, limited range, pain or no pain. The end-feel is gauged; the normal joint possesses an unmistakable free feel at extreme of elevation. Range of passive movement is compared with the range attained on the previous active movement.

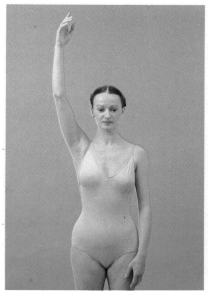

3.5

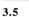

3.6

Limitation and pain on passive elevation is part of the capsular pattern; arthritis is accompanied by a hard end-feel. Pain at full elevation can be a localising sign in infraspinatus or supraspinatus tendinitis.

The patient then actively elevates her arm again and is asked to state at what moment (if any) the pain starts and whether it ceases on further elevation. A painful arc (*Figure 3.7*) is a secondary localising sign indicating the lesion lies in a pinchable position between the acromion and the tuberosities. Elevation beyond the painful arc may have to be accomplished in defiance of the patient's inclination in order to verify that the pain does in fact cease.

Fig 3.5 *Active elevation.*

Fig 3.6 *Passive elevation.*

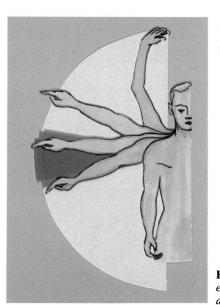

3.7

Fig 3.7 *A painful arc. The pain ceases on either side of the horizontal. It is an accessory sign.*

The exact amount of glenohumeral range can be established by testing passive abduction. The examiner fixes the lower angle of the scapula with his thumb, applying the heel of his hand to the patient's mid-thorax (*Figure 3.8*).

The patient's elbow is lifted upwards with the physician's other hand until he feels the scapula start to rotate. In a normal joint this happens when the arm arrives at the horizontal; it is at this point glenohumeral movement has attained its full extent and the physician's thumb starts to shift (*Figure 3.9*).

The two other passive movements for the joint are passive lateral rotation (*Figure 3.10*) and passive medial rotation (*Figure 3.11*). The capsular pattern at the shoulder will be evident by limitation in a fixed proportion of these two movements coupled with corresponding proportionate limitation of elevation. But an affection of the acromioclavicular joint throws up inexplicable pain on all three passive movements and its involvement can only be confirmed by checking whether passive horizontal adduction hurts as well.

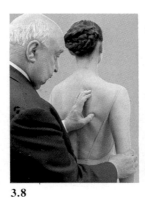
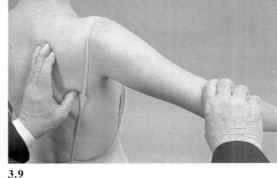

3.8   **3.9**

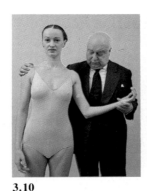
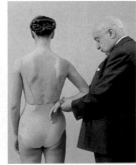

3.10   **3.11**

Figs 3.8, 3.9 *Passive elevation. The physician places his thumb on the angle of the shoulder blade to detect the point at which scapular rotation commences.*

Fig 3.10 *Passive lateral rotation.*

Fig 3.11 *Passive medial rotation.*

The mechanism of arm elevation

The first 90° of elevation take place at the glenohumeral joint. The scapula does not move appreciably in this phase.

The muscles controlling this movement are the supraspinatus and deltoid.

The next 60° of elevation result from rotation of the scapula. Even if the shoulder is ankylosed, 60° of passive abduction are possible; 60° of arm elevation always consists of scapular rotation.

The muscles concerned during this phase are the serratus anterior and the upper half of the trapezius muscle.

During the last 30° the scapula is stationary. The motion again takes place at the glenohumeral joint as a result of adduction of the humerus; the pectoralis major is responsible (*Figure 3.12*).

Diagnostic implications
The range of arm elevation possible at the shoulder is thus the 60° of scapular rotation always attainable plus the amount of glenohumeral movement whether occurring at the first or third stage of elevation.

The range of arm abduction must come to the amount of glenohumeral movement plus 60° (*Figure 3.13*). Thus if on active elevation

Fig 3.12 *Arm elevation, full. Only the first 90° and the last 30° take place at the glenohumeral joint.*

Figs 3.13, 3.14 *Arm elevation, restricted. Sixty degrees always consist of scapular rotation. This makes neurosis easy to detect.*

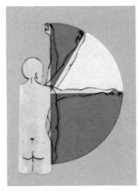
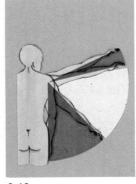
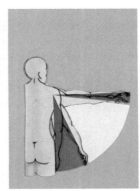

3.12   **3.13**   **3.14**

the patient alleges elevation beyond the horizontal is not feasible, it follows that her scapula should start to rotate at 30° (*Figure 3.14*). If, in fact, scapular rotation does not begin until 90°, the diagnosis is of neurosis or malingering, since there must always be at least a further 60° of elevation after commencement of scapular rotation.

Resisted movements

The resisted movements follow, evaluating contractile structures. Pain indicates a lesion to the muscle or tendon; a finding of weakness can most often be put down to one of the neuritises or, more likely, to a cervical root palsy.

Resisted abduction with the doctor correctly positioned (*Figure 3.15*) with his hand on the far side of the patient's trunk tests the deltoid (rarely affected) and supraspinatus, commonly injured at one of four sites. The patient presses outwards and the movement is thwarted at or above the elbow.

The doctor must not stand so the patient brings other muscles into play and topples over (*Figure 3.21*).

Resisted adduction (*Figure 3.16*) tests the pectoralis major, the latissimus dorsi and both the teres—lesions to any of these are rare. Counterpressure at the hip ensures muscle activity is limited to the shoulder joint.

The patient presses outwards and lateral rotation is resisted (*Figure 3.17*). Pain on this movement alone implies a lesion of the infraspinatus, but if resisted abduction hurts as well then the lesion lies in the supraspinatus. Very occasionally, both resisted lateral rotation and resisted adduction are painful, showing the teres minor to be at fault.

Resisted medial rotation (*Figure 3.18*) principally tests the subscapularis; the patient pulls inwards. In theory the pectoralis major, teres major or latissimus dorsi may be involved but in practice they are seldom injured.

Finally, two movements are performed for muscles which, although they control the elbow, extend to the shoulder. Resisted elbow flexion (*Figure 3.19*) assesses the biceps, frequently affected at any one of five sites. The patient pushes upwards.

Lastly, resisted elbow extension (*Figure 3.20*) puts strain on the triceps (rarely at fault). The patient forces her arm downwards.

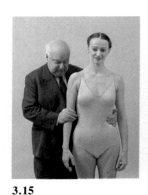
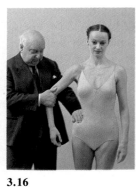
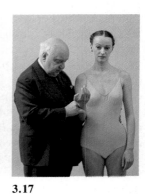

3.15 **3.16** **3.17**

Fig 3.15 *Resisted abduction, correct.* **Fig 3.16** *Resisted adduction.* **Fig 3.17** *Resisted lateral rotation.*

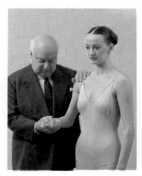
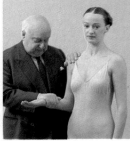
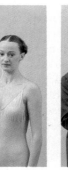
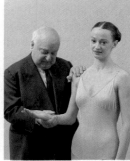

3.18 **3.19** **3.20**

Fig 3.18 *Resisted medial rotation.* **Fig 3.19** *Resisted elbow flexion.* **Fig 3.20** *Resisted elbow extension.*

Although the triceps are of C7 derivation, normally the pain from this movement will be felt in the C5 dermatome, thus exculpating the triceps.

Such symptoms are attributable to upward movement of the humerus against the tissues under the acromion (i.e. patients with a painful arc).

Double lesions are an occasional feature of the shoulder and the examination should never be relinquished until all 12 movements have been performed.

Fig 3.21 *Resisted abduction, incorrect.*

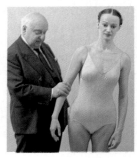

3.21

Findings

Capsular lesions

There are about a dozen separate disorders characterised by limitation of movement in the capsular pattern, but the three commonest are traumatic arthritis, steroid sensitive arthritis and osteoarthrosis. This last is often painless of itself although the joint becomes more sensitive and thus liable to develop a superimposed traumatic arthritis; crepitus is palpable.

The capsular pattern is designated by a hard end-feel and limitation of all three passive movements in fixed proportions. Limitation of medial rotation (*Figure 3.22*) is slight; the patient cannot fully put her arm behind her back. There is greater restriction of glenohumeral abduction (*Figure 3.23*) but it is impairment of lateral rotation that is the most marked (*Figure 3.24*).

In a case of medium severity, medial rotation is cut back by some 10°–15°, glenohumeral abduction by about 45° and lateral rotation by 60° to 70°. In a very mild attack, medial rotation is full but painful and the other limitations amount to between 10° and 30° and to about 45° respectively.

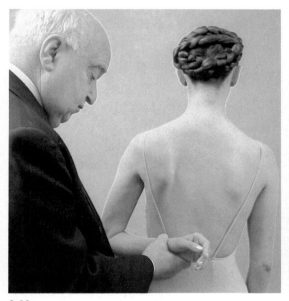

3.22

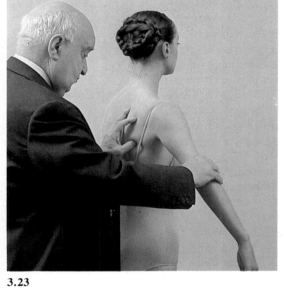

3.23

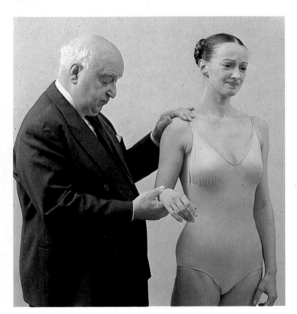

3.24

Figs 3.22, 3.23, 3.24 *Arthritis. The capsular pattern is a matter of proportion—maximum attainable range is shown in a mild case. Medial rotation (top left) is less limited than glenohumeral abduction (top right) which, in turn, is less limited than lateral rotation (left).*

Traumatic arthritis

The patient is aged 45 or over. The causative trauma is often slight and the pain only starts a week later when it gradually spreads down the arm. If untreated, the pain and limitation fill out together, reaching their maximum after about three months with symptoms extending to the wrist. The pain wears off as it recedes up the arm over the next four months, but full range will not return for a year from onset.

Treatment varies according to the stage the condition has reached. Immobilisation arthritis can be avoided by use of the joint daily; if stiffness has already set in, the treatment is stretching as for traumatic arthritis.

Stage 1

During the first four or five weeks the traumatic arthritis can be aborted by stretching the capsule (*Figure 3.25*); in this period the end-feel should be elastic.

Short-wave diathermy is administered as an analgesic immediately before the treatment commences. Then the joint is repeatedly pushed towards the extreme of elevation with one hand on the patient's sternum to prevent her back arching (*Figure 3.26*). The movement is gentle but pressure does not cease until pain rather than discomfort is evoked, and the physiotherapist must expect to overcome appreciable resistance to movement (which is encountered before painful range is reached). The stretching is not a matter of sharp jabs; it is by careful and sustained pressure that gross muscle spasm is avoided.

If the ache engendered by treatment persists for more than a couple of hours, subsequent attempts are called off. Otherwise the sessions last 15 minutes three times a week until full range is restored in a month or so. When some progress has been made, stretching of abduction and rotation can be cautiously added.

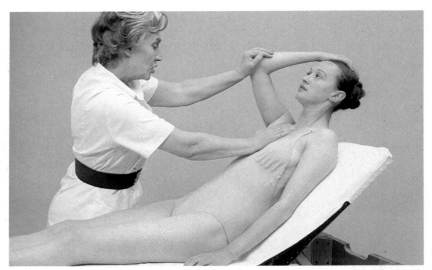

3.25

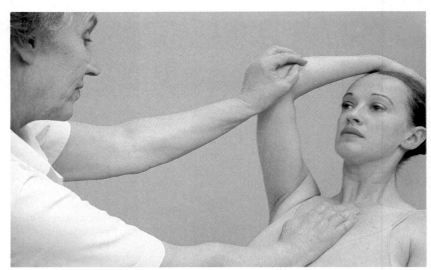

3.26

Fig 3.25 *Stretching the shoulder joint is called for in all cases of recent capsular trauma.*

Fig 3.26 *Elevation is forced by upwards pressure against the patient's elbow. Active exercises in every direction follow each treatment.*

Stage 2

If untreated for the first month, the joint becomes too irritable to be stretched. This phase is definitely under way when all the following hold true:

(1) The pain has spread below the elbow.
(2) The arm is painful even when still.
(3) The patient cannot lie on her bad side at night.

If only one or two of the above indicators are present, stretching may be tried cautiously but the treatment must be halted immediately on any adverse response.

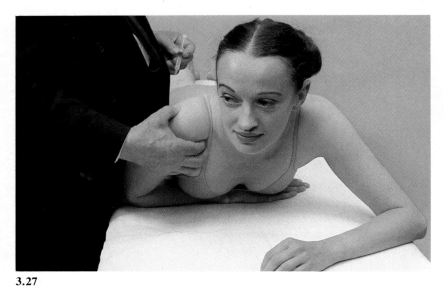

3.27

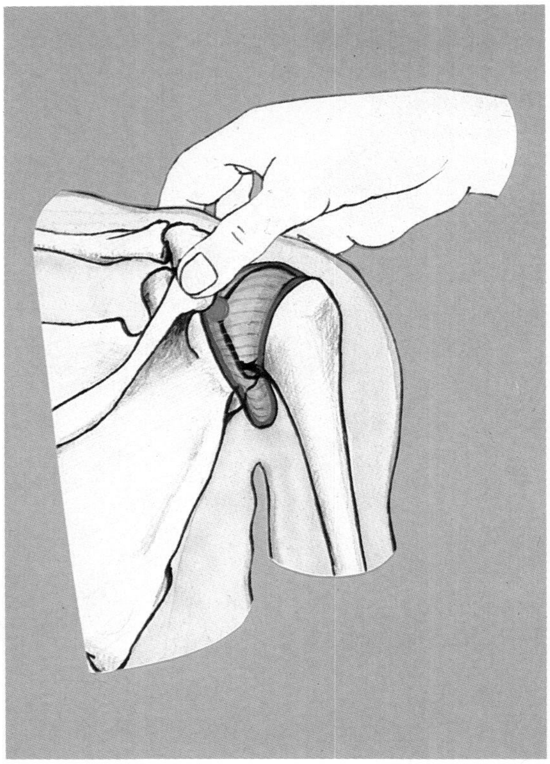

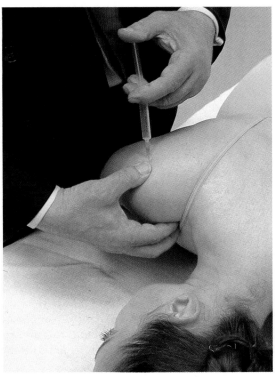

3.28

Fig 3.27 *Capsular injection. The glenoid cavity lies between the operator's thumb and index finger.*

Fig 3.28 *The injection is given when impingement against cartilage is felt.*

Treatment during the second stage consists of an injection of steroid suspension 2ml using a 5cm needle. The patient lies prone with her forearm under her stomach, thus turning the articular surface of the humerus to face posteriorly. The index finger of the operator's free hand is on the tip of the coracoid process with his thumb where the acromion and the spine of the scapula join at right angles. An imaginary line linking the fingers would cross the glenoid cavity (*Figure 3.27*).

The needle punctures the skin at the physician's thumb and is aimed just lateral to the tip of his index finger (*Figures 3.28; 3.29*).

The joint capsule offers clear and characteristic resistance at about 4cm. When impingement against cartilage is felt, the needle is withdrawn 0.5mm and the injection given. The constant pain goes in 36 hours and the injection is repeated after a week. Further injections follow at increasing intervals to forestall the return of pain; four is the least and ten the greatest number of injections to expect. Range of movement does not start to come back until after the first four.

3.29

Fig 3.29 *Both traumatic and monarticular rheumatoid arthritis respond well to intra-articular steroid suspension.*

Alternatively, in the second stage, the joint can be distracted. Each aspect of the joint capsule is relaxed by maintaining the patient's arm in slight flexion and medial rotation (*Figure 3.30*).

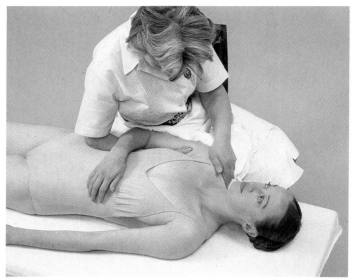

3.30

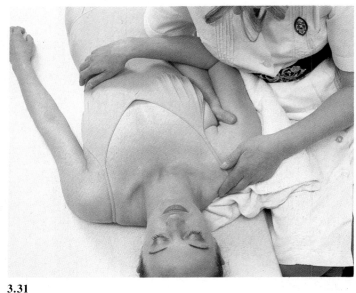

3.31

The physiotherapist strives to pull the head of the humerus away from the glenoid cup. Abduction must not occur and is curbed by the physiotherapist's exerting counterpressure via a rolled towel at the patient's elbow. This ensures that the whole of the patient's upper arm is moved away from the thorax while remaining parallel to the axis of her body. The pressure is directed outwards, with the physiotherapist's hand slotted into the axilla

(*Figure 3.31*). Pressure is intermittent and only minimal distraction, for example, 1cm, can be coaxed. Sessions last half an hour, initially daily, and in a severe case the muscles will not relax until the second or third treatment, with no distraction attained at the first. As pain abates over succeeding sessions greater distraction is employed until in due course the end-feel becomes elastic. Then the joint may be stretched in the ordinary way.

Figs 3.30, 3.31
Distraction techniques are an alternative when the joint is too irritable for stretching. The hand in the axilla does all the work.

Stage 3
Recovery can be expedited by stretching. The three diagnostic indicators will be absent. Normally this phase sets in some five months after onset, and thereafter stretching can lop up to several months off recovery time which might otherwise run to a full year.

Steroid sensitive arthritis
The patient is aged between 30 and 70, more commonly between 45 and 60. There is no trauma. Over a span of three months pain spreads down the arm to the forearm and wrist; the ache is constant with marked limitation in the capsular pattern. Spontaneous recovery takes up to two years, and limitation persists after the ache has gone. Sometimes there is recurrence at the other shoulder.

Steroid suspension 2ml is injected into the joint using the same technique as for traumatic arthritis; the pain disappears by the next day. The injection is repeated weekly at first and thereafter at widening intervals, but in any event before the onset of pain. Six to 12 injections are the rule.

Arthritis complicating psoriasis, lupus erythematosus and ankylosing spondylitis also benefit from this treatment, but not Reiter's disease.

Non-capsular lesions

Acute subdeltoid bursitis

Acute subdeltoid bursitis limits passive movement but not in the capsular pattern. Without injury, the whole bursa (*Figure 3.32*) becomes badly inflamed and in the course of two or three days the patient loses almost all capacity to abduct the arm; the pain reaches the wrist. Other passive movements retain very nearly full range, the resisted movements are painless, and the painful arc appears only as the condition abates because initially arm elevation is out of the question. There is often a history of previous attacks.

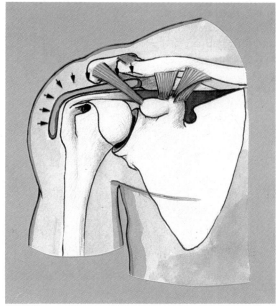

3.32

Fig 3.32 *The whole extent of the bursa is extremely tender and often thickened. A large portion of the lesion may lie in the restricted space under the acromial arch.*

Stage 1

The acute pain lasts seven to ten days and it is worth injecting only in this period. The physician palpates for tenderness to outline the tender area, but he will bear in mind that part of the bursa is shielded by the acromion.

Morphine is injected as a preliminary measure. Then the accessible extent of the bursa receives a cluster of little infiltrations using steroid suspension 5ml and a 5cm needle (*Figure 3.33*).

The site and angle of insertion are altered; a further injection of steroid suspension 5ml is given by multiple insertions into the subacromial extent of the bursa (*Figure 3.34*). The physician locates the point of the acromion with his thumb and slides the needle under it so that the approach is horizontal (*Figure 3.35*). Following infiltration, more morphine is administered and by the next day the patient is sore but mobile.

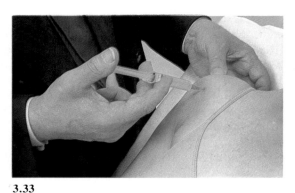

3.33

Fig 3.33 *Steroid suspension 5ml is injected throughout the accessible extent.*

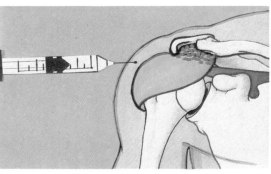

3.34

3.35

Figs 3.34, 3.35 *Another 5ml is directed into the part of the bursa under the acromion.*

Stage 2

After the first week the patient is on the mend and injection is not warranted. Instead a figure of eight bandage (*Figure 3.36*) is needed at night to stop the arm drifting into painful range. Analgesics are prescribed for a week or so.

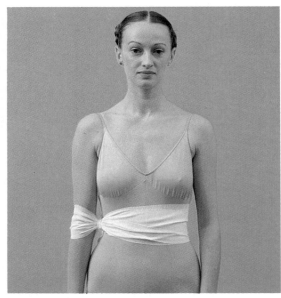

3.36

Fig 3.36 *Acute bursitis recovers spontaneously in six weeks. After the first phase, only a nocturnal bandage is needed.*

Chronic subdeltoid bursitis

Chronic subdeltoid bursitis may continue indefinitely. Unlike acute bursitis, only a sector of the bursa is affected.

The condition is hard to distinguish from minor tendinitis and can be the cause of otherwise incomprehensible shoulder pain. Often a painful arc is the only symptom and all resisted and passive movements are painless.

The sensitive spot is sought by palpation and, if found, is injected. If it cannot be traced, the inflammation must lie concealed under the acromion and a likely area is infiltrated. A solution of 0.5% procaine 5–10ml (depending on the size of the lesion) is injected in droplets all over the inflamed area. A couple of infiltrations into the correct spot are usually curative; if not, steroid suspension 5ml is substituted.

Differential diagnosis

Other causes of limitation of passive movements in the non-capsular pattern include:

(1) Pulmonary neoplasm: muscle spasm restricts elevation beyond the horizontal; the scapula is mobile with a full range of movement at the shoulder joint.
(2) Capsular adhesion: localised capsular scarring. Treatment is by stretching.
(3) Subcoracoid bursitis: isolated limitation of lateral rotation. Steroid suspension 2ml should be injected.
(4) Contracture of the costocoracoid fascia: gradually intensifying pectoroscapular pain, slight limitation of elevation of scapula. No treatment avails.
(5) Fracture of the first rib: the pain is brought on by neck and scapular movements. Active elevation of the arm is limited but passive elevation is full; an X-ray is diagnostic.
(6) Psychogenic pain.

All except the last are rare.

Contractile structures

Tendinous lesions abound at the shoulder. Although active range may often be limited by pain, passive movement is full. One resisted movement brings on the pain. In all cases—with the exception of the musculotendinous junction of the supraspinatus and the glenoid origin of the biceps—the tendinitis responds to either massage or steroid injection.

Often localising signs indicate the particular site of the lesion in the tendon. As a rule the disorders are brought on by over-use or repeated strain rather than by a single causative strain.

Recurrence is rare and should be disposed of by further injection or massage.

Supraspinatus tendinitis

This is the most prevalent tendinous lesion at the shoulder, and is signalled by painful resisted abduction sometimes coupled with painful resisted lateral rotation. The lesion can lie at any one of four different sites (*Figures 3.37*) readily differentiated by the presence or absence of a painful arc and/or pain on full elevation. The musculotendinous site can be put right by massage; the other three benefit from massage or alternatively an injection of steroid suspension.

A very painful arc suggests calcification (uncommon), which shows on the X-ray. This makes massage redundant and 5ml of 2% procaine is exchanged for the steroid infiltration.

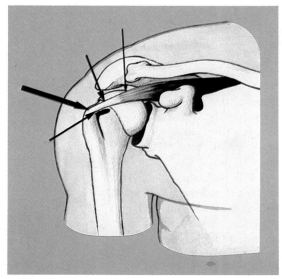

3.37a

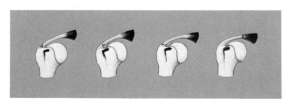

3.37b

Figs 3.37a, 3.37b *Supraspinatus tendinitis. The lesion may lie at one of four sites. They must be distinguished if treatment is to be effective.*

The tenoperiosteal site

If painful resisted abduction is accompanied by a painful arc, that demonstrates the lesion lies in a pinchable position between the acromion and the greater tuberosity, that is, at the superficial aspect of the tenoperiosteal junction. The momentary pain is caused as the inflamed area squeezes under the acromial arch on arm elevation (*Figures 3.38; 3.39; 3.40*).

The treatment is either massage or injection, but in both cases the same obstacle must be overcome: the tendon in its horizontal course is masked from above by the acromion (see *Figure 3.37a*).

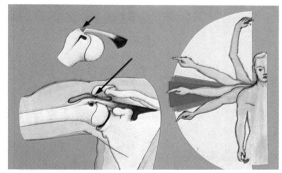

3.38, 3.39, 3.40

Figs 3.38, 3.39, 3.40 *The tenoperiosteal site gives rise to a painful arc. After attaining the horizontal, the head of the humerus starts to drop slightly in the glenoid cavity.*

The lesion can be reached if the patient arranges her arm behind her back with the elbow bent (*Figure 3.41*). Medial rotation of

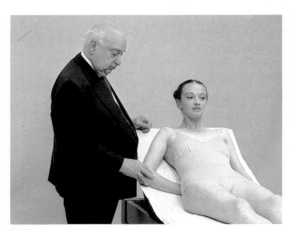

3.41

the shoulder brings the greater tuberosity forwards; adducting the elbow as the arm moves across behind the back further exposes the tendon which can now be felt just lateral to the bicipital groove, climbing almost vertically upwards from the tuberosity (*Figures 3.42; 3.43*).

The needle is thrust downwards and the lesion infiltrated with steroid suspension 1ml (*Figure 3.44*). No resistance is felt until the tip reaches the tendon, and provided the needle lies correctly, it encounters tough tendinous resistance as the injection proceeds.

About 20 droplets are distributed throughout the cubic extent of the lesion by a series of half-withdrawals and reinsertions; the tendon is about 1.5cm wide. Normally one or two injections are curative.

For massage, the patient's position is similar, with her arm behind her back (*Figure 3.45*). Sessions last 20 minutes twice weekly for two to five weeks. Counterpressure is supplied by the thumb on the deltoid and the greatest strength of the physiotherapist is hardly enough to break up the scar tissue. The amplitude of sweep is 2cm with the fingers moving horizontally (*Figure 3.46*) across the near-vertical tendon.

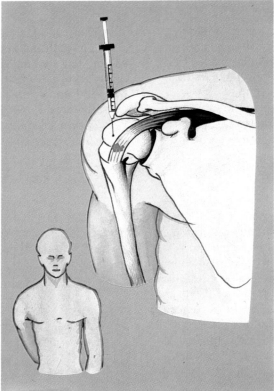

3.42, 3.43

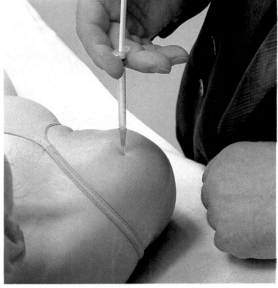

3.44

Fig 3.41 *Injection. The patient's arm is placed right behind her back.*

Figs 3.42, 3.43 *In this position the tendon passes forwards over the head of the humerus. This makes it emerge from under the acromion.*

Fig 3.44 *About half the cases are cured by one injection. Most of the rest get well with two or three.*

Figs 3.45, 3.46 *Massage is the alternative. On average the patient is better in a month.*

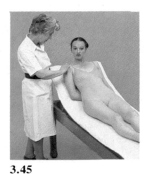

3.45

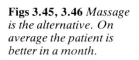

3.46

The tenoperiosteal junction, deep aspect
Painful resisted abduction linked with pain on
full passive elevation shows that the lesion is
disposed where the greater tuberosity and the
glenoid rim pinch the tendon at the deep aspect
of the tenoperiosteal junction (*Figures 3.47;
3.48*).

Both injection and massage conform to the
pattern at the superficial aspect except:
(1) The needle must penetrate more deeply.
(2) Recovery by massage is slower because the
thickness of the tendon intervenes between
the physiotherapist's digit and the lesion.

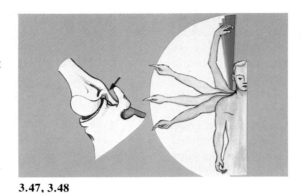

3.47, 3.48

Figs 3.47, 3.48 *Full
passive elevation hurts if
the scar lies deeply at the
distal end of the tendon.*

The distal end of the tendon
Painful resisted abduction accompanied by
both a painful arc and pain on full elevation
argues that the lesion must occupy both the
superficial and the deep aspect of the tendon;
that is, it runs right through (*Figures 3.49;
3.50*).

Again both injection and massage are
effective. The injection must reach both
aspects of the tendon.

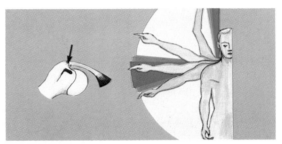

3.49, 3.50

Figs 3.49, 3.50 *If both
signs are found, the
distal end of the tendon
is clearly traversed by the
lesion.*

The musculotendinous junction
If resisted abduction hurts with neither a
painful arc nor pain on full elevation, attention
is drawn to the proximal end of the tendon
(*Figure 3.51*).

At this site only massage works. With the
arm dependent, the lesion is completely
sheltered by the acromion; but if the patient
sits with her arm supported horizontally, the
musculotendinous junction slides proximally to
within reach of the physiotherapist's finger.

The physiotherapist is stationed behind and
to the side of the patient (*Figure 3.52*). The
reinforced middle finger is pressed deeply into
the angle formed by the spine of the scapula
and the back of the outer part of the clavicle,
while the friction is imparted by rotating the
forearm to and fro (*Figures 3.53; 3.54*). Eight
quarter-of-an-hour treatments on alternate
days should suffice.

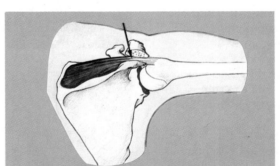

3.51

Fig 3.51 *Musculotendinous junction.
Diagnosis at this site may have to be
verified by local anaesthesia.*

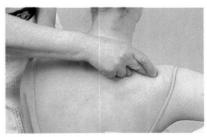

3.52

Fig 3.52 *Massage. This posture brings
the lesion within reach.*

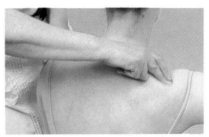

3.53

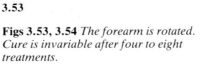

3.54

Figs 3.53, 3.54 *The forearm is rotated.
Cure is invariable after four to eight
treatments.*

The infraspinatus

Pain on resisted lateral rotation incriminates the infraspinatus tendon, but the localising signs for the various sites (*Figure 3.55*) are not so plain. A painful arc suggests that the lesion lies at the superficial aspect of the distal end of the tendon, and pain on full elevation focuses attention on the deep aspect of the distal end. In default of these signs the body of the tendon (not the musculotendinous junction) contains the lesion; the physician searches for the point of maximum tenderness. The lesion is rather difficult to pinpoint and if in doubt local anaesthetic should be used diagnostically.

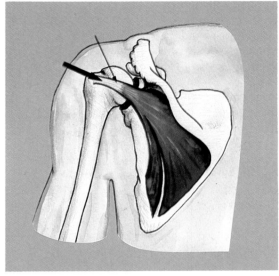

3.55

Fig 3.55 *The sites. The painful scar lies either close to or at the insertion of the tendon into the greater tuberosity.*

For injection or massage the patient lies prone, propped up on her elbows. This pushes the scapula upwards and uncovers the head of the humerus. The patient's arm is in flexion and slight lateral rotation; then it is put into slight adduction (*Figure 3.56*) to draw out the humeral tuberosity from under the acromion.

This ensures that the infraspinatus is easily found just below the most lateral extent of the spine of the scapula as it runs in its course towards the head of the humerus.

The injection of 1ml steroid (*Figure 3.57*) is delivered in 20 droplets to the cubic extent of the affected area both deeply and superficially. A back-up injection may subsequently be required.

The massage position is identical. While the fingers supply counterpressure, the thumb is alternately abducted and adducted across the lesion (*Figure 3.58*) for 20 minutes at a time every other day. Recovery is to be anticipated in about three weeks.

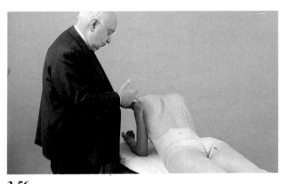

3.56

Fig 3.56 *Injection. The patient adopts a special position.*

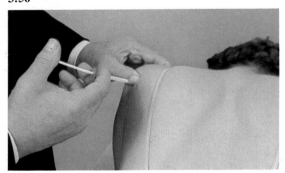

3.57

Fig 3.57 *Most cases are well after one or two injections.*

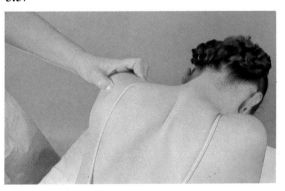

3.58

Fig 3.58 *Massage. The main difficulty is to ensure the treatment is given to the exact spot.*

The subscapularis

Pain on resisted medial rotation can be ascribed to the subscapularis but in the unlikely event that resisted adduction also hurts, one of the other members of the group—the pectoralis major, latissimus dorsi or teres major—is to blame. There are two sites for a lesion to the subscapularis (*Figure 3.59*), both at the insertion into the humerus.

A painful arc argues that the tendon is injured at the uppermost site. But if full passive adduction of the arm across the front of the chest hurts then the lesion is situated at the lower extent along the shaft of the humerus, where it can be pinched against the point of the coracoid.

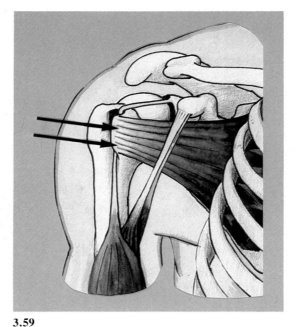

3.59

Fig 3.59 *The tendon is affected at the insertion into bone. There are two sites.*

For the injection of steroid suspension 1ml the patient lies with her hand on her thigh so the bicipital groove faces directly anteriorly. To palpate, the thumb is laid on the head of the humerus and guided laterally until it encounters the bicipital groove, identification of which is facilitated by an assistant rotating the patient's arm. This shifts the two edges under the physician's stationary thumb (*Figure 3.60*).

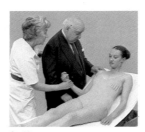

3.60

Fig 3.60 *Identification of the bicipital groove.*

The subscapularis is immediately medial to the inner edge of the groove; the tendon is extremely thin and feels as hard as the bone it overlies. The point of maximum tenderness is sought. As the needle proceeds it can be felt to pierce tendon and then hit bone. The tendon is infiltrated with about 20 droplets at points 0.5 to 1cm medial to the edge of the groove (*Figure 3.61*). Results are good; one injection is curative.

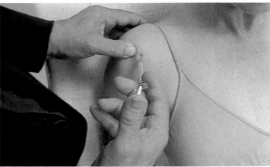

3.61

Fig 3.61 *Steroid suspension is extremely successful.*

For the massage, the physiotherapist locates the tendon and hooks her thumb round the medial edge of the upper part of the deltoid. She draws the belly laterally, letting the short head of biceps slip under her finger, so that her thumb can connect directly with the subscapular tendon (*Figure 3.62*) without the intervening mass of deltoid belly.

Her thumb moves vertically up and down while counterpressure is maintained by her fingers at the back of the shoulder. The therapy is very painful for the patient, so treatment is limited to two sessions a week; recovery takes about a month.

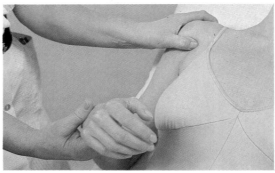

3.62

Fig 3.62 *Massage is the alternative, but not more than two-thirds of patients achieve full relief. The treatment is very painful.*

The biceps

There are five sites (*Figure 3.63*). The two at the lower extent are dealt with as elbow structures on page 52.

Two movements are painful—resisted elbow flexion and resisted supination. But if resisted supination does not hurt, the brachialis (rarely affected) is at fault.

The lesion may be at either the glenoid origin or the upper part of the tendon where it lies recessed in the bicipital groove. This latter site is accessible to palpation and the pain is at the front of the upper arm.

By contrast the glenoid origin is sheltered by the acromion and the coracoid, and the pain is confined to the front of the shoulder.

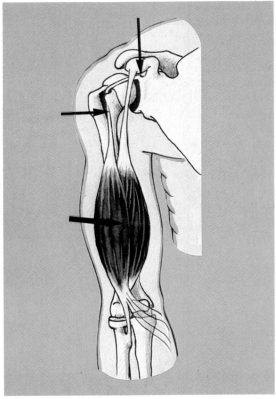

3.63

Fig 3.63 *There are three upper sites. Only when the forearm is held supinated will a bicipital lesion cause pain on resisted flexion.*

The glenoid origin

Massage is impossible. For the injection (*Figure 3.64*) the patient is in the half-lying position, the arm fully abducted and gripped by an assistant at about 45° short of full lateral rotation. This ensures the bicipital groove is level with the anterior edge of the acromion.

The physician places his left thumb at the gap between the tuberosities either side of the tendon and the needle is thrust in 1cm distally (*Figure 3.65*).

As the tip passes backwards and medially between the two tuberosities, it runs into the resistance of the tendon at a depth of about 3cm (*Figure 3.66*) and steroid suspension 2ml is discharged in 20 droplets. As a rule, one injection is curative.

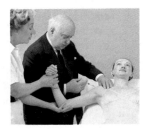

3.64

Fig 3.64 *Injection. The patient's arm is fully abducted and in lateral rotation. At this rare site resisted adduction can be the only movement that hurts.*

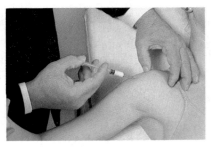

3.65

Fig 3.65 *The injection is difficult technically as the point of entry is distant from the lesion and the position of the patient's arm is critical.*

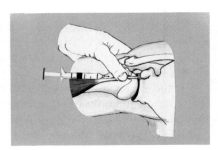

3.66

Fig 3.66 *Correctly placed infiltration is curative.*

The bicipital groove

Massage succeeds so quickly that injection is an unnecessary luxury. The physiotherapist identifies the biceps tendon in the groove of the humerus and presses her fingers down hard on the lesion. She then rotates the humerus to and fro using the patient's flexed forearm as a lever (*Figures 3.67; 3.68*); if the massage is kept up in this way for some 20 minutes on alternate days the patient should be well in two weeks.

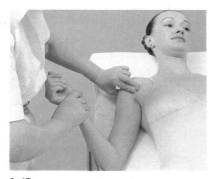
3.67

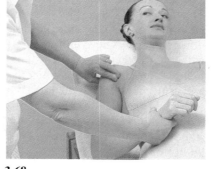
3.68

Figs 3.67, 3.68 *Massage, by rotating the tendon under the pad of the stationary index finger. An alternative approach is to move the thumb over the tendon.*

The belly

Normally the lesion lies deeply about half-way down the belly and can be traced by pinching the deep aspect of the muscle between fingers and thumb, although in awkward cases local anaesthesia furnishes useful corroborative evidence. Palpation from in front is of no help as the lesion does not lie anteriorly.

The treatment is massage; the physiotherapist squeezes the tender area between fingers and thumb. Pressure is maintained while the friction is imparted by the physiotherapist pulling her whole hand vigorously to and fro by a good inch (*Figures 3.69; 3.70*).

The sessions last 20 minutes on alternate days for two or three weeks. Steroids will fail.

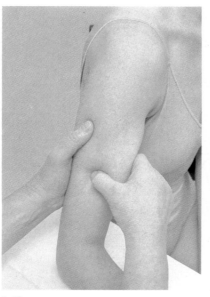
3.69

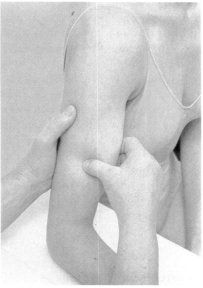
3.70

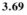

Figs 3.69, 3.70 *Massage, belty. Note the amount of pull. Only very chronic cases prove intractable.*

Weakness

Painless weakness in the arm may result from:
(1) A cervical root palsy with impaired conduction (see pages 164–166).
(2) Rupture, usually of the supraspinatus. The painful arc can be abolished by injection of steroid suspension 1ml to the frayed ends of the tendon.
(3) Neuritis. A long thoracic neuritis or spinal accessory neuritis is denoted by incapacity fully to elevate the arm actively. Passive elevation is full and painless. Suprascapular neuritis is marked by very weak resisted lateral rotation and weak abduction.

In all three neuritises the pain goes on for three weeks and muscle power returns in four to eight months. Treatment does not accelerate the spontaneous recovery.
(4) Malignant deposits in the acromion.

The acromioclavicular joint

The acromioclavicular joint is a C4 structure and therefore is incapable of referring pain down the arm. The symptoms are purely local whatever the cause and are usually elicited by the extreme of passive movement of scapula and arm; that is, since the joint is minimally shifted by all shoulder movements they all tend to hurt, although passive horizontal adduction stands out as the most painful. There is no limitation.

The condition is usually traumatic and is prevalent among athletes after a fall on the shoulder; osteoarthrosis with much the same symptoms also occurs. Spontaneous recovery normally takes one to two months but the symptoms, whether traumatic or osteoarthritic, may be eliminated within 24 hours by an injection of steroid suspension. Alternatively, massage alleviates the discomfort in a few weeks but the treatment is only successful if the superior ligament alone is affected.

Fig 3.71 *Injection. One to two ml of steroid suspension get rid of the post-traumatic inflammatory reaction. The injection is viewed from above.*

Fig 3.72 *Both the superior and inferior ligaments are injected. The joint line is tiny and difficult to palpate.*

For the injection (*Figure 3.71*) the lateral edge of the acromion is identified; 2cm medial to this line is the gap between acromion and clavicle.

The physician palpates for tenderness. Steroid suspension 1ml is sufficient if just the inferior ligament needs infiltration, but if the superior ligament is to be tackled as well the dosage is 2ml.

The needle is thrust vertically downwards (*Figure 3.72*); should bone be encountered at a depth of less than 1cm, the tip does not rest intra-articularly and must be adjusted until it slips in to about 2cm. The deep ligament is infiltrated by 5 or 10 drops distributed fanwise and the superior ligament is similarly injected along each side of the joint line.

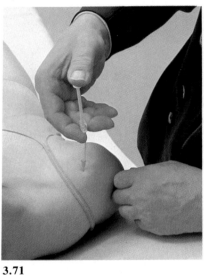

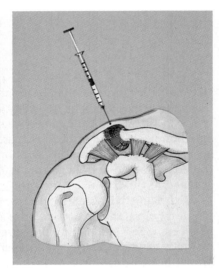

3.71

3.72

The sternoclavicular joint

The pain is felt locally at the front of the base of the neck. The condition is nearly always traumatic. Both active and passive scapular elevation and elevation of the arm are painful, and passive neck extension and resisted neck flexion hurt too. This combination of pain on both neck and scapular movement directs attention towards the sternoclavicular joint, which proves tender. The symptoms are inclined to continue indefinitely if untreated, but they may be despatched by infiltration (*Figure 3.73*) of steroid suspension 1–2ml. The point of entry is between the clavicle and the sternum; the injection is made intra-articularly (*Figure 3.74*).

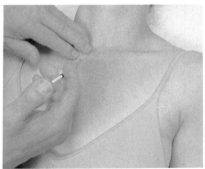

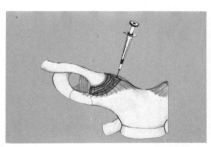

3.74

3.73

Figs 3.73, 3.74 *The joint responds so well to steroid suspension that other methods of treatment are not worth considering.*

CHAPTER FOUR

THE
ELBOW

Although the elbow is a complicated joint, the lesions are relatively simple to identify. As at the shoulder, history is of little assistance diagnostically but the clinical findings are clear-cut and easy to interpret.

Symptoms can of course be referred from the shoulder or neck, but the patient generally distinguishes pain of local origin. Lesions of the elbow itself cause pain felt locally.

The normal end-feel at the elbow is hard on extension and leathery on rotation. Flexion is marked by tissue approximation.

The elbow joint proper and the superior radioulnar joint are considered as an entity.

Referred pain

The front of the elbow is within the C5 and C6 dermatomes (*Figures 4.1; 4.2*) so the symptoms may arise from the shoulder or cervical nerve roots. At the posterior aspect the dermatome is C7 (*Figure 4.3*). Referred pain is characterised by its indefinite extent.

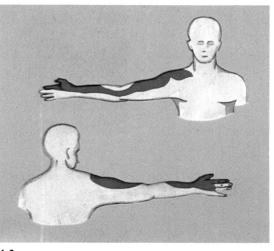

4.2

Fig 4.2 *Note the C6 dermatome includes part of the hand.*

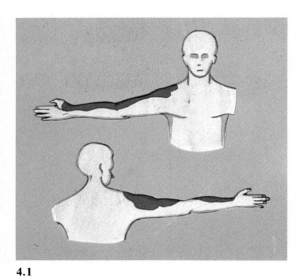

4.1

Fig 4.1 *The C5 dermatome.*

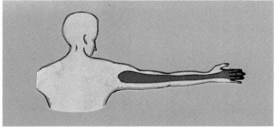

4.3

Fig 4.3 *The most likely cause of a C7 pain is a C6 disc lesion.*

Examination

After a careful history, and preliminary examination of the neck and shoulder if necessary, the elbow is evaluated by 10 movements.

Passive movements
The primary movements are passive flexion (*Figure 4.4*) and passive extension (*Figure 4.5*). Early arthritis declares itself as limitation in the capsular pattern of these two movements alone. A soft end-feel on extension suggests a loose body, and a hard end-feel on flexion indicates arthritis.

Passive pronation (*Figure 4.6*) and supination (*Figure 4.7*) test the upper radioulnar joint; the elbow is held flexed to avoid rotation at the shoulder. Painful limitation may arise in severe arthritis at the elbow; again the end-feel would be hard. It will be remembered that the source of pain on passive pronation can be a lesion of the biceps tendon at the tuberosity (see page 53).

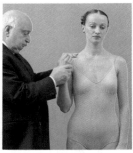
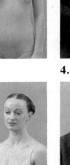
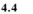

4.4

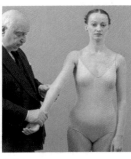
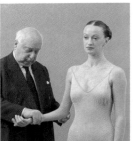

4.5

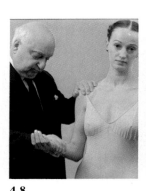

4.6

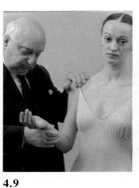

4.7

Fig 4.4 *Passive flexion.*

Fig 4.5 *Passive extension.*

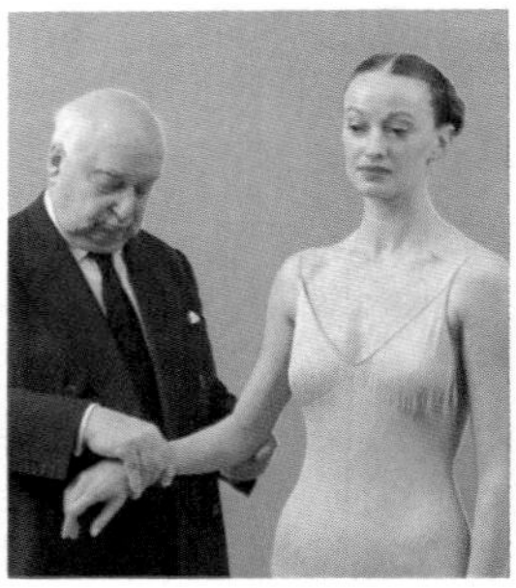

Fig 4.6 *Passive pronation.*

Fig 4.7 *Passive supination.*

Resisted movements
Resisted movements follow to assess the contractile structures. The resistance is applied to the lower forearm to preclude involvement of the wrist.

Pain on resisted flexion (*Figure 4.8*) incriminates the biceps (common) or brachialis (rare). The patient presses upwards.

Pain on resisted extension (*Figure 4.9*) suggests, theoretically, a lesion of the triceps (rare). But pain is more likely to be evinced by the impinging of the humerus on the underside of the acromion as the result of upward movement.

Resisted pronation (*Figure 4.10*) puts strain on the pronator teres. But on the whole, pain on this movement is an accessory sign for a golfer's elbow.

Resisted supination (*Figure 4.11*) tests the supinator brevis (rare) and the biceps (common); a lesion of the latter also produces pain on resisted flexion.

Pain on resisted wrist flexion (*Figure 4.12*) points to a golfer's elbow; the patient presses her hand downwards. For both the resisted movements at the wrist, the elbow joint is held in full extension.

Pain on resisted wrist extension (*Figure 4.13*) is normally due to a lesion of the extensores carpi radialis—a tennis elbow.

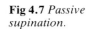

4.8

Fig 4.8 *Resisted flexion.*

4.9

Fig 4.9 *Resisted extension.*

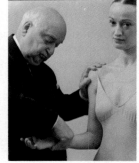

4.10

Fig 4.10 *Resisted pronation.*

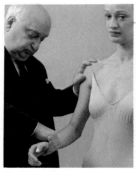

4.11

Fig 4.11 *Resisted supination.*

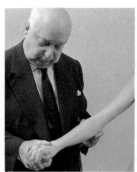

4.12

Fig 4.12 *Resisted wrist flexion.*

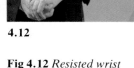

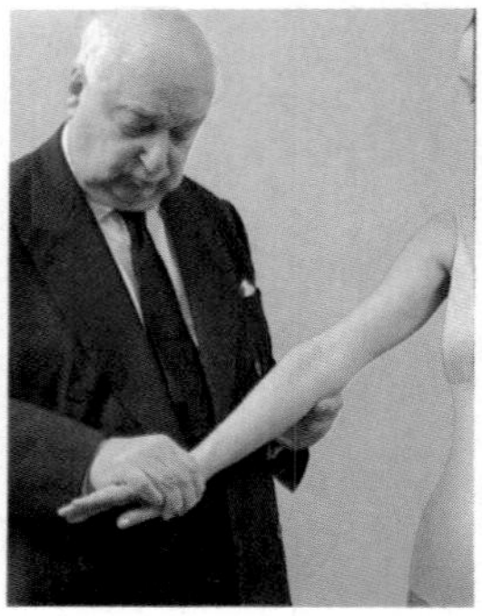

4.13

Fig 4.13 *Resisted wrist extension.*

Findings

Capsular lesions

Both traumatic arthritis and rheumatoid arthritis are common and both respond well to treatment by steroid infiltration. But osteoarthrosis requires no treatment, as it is almost entirely without symptoms unless over-use has superimposed a traumatic arthritis.

The capsular pattern is greater limitation of flexion (*Figure 4.14*)—the patient cannot bend her elbow fully—than of extension where it cannot be fully straightened (*Figure 4.15*).

Thirty degrees limitation of flexion would correspond to about 10° restriction of extension; occasionally the amounts of

limitation are about equal. The pictures illustrate the early capsular pattern. Because arthritis initially shows itself as an isolated affection of the humeroulnar joint, the rotations stay free.

But in advanced cases both pronation and supination will be slightly limited (*Figures 4.16; 4.17*), a finding most easily made by comparison with the good arm.

Palpation may reveal warmth and/or synovial thickening. Fluid may be present; aspiration will determine whether it is blood (aspirate *stat.*) or clear, in which case the cause must be found and dealt with.

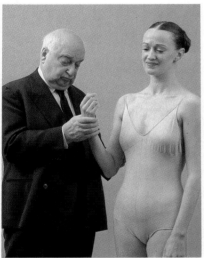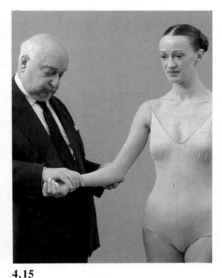

4.14 **4.15**

Figs 4.14, 4.15 *The capsular pattern is rather variable, but flexion (Fig 4.14) is usually more limited than extension (Fig 4.15).*

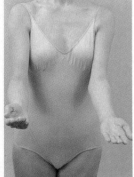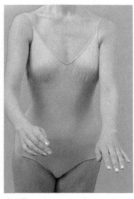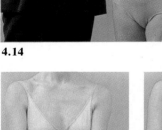

4.16 **4.17**

Figs 4.16, 4.17 *Only in severe cases will rotations be limited.*

Myositis ossificans: Caution

It is widely held that myositis ossificans results from improper treatment of a damaged elbow. Therefore forced movement towards extension is most ill-advised and must be avoided for fear

of medicolegal consequences.

The only conditions at the elbow that call for manipulation are a loose body and sometimes an epicondylar tennis elbow.

Arthritis

Arthritis, whether of traumatic or rheumatoid origin, can be effectively treated by an injection of steroid suspension 2ml. In rheumatoid-type cases the injection is repeated as the symptoms warrant, but although the pain is stopped range of movement is not much enhanced. Reiter's disease does not benefit.

With traumatic arthritis, any blood is aspirated before the first injection and a follow-up injection is required two weeks later. If rotation is painful in recent/acute traumatic arthritis, the head of the radius is almost certainly chipped in which case an X-ray is diagnostic.

For the injection the patient lies prone with her arm fully supinated and in full extension by her side. Now the groove between the humerus and the head of the radius can easily be felt posteriorly (*Figure 4.18*).

The needle is accurately introduced into the gap (*Figure 4.19*). At 2.5cm the tip must repose intra-articularly and the injection of steroid suspension 2ml is made there (*Figure 4.20*). With traumatic (but not rheumatoid) arthritis the arm is kept in a sling for about a week.

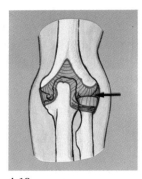

4.18

Fig **4.18** *The crack between capitellum and the head of the radius is identified.*

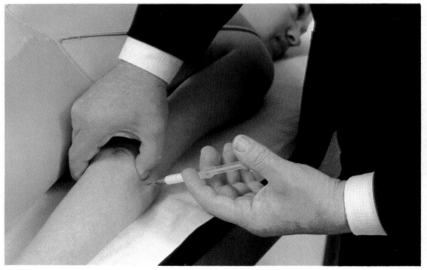

4.19

Fig **4.19** *The needle is inserted at the interval between the humerus and radius.*

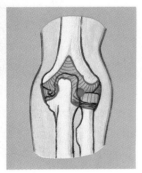

4.20

Fig **4.20** *All that is required is two injections a week apart into the joint. Point of delivery is marked.*

Rest in increasing flexion in a collar-and-cuff bandage is also effective for traumatic arthritis. But it is not as swift a remedy as steroid injection. The elbow is supported in the maximum attainable flexion and the bandage adjusted upwards each day as range towards flexion returns (*Figures 4.21; 4.22*).

Support in full flexion must be maintained for about two weeks before the bandage can be lengthened in stages to allow extension. Enough range is gained in about six weeks for the patient to progress to an ordinary sling.

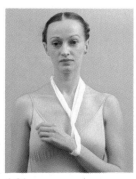

4.21

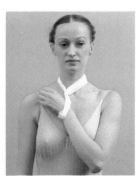

4.22

Figs **4.21, 4.22** *Rest in flexion. The bandage is shortened in stages until attainment of full flexion.*

Non-capsular lesions

Displacements

A displaced loose body blocks the joint, preventing either full flexion or full extension, but not both. In adolescence, osteochondritis dissicans leads to exfoliation of a fragment of bone covered by cartilage. Attacks of internal derangement follow, marked by sudden twinges at irregular intervals and abrupt fixation abating in the course of some days. The loose body will grow so it should be taken out; often there are several fragments. Manipulative reduction (see below) is the short-term measure.

In adults, an impacted loose body causes a constant ache, intermittent attacks or pain whenever the elbow is moved.

Osteoarthrosis may well be accompanied by a loose body; the history is indicative. A middle-aged or elderly patient describes a slight long-standing ache in the elbow (the osteoarthrosis), punctuated by attacks developing over some hours and subsiding even more gradually (the displacement), during which time the elbow is divested of most of its movement.

The displacement may be lodged either:

(1) Between humerus, ulnar and radial head. This limits extension.
(2) Between the coronoid process and the anterior aspect of the humerus. This restricts flexion; the end-feel is hard.

Manipulation is effective only if the displacement limits extension. Hence if flexion is blocked, treatment is removal of the loose body or nothing.

Figs 4.23, 4.24, 4.25, 4.26, 4.27, 4.28
Reduction of a loose body is only practicable if extension is limited. The elbow is swung towards extension. Meanwhile the patient's forearm is rotated quickly to full supination and, at the next attempt, full pronation.

Two assistants team up for the manipulation. One anchors the patient's trunk and the other secures the patient's arm against the pull of the operator (*Figure 4.23*).

The manipulator holds the patient's arm in as much extension as is painless, and to underline the traction he leans heavily backwards, bracing his foot against that of the physiotherapist (*Figure 4.24*).

He pulls hard, takes his free foot off the ground and pivots round. This swings the elbow towards further extension; as he turns, the manipulator takes the arm as far as it will go and then forces extension a little bit further (*Figures 4.25; 4.26*).

Meanwhile he repeatedly pronates (*Figure 4.27*) and supinates the patient's forearm giving a final jerk (*Figure 4.28*) towards one of the rotations as maximum extension is reached. Full extension should not be sought at first.

The patient is reappraised and the remedy repeated as necessary up to, say, ten times in a single session. It is the clinician's judgement whether the final jerk towards pronation or supination is the more beneficial.

Since the elbow may remain the site of traumatic arthritis consequent upon the original subluxation, the joint does not recover its full range immediately; if the traumatic arthritis persists, injection is required.

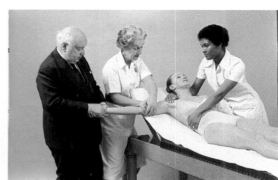

4.23

4.24

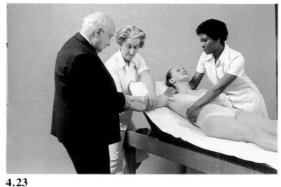

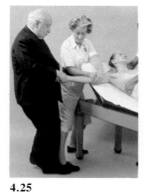

4.25 **4.26**

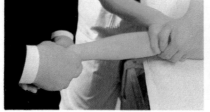

4.27 **4.28**

Contractile structures

There are three main contractile structures to be considered. The biceps is dealt with below; the tennis and golfer's elbows are described on pages 54–58.

Occasionally the triceps (painful resisted extension) or supinator brevis (painful resisted supination without painful resisted flexion) are strained. Deep massage is quickly curative.

The biceps

There are five sites. The three at the upper extent are treated as part of the shoulder on page 44. The other two sites (*Figure 4.29*) are discussed here. They are only about a couple of centimetres apart but as one is situated in the lowest extent of the belly it responds only to massage. In either case there are two painful movements—resisted elbow flexion and resisted supination. But if resisted supination does not hurt, suspicion falls on the brachialis (rare).

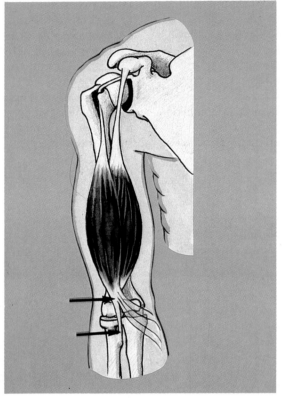

Fig 4.29 *The two sites. There is a distinct localising sign at the tenoperiosteal junction.*

4.29

The lower musculotendinous junction
The lesion is readily delineated by palpation for tenderness. Steroid suspension is ineffective. The treatment is massage, imparted by grasping the lesion between thumb and one finger and pinching the affected area time and again (*Figures 4.30; 4.31*).

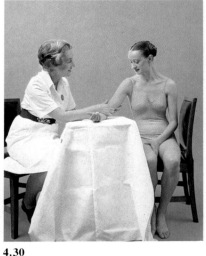 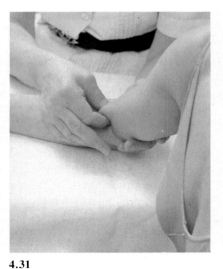

Figs 4.30, 4.31 *Deep friction, group and detail. There is no alternative to proper massage; without it, the pain may persist indefinitely.*

4.30   4.31

The lower tenoperiosteal junction
At this site the patient complains of pain starting at the centre of the front of the elbow and radiating down as far as the wrist. Full passive pronation also hurts as the lesion is caught between the radial tuberosity and the shaft of the ulna. No particular tenderness is found.

Treatment by injection (*Figure 4.32*) is preferable to massage. The patient lies prone and her elbow is arranged in extension and full pronation; in this position the tubercle and the insertion of the tendon are both rotated backwards and thus become accessible to a posterior approach. The groove between the head of the radius and the capitellum is identified posteriorly.

The needle is steered vertically downwards 2cm distal to the groove until it penetrates the tendon before hitting bone. Steroid suspension 2ml is delivered in a series of droplets (*Figure 4.33*). Up to three injections may be required.

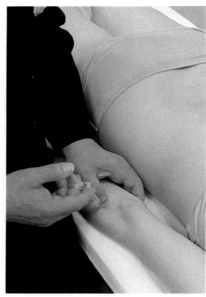

4.32

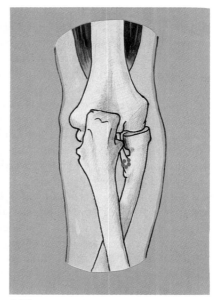

4.33

Fig 4.32 *The free hand identifies the groove. It is difficult to infiltrate the scar accurately in the absence of tenderness.*

Fig 4.33 *A series of droplets are injected at the insertion into the tuberosity.*

For the massage (*Figure 4.34*) the physiotherapist sits facing the patient. The tip of her flexed thumb is applied anteriorly to the radial tuberosity. The counterpressure is supplied by her fingers at the back of the forearm. Then with her other hand she alternately supinates and half pronates the patient's forearm (*Figures 4.35; 4.36*) sensing the tendon slip to and fro under her stationary thumb. Sessions are painful and last 20 minutes twice a week with recovery in about a month.

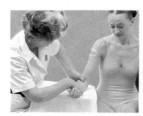

4.34

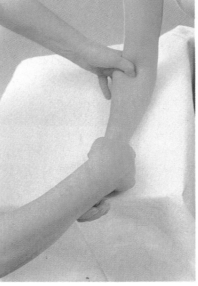

4.35

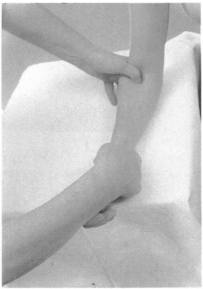

4.36

Fig 4.34 *Deep friction, group. The treatment is an alternative but it is painful and takes several weeks.*

Figs 4.35, 4.36 *The massage is imparted by repeatedly rotating the patients' arm between full supination and half-pronation, as beyond that point the tuberosity is out of reach.*

Tennis elbow

A lesion of the extensores carpi radialis longus and brevis is popularly known as a tennis elbow. Resisted extension at the wrist is the painful movement and hurts at the elbow; usually the pain is referred along the back of the forearm as far as the wrist and dorsum of the hand. At the moment of strain the patient feels nothing; some days later an ache comes on and within two weeks the symptoms are fully developed. Sudden paralysing twinges are not uncommon. The patient is always over 25 and generally between 40 and 60.

There are four sites (*Figure 4.37*), each responsive to a different treatment; the physician palpates, but he will disregard the associated tenderness often found at the posterior half of the lateral humeral epicondyle. Likewise, pressing the muscle bellies against the radius is normally painful so they are palpated from the side and not from above.

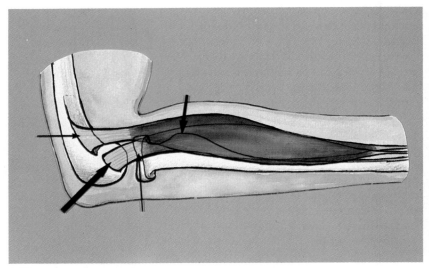

4.37

Fig 4.37 *The four sites. Ninety per cent of cases occur at the anterior aspect of the lateral humeral epicondyle.*

The epicondyle

About nine lesions out of ten lie at the tenoperiosteal junction at its origin from the lateral epicondyle. At the other sites there is no spontaneous recovery; here the patient is better in one year, or two if he is over 60. Pain on resisted extension is so pronounced that the patient usually winces and lets his hand go.

The physician's armoury consists of a progression of three treatments.

Injection

Steroid suspension 1ml is injected in droplets (*Figure 4.38*). The patient sits with her elbow supported in mid-flexion and fully supinated while the physician ascertains the precise extent of the lesion.

The needle (2cm) is aimed vertically downwards until it touches bone. A droplet is injected here and then the entire cubic extent of the lesion is infiltrated by a series of half-withdrawals and reinsertions (*Figure 4.39*). The tendon is as thick as the little finger and great care is always taken to cover the area both deeply and superficially with multiple punctures. The operator's thumb can monitor each droplet as it goes in.

The injection is painful for a day and *must* be repeated within two weeks unless *all* symptoms, even on exertion, have been abolished. Failure or repeated relapse are treated by a combination of massage and Mills's manipulation.

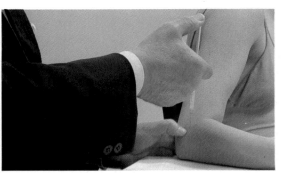

4.38

Fig 4.38 *Steroid suspension only helps at the epicondylar site.*

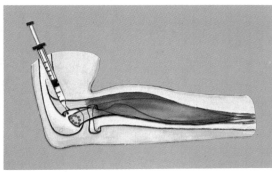

4.39

Fig 4.39 *The exact limits of the tender area are infiltrated by a series of punctures.*

Massage and Mills's manipulation

The object is to pull apart the two surfaces joined by the painful scar so that the rest of the tendon takes the strain instead. In due course, this fresh tear is bridged by new fibrous tissue under no tension. This tactic can be tried first if there is no-one to give the injection.

First the patient receives strong, deep friction (*Figure 4.40*) for 15 minutes to engender hyperaemia. Counterpressure is afforded by the fingers at the medial side of the joint while the thumb crosses to and fro over the tendon.

Mills's manipulation follows immediately after the preliminary massage while hyperaemia is at its height. The operator takes up position behind the seated patient, who lifts her arm to a right angle, internally rotates her shoulder and pronates her forearm (*Figure 4.41*).

The operator clamps the patient's wrist into fullest flexion and rests her other hand lightly on the patient's flexed elbow (*Figure 4.42*).

The elbow is then snapped smartly into full extension (*Figure 4.43*). Provided full wrist flexion has been maintained, sharp strain falls on the extensor carpi radialis tendon. This is because the muscle spans both elbow and wrist; thus it is only fully stretched when the elbow is in extension and the wrist in flexion.

The manipulation is extremely painful momentarily. It is repeated twice a week—once on each visit—for a month or more. If traumatic arthritis supervenes, inadequate maintenance of flexion at the wrist is the probable cause: strain has been taken by the joint not the tendon. The next session is deferred pending subsidence of the arthritis.

Mills's manipulation is useless if full extension is not attainable and strongly contraindicated by signs of capsular disorder.

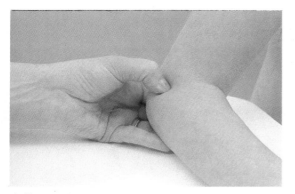

4.40

Fig 4.40 *First analgesia is produced by deep massage.*

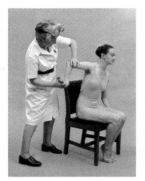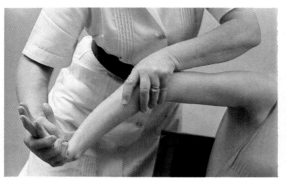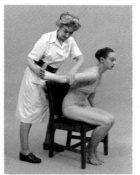

4.41   **4.42**   **4.43**

Figs 4.41, 4.42, 4.43 *Mills's manipulation may succeed at the epicondyle should injection fail, but the procedure is valueless unless the patient's wrist is fixed in fullest flexion throughout.*

Tenotomy

If Mills's manipulation fails, one injection of sclerosant solution 1ml (P2G, see page 181) may provoke dense adhesions to engulf the scar. Alternatively, tenotomy may produce the desired result (*Figure 4.44*) by dividing the tendon across its full width down to the bony epicondyle.

Procaine 2ml is first injected and Mills's manipulation immediately follows the tenotomy. If this approach comes to nothing, steroid infiltration will now succeed.

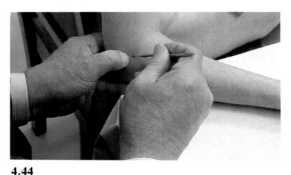

4.44

Fig 4.44 *Tenotomy is reserved for obstinate cases.*

The bellies

The tender spot is deep to the brachioradialis muscle and level with the neck of the radius. About 10% of tennis elbows occur here; the great difficulty is to find the right point and infiltrate it thoroughly. The physician palpates for tenderness by squeezing the belly of the muscle between his finger and thumb.

For the injection (*Figure 4.45*) the elbow is bent to a right angle and 10ml 0.5% procaine is injected, the fingers pinching up the lesion.

Delivery commences when the tip of the needle (5cm) lies between the operator's fingertips, and as it continues the needle is repeatedly half-withdrawn and reinserted at different angles and depths to saturate the entire lesion at and around the point of maximum sensitivity (*Figure 4.46*). If the correct spot has been found resisted extension will prove painless a few minutes later. Two or three well placed weekly injections afford lasting relief. Massage is disappointing.

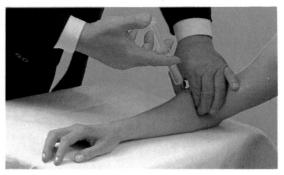

4.45

Fig 4.45 *The fingers feel the belly expand as the fluid is forced in.*

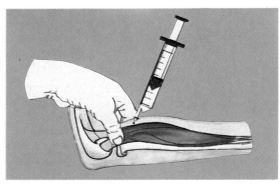

4.46

Fig 4.46 *Local anaesthesia produces permanent cure even in longstanding cases.*

The tendinous and supracondylar sites

The sprain may lie either at the body of the tendon by the head of the radius or at the origin of the extensor carpi radialis longus at the supracondylar ridge.

A lesion at either site is very rare but responds swiftly to massage. Steroids do not work.

For the supracondylar variety (*Figure 4.47*) the massage is imparted by drawing the thumb upwards and downwards along the line of origin from the supracondylar ridge. The fingers apply counterpressure; the patient's hand is clasped in supination.

For the tendinous variety (*Figure 4.48*) the massage is given by drawing the thumb to and fro across the tendon. The forearm is half extended and nearly fully pronated; in this position the tendon is directly over the head of the radius which provides a firm basis against which to massage.

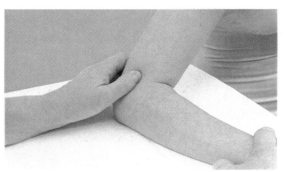

4.47

Fig 4.47 *Massage, supracondylar site. This is the easiest tennis elbow to relieve.*

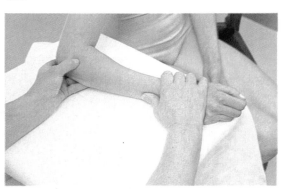

4.48

Fig 4.48 *Massage, tendinous site. Four to eight sessions suffice.*

Golfer's elbow

This is both less common and less disabling than a tennis elbow. It is a lesion of the common flexor tendon at the medial epicondyle; resisted wrist flexion is the one painful movement. The pain is felt clearly at the inner side of the elbow and does not radiate far, seldom straying beyond the ulnar side of the mid-forearm. The patient is normally aged 40–60.

There are two sites for the lesion, only 5mm apart (*Figure 4.49*). At the musculotendinous junction, injection does not avail.

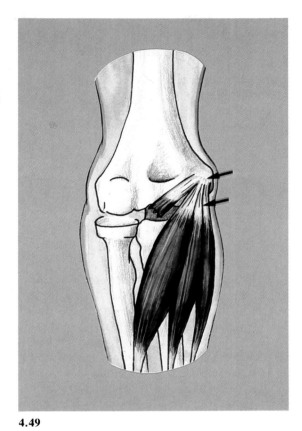

Fig 4.49 *The two sites. Wrist flexion should be tested with the elbow in extension.*

4.49

The tenoperiosteal site

The lesion responds to either massage or steroid infiltration. For the injection (*Figure 4.50*) the thumb locates the most tender point and the entire cubic extent of the lesion is infiltrated with steroid suspension 1ml in a series of droplets (*Figure 4.51*). One to two injections suffice and in the event of failure massage is called for.

For massage (*Figure 4.52*) the elbow is supported in full extension and supination; this provides a firm, bony foundation against which to rub the tendon. The thumb applies counterpressure on the outer side of the arm, and the movement of the finger is not vertical but almost horizontal as it follows the contour of the epicondyle. The very strongest friction is scarcely powerful enough. Sessions last 15 minutes on alternate days and secure relief in a month or less.

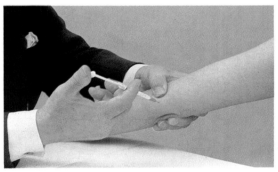

4.50

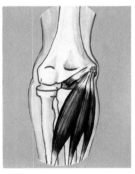

4.51

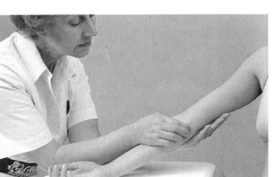

4.52

Figs 4.50, 4.51 *Some 20 droplets are injected all over the affected area of tendon. The tip of the needle is against bone.*

Fig 4.52 *Massage is an alternative. The motive force is flexion and extension of the physiotherapist's wrist.*

The musculotendinous site
At this site only massage works (*Figure 4.53*).
The lesion lies about a quarter-of-an-inch distal
to the medial epicondyle, that is just below the
previous site. Again the patient's arm is held in
extension and supination over a firm support.

The thumb applies counterpressure; strong
friction is required. Considerable pain is
provoked but recovery in four to eight sessions
is the rule.

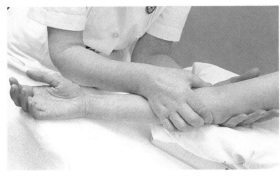

Fig **4.53** *Massage is both tiring and painful, but there is no alternative.*

4.53

Other symptoms

Weakness of the resisted movements may be
caused by a cervical root palsy (see pages
164–166). In Volkmann's ischaemic
contracture, finger extension is impossible
without wrist flexion.

Lesions of the brachialis, triceps or supinator
brevis are rare. All three can be cleared up by
massage; in addition, the tendon of the triceps
responds to steroid infiltration (1ml).

Paraesthesia at the fourth and fifth fingers
may result from interference with the ulnar
nerve; friction against bone at the medial
humeral condyle is responsible. An injection of
steroid suspension 1ml not into but along the
nerve can afford lasting relief, but postural
strain must be forestalled by avoidance of
prolonged flexion. If this fails, transposition of
the ulnar nerve is curative.

The reader is referred to Appendix II for a
summary of the causes of pins and needles in
the fingers.

CHAPTER FIVE

THE
WRIST AND HAND

Lesions at the wrist are most often due to injury or rheumatoid arthritis, although they may be induced by over-use. The fingers are commonly afflicted by arthritis, whether osteoarthrosis, rheumatoid or traumatic.

Symptoms of local origin are not referred appreciably and the patient can normally tell where the pain comes from. A more misleading referred phenomenon is pins and needles, which seldom arise locally.

The C5 dermatome extends to the radial side of the wrist. The sixth, seventh, eighth cervical and first thoracic dermatomes cover the hand and fingers at their distal extent. Cervical discs (commonly at C6) compressing a nerve root can give both pain and paraesthesia in this region, whereas the carpal tunnel syndrome and thoracic outlet syndrome may explain painless pins and needles.

Examination sticks to the standard principles of assessment of function by passive and resisted movements. But at the wrist many joints have to be handled simultaneously, so the final diagnosis may depend on palpation for tenderness. Lesions of the radioulnar joint are rare, but must not be overlooked.

Lesions of the many joints in this region can easily be distinguished, providing the examination sequence is strictly followed.

Inspection

After a careful history, the joints are inspected in good light. Swelling may be discernible at the wrist. If it is diffuse, rheumatoid arthritis should be considered but localised swelling is more likely to result from a ganglion or ostephytes secondary to an old fracture. At the finger, smooth swelling of the joints points to rheumatoid or traumatic arthritis but a knobbly texture implies osteoarthrosis. Variations in colour denote circulatory changes. A white hand suggests Raynaud's phenomenon, and a red hand may be engendered by gout or—sometimes—liver disease.

Wasting of the abductor pollicis is nearly always attributable to pressure on the nerve trunk by a cervical rib which may also cause disappearance of the pulse on scapular elevation. Crepitus is one of the classical signs of tenosynovitis, common only at the abductor and extensor tendons of the thumb where they curl round the wrist.

Examination

The radioulnar joint

The opening moves are passive pronation (*Figure 5.1*) and passive supination (*Figure 5.2*) to evaluate the capsule of the radioulnar joint. The grip is above the wrist to stop any strain from reaching the carpal joints.

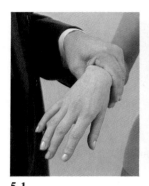

Fig 5.1 *Passive pronation.*

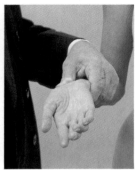

Fig 5.2 *Passive supination.*

5.1   5.2

The wrist

Examination now passes to the wrist joint. Four passive movements are executed. Passive wrist flexion (*Figure 5.3*) and passive wrist extension (*Figure 5.4*) both test the capsule, but passive flexion also stretches the ligaments at the dorsum of the wrist.

Passive radial deviation (*Figure 5.5*) puts strain on the ulnar collateral ligament; conversely, passive ulnar deviation (*Figure 5.6*) puts strain on the radial collateral ligament, rarely affected.

The same four movements are now re-enacted against resistance to assess the contractile structures about the wrist. The patient pushes downwards and resisted wrist flexion (*Figure 5.7*) tests the flexor tendons of both the wrist and the fingers. Lesions of either are unusual. Similarly, resisted wrist extension (*Figure 5.8*) puts strain on the extensor tendons of both the wrist and theoretically the fingers. The patient presses upwards.

Resisted ulnar deviation (*Figure 5.9*) assesses the ulnar deviators. The patient presses her hand towards the operator.

Pain on resisted radial deviation (*Figure 5.10*) with the patient pressing her hand towards herself can be ascribed to the radial deviators.

Figs 5.3, 5.4, 5.5, 5.6 *Passive wrist movements. Flexion, extension, radial and ulnar deviation (left to right).*

Figs 5.7, 5.8, 5.9, 5.10 *Resisted wrist movements. Flexion, extension, ulnar and radial deviation (left to right).*

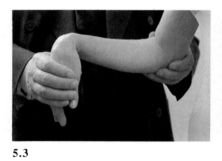

5.3

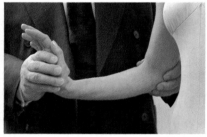

5.4

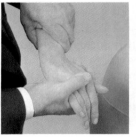

5.5

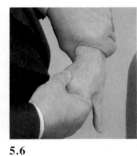

5.6

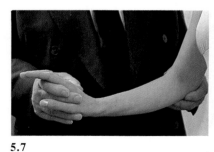

5.7

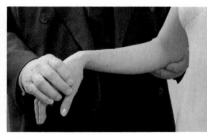

5.8

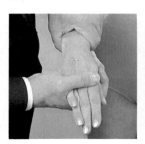

5.9

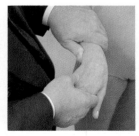

5.10

The thumb

The thumb can give rise to pain felt at the wrist. Only one passive movement is necessary: extension (*Figure 5.11*). As maximum range is reached the thumb is pressed backwards to stretch the anterior aspect of the capsule—it is this movement that always hurts in arthritis of the trapezio-first-metacarpal joint.

The resisted movements at the thumb come next. Painful resisted extension (*Figure 5.12*)—the patient pushes up—is nearly always associated with pain on resisted abduction which tests the abductor longus and extensor brevis pollicis.

Resisted thumb flexion (*Figure 5.13*) puts strain on the flexor pollicis longus.

The patient pushes her thumb outwards; abduction is resisted (*Figure 5.14*). This tensions the abductor longus and extensor brevis which are often at fault.

Resisted adduction (*Figure 5.15*) tests the adductor of the thumb, an unusual cause of trouble. The patient pulls her thumb in towards her fingers.

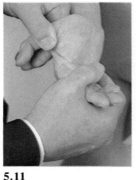
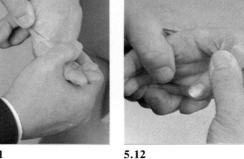

5.11　　　　　**5.12**

Fig 5.11 *Passive thumb extension.*

Fig 5.12 *Resisted thumb extension.*

Fig 5.13 *Resisted thumb flexion.*

Fig 5.14 *Resisted thumb abduction.*

Fig 5.15 *Resisted thumb adduction.*

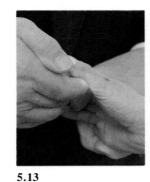
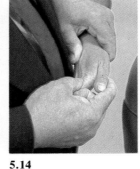
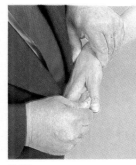

5.13　　　　　**5.14**　　　　　**5.15**

The fingers

The intrinsic muscles of the fingers are examined by resisted finger abduction (*Figure 5.16*) and by resisted adduction (*Figure 5.17*) when the fingers are squeezed together. A strained interosseous muscle can precipitate pain felt at the wrist if the proximal part of the muscle is affected.

Resisted extension and flexion of each finger checks the integrity of the flexor and extensor muscles in the palm and fingers, but for convenience all the fingers may be assessed simultaneously (*Figure 5.18*).

Finally, the passive movements of flexion and extension can be performed for each joint of each digit. In arthritis both movements tend to be equally limited and painful. Again, all the digital joints may be assessed in one fell swoop.

Throughout the examination the physician listens and feels for crepitus, a sign of tenosynovitis or osteoarthrosis. Dupuytren's contracture leads to a fixed flexion deformity of the fingers, and a trigger thumb or finger causes fixation in flexion of one or two digits which can be overcome by stretching out with the patient's other hand.

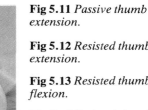

5.16

Fig 5.16 *Resisted finger abduction.*

Fig 5.17 *Resisted finger adduction.*

Fig 5.18 *Resisted finger extension.*

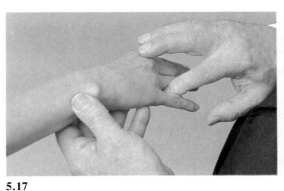
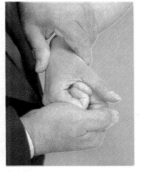

5.17　　　　　**5.18**

The radioulnar joint

Lesions of the radioulnar joint are out of the ordinary and only set up pain at the wrist: the one outstanding condition is arthritis. The capsular pattern is pain (but no limitation) on both passive rotations.

A single injection of steroid suspension 1ml is effective unless the condition is of rheumatoid origin, in which case repetition is called for as the symptoms warrant.

The patient's forearm is fully pronated; by moving the ulna backwards and forwards on the radius, the line of cleavage between them can be identified (*Figure 5.19*). A point is chosen on this line and the insertion made at the mid-point of the joint about 5mm proximal to the sharp lower edge of the ulna (*Figure 5.20*).

The needle is thrust down until it hits bone at about 1.5cm and is then nudged into the joint. Use of a 2cm needle will prevent the tip emerging at the far side.

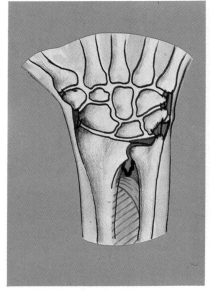

5.19

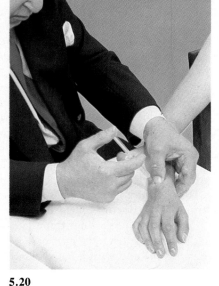

5.20

Figs 5.19, 5.20 *The joint (red) is seldom tender but it can be identified by pushing the radius and ulna backwards and* *forwards on each other. The only effective conservative treatment is steroid suspension injected into the joint.*

The wrist

The capsular pattern at the wrist (*Figure 5.21*) is denoted by roughly the same amount of limitation of flexion as of extension—ultimately fixation in the mid-position encroaches. Both deviations are slightly limited.

(1) Traumatic arthritis results from a carpal fracture, generally of the scaphoid. The whole wrist is swollen, with both passive flexion and extension cut short by muscle spasm; the radiograph may disclose no lesion for the first two weeks. A plaster cast should be applied immediately.

(2) Rheumatoid arthritis usually attacks both wrists. In the acute stage the entire wrist in inflamed and swollen, limitation is very pronounced and immobilisation in plaster may be the only option. In the sub-acute or chronic stage, the tender and swollen area is normally better defined and the entire extent of capsulo–ligamentous thickening can be infiltrated with steroid suspension 2ml (*Figure 5.22*). The injection is painful, but the results are worthwhile.

(3) Osteoarthrosis engenders little pain and no treatment has appreciable effect. The symptoms seldom merit arthrodesis.

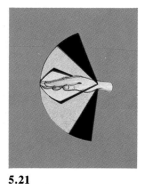

5.21

Fig 5.21 *The capsular pattern.*

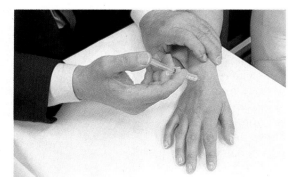

5.22

Fig 5.22 *Rheumatoid arthritis, injection. It is the area of capsular thickening and not the joint that is infiltrated.*

Carpal capitate subluxation

Passive extension is limited by 5 or 10°. Passive flexion is full and painful (*Figure 5.23*). The pain is localised to the dorsum of the wrist.

The X-ray is uninformative, but with the wrist held in flexion the projection can be seen and felt with ease and the strained ligaments about the capitate bone (*Figure 5.24*) are tender.

Manipulative reduction can be readily engineered during traction and is accomplished by separating the proximal from the distal row of bones and then gliding them anteroposteriorly.

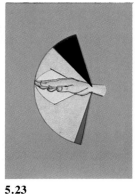
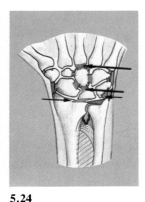

5.23   5.24

Fig 5.23 *Persistent subluxation. The sign that draws immediate attention is limitation of movement in one direction only.*

Fig 5.24 *Ligaments likely to be affected by a carpal subluxation or sprained wrist.*

For the manipulation, the patient half-lies. A physiotherapist grips the patient's arm just above the elbow while the operator grasps the patient's forearm and hand and leans backwards, his foot braced against the assistant's foot (*Figure 5.25*).

One of the operator's thumbs lies just above and the other just below the wrist. Traction is obtained by pulling only with the hand below the wrist (*Figure 5.26*).

The operator's hands are moved vertically up and down in opposite directions while his little finger presses up against the patient's palm (*Figure 5.27*) emphasising an anteroposterior glide that is bereft of both flexion and extension. The patient is reassessed and the process repeated if necessary.

One session usually affords full relief, and any residual symptoms from ligamentous strain can be cleared up by massage to the ligament. A variant of the manipulation involves assuming the same position, except that the operator's upper hand is used to squeeze the wrist as hard as possible during traction. A little click is felt on reduction.

If a ligament has actually ruptured, the joint is unstable and manipulative reduction cannot last. Accordingly, a sclerosant solution is injected at the point of rupture immediately following successful manipulation; the procedure is painful and not always fruitful. Usually the capitate-third-metacarpal ligament is involved.

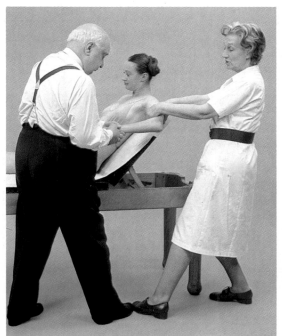

5.25

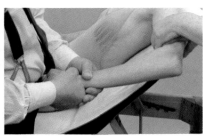
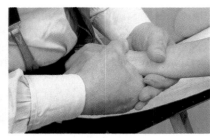

5.26   5.27

Fig 5.25 *Reduction is easy and immediate relief follows even in cases that have lasted years.*

Figs 5.26, 5.27 *Traction is negated if the manipulator pulls with the hand lying above the patient's wrist. The physician's near hand glides the carpal joints up and down. Maximum upwards lift is shown in Fig 5.27.*

Ligamentous sprains

There are several sites; the preferred is sprain to the lunate-capitate ligament which responds to massage, as does the radial collateral ligament.

But at the ulnar collateral ligament the only successful measure is injection.

The lunate-capitate ligament

Passive wrist flexion at the extreme of range is the one painful movement, with the symptoms concentrated at the dorsum of the wrist. Sprain and/or adhesions may occur with or without accompanying capitate subluxation; if untreated the condition can drag on for years. Other ligaments (e.g. the radiolunate, capitate-third-metacarpal, ulnar-triquetral) may be affected at the same time and the physician palpates for tenderness (see *Figure 5.24*).

Steroids are ineffective. Massage is the treatment of choice (*Figure 5.28*) both for strains and adhesions but to ensure recovery *all* the sprained ligaments must be treated. Manipulative rupture, forced movements, and so on, are contraindicated.

The wrist is held fully flexed with one hand. The digital extensor tendons must be pushed aside so the thumb can connect directly with the ligament to apply the transverse friction (*Figure 5.29*).

Counterpressure is maintained by the fingers at the front of the wrist. Full recovery is invariable and is rapidly established after two to six sessions.

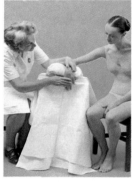 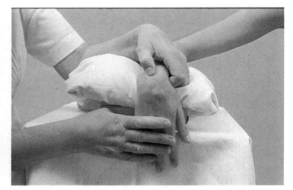

Figs 5.28, 5.29 *Massage. The tender spots lie superficially and are easily found if the wrist is kept flexed. The thumb moves to and fro over the ligament.*

5.28   **5.29**

The radial collateral ligament

Sprain of the radial collateral ligament is highly unusual. Although passive ulnar deviation is the only painful movement, hurting at the extreme of range, the disorder is often confused with tenovaginitis of the thumb.

Both infiltration of steroid 1ml and massage are successful, although the latter measure requires several sessions.

The ulnar collateral ligament

Sprain to the ulnar collateral ligament (rare) may be the legacy of imperfect reduction of a Colles's fracture or fracture of the styloid process of the ulna. Only radial deviation hurts.

Although injection of steroid suspension 1ml (*Figure 5.30*) into the tender area is rapidly curative, massage does not work.

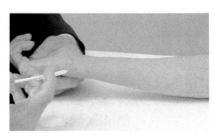

Fig 5.30 *Spontaneous recovery takes a year in default of injection.*

5.30

The carpal tunnel syndrome

Pressure exerted at the distal part of the median nerve gives rise to pins and needles which are perceived at the front of the outer three-and-a-half digits (i.e. excluding the little finger) of, usually, the right hand (*Figures 5.31; 5.32*). The condition should be distinguished from a cervical disc lesion and the thoracic outlet syndrome.

The symptoms may be evoked by:

(1) The physician pressing at the front of the wrist while the patient flexes and extends her fingers.
(2) Keeping the wrist flexed for a minute and abruptly extending it.

There is a wealth of possible causes. Some are listed below, together with the appropriate treatment:

(1) Subluxation of the lunate bone—operation.
(2) Rheumatoid-type arthritis—division of the carpal ligament.
(3) Swelling on a digital flexor tendon—acupuncture of the swelling.
(4) Colles's fracture—await spontaneous recovery.

However there are various other contenders, many of which respond to steroid therapy. In any event (except with a carpal subluxation) steroid suspension should be injected diagnostically. If the diagnosis is well founded, the relief may last for some weeks and in some cases—about half the total, being those where no abnormality is palpable—the injection is curative.

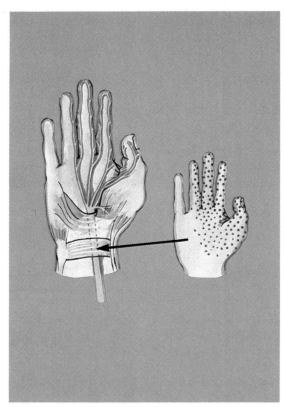

5.31, 5.32

Figs 5.31, 5.32 *Pins and needles. They are brought on by pressure on the nerve as it passes under the transverse carpal ligament, and are increased by use of the hand.*

For the injection of steroid suspension 2ml the patient sits with her forearm supported in full supination with the wrist extended. The point of entry is about 4cm above the wrist (*Figure 5.33*).

The needle is angled almost horizontally and passes its full length into the carpal tunnel without piercing either the tendon or the nerve. The entire suspension is discharged under the transverse ligament (*Figure 5.34*). Should the symptoms return only after months or years the injection is repeated as needs be.

Figs 5.33, 5.34 *The diagnosis is confirmed by injection. Note the angle of entry; the needle travels parallel to the tendons and nerve.*

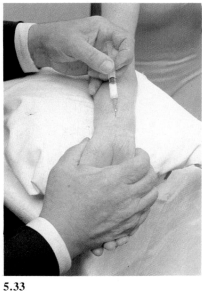

5.33

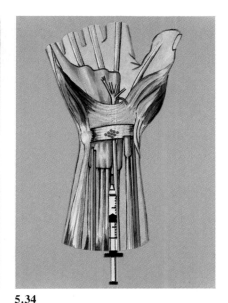

5.34

Contractile structures at the wrist

Two structures may malfunction—the extensor carpi radialis and the common flexor tendon. The lesion may lie at the elbow (golfer's or tennis elbow–see pages 54–58) or at the wrist itself, but the patient is almost sure to know which end is affected.

Resisted wrist extension

Pain felt at the wrist on resisted wrist extension incriminates the extensor tendons. Resisted radial and ulnar deviation will ascertain whether the extensores carpi radialis or extensor carpi ulnaris are involved; in both cases the lesion is rare and inclined to result from over-use. Either massage or injection is effective, unless the inflammation is rheumatoid in which case the wrist is palpably warm, swollen or nodular. Massage is then out of court. The long extensors can be exculpated by testing extension with the fingers flexed.

The extensores carpi radialis

The lesion is somewhere in the distal inch of the tendons, frequently at their insertion into the bases of the second and third metacarpal bones (*Figure 5.35*). Palpation is conducted with the wrist gripped in full flexion; usually it will be found that both radial extensor tendons are inflamed. The pain is accurately localised at the dorsum of the wrist. One injection of steroid suspension 1ml delivered in droplets does the trick (*Figure 5.36*).

For the alternative treatment, massage, the wrist is held in full flexion to stretch the tendons (*Figure 5.37*) and one finger reinforced by another is rolled hard across the lesion. Twenty-minute sessions are given on alternate days and usually result in recovery in about two weeks.

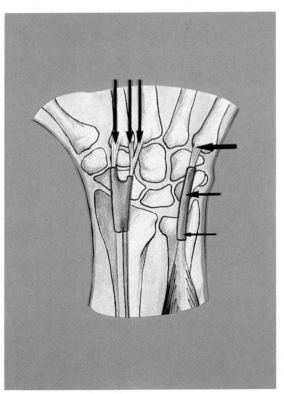

Fig 5.35 *Right wrist, posterior view. Possible sites of a lesion of the extensores carpi radialis (left) and ulnaris (right).*

5.35

Fig 5.36 *Injection. Tenosynovitis here results from over-use.*

Fig 5.37 *Massage. Usually both tendons are affected, but the tender spot is easy to locate.*

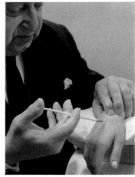

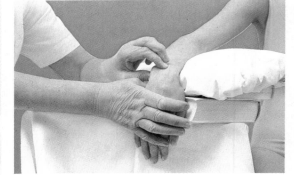

5.36   5.37

The extensor carpi ulnaris

The lesion may be at one of three sites (see *Figure 5.35*). There is a localising sign if it is at the tendon at the groove in the lower extremity of the ulna: pain is then elicited at the extreme of passive supination of the forearm. The two other favoured locations are between the ulna and the triquetral or at the base of the fifth metacarpal bone; the physician palpates with the wrist in full radial deviation.

An injection of steroid suspension 1ml (*Figure 5.38*) delivered in droplets into the affected area is normally efficacious.

If treatment is by massage the wrist is maintained in flexion and radial deviation (*Figure 5.39*). This divides the base of the metacarpal bone from the cuneiform bone and the head of the ulna.

One finger is placed squarely on the lesion and, using the thumb as a fulcrum, the wrist is flexed and extended across the tendon. Sessions take 20 minutes on alternate days with recovery in about two weeks.

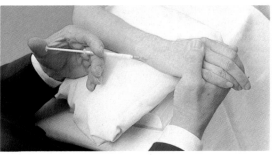

5.38

Fig 5.38 *Injection. The tender area is sought and infiltrated with the wrist in radial deviation.*

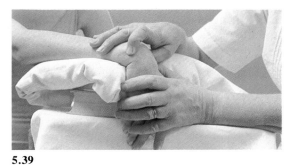

5.39

Fig 5.39 *Massage. The tendon is maintained on the stretch by wrist flexion.*

Resisted wrist flexion

The normal inference to be drawn from pain at the wrist on resisted flexion is a lesion of the flexor carpi radialis or flexor carpi ulnaris, although the flexor digitorum occasionally give rise to symptoms at the wrist. Rheumatoid tenovaginitis can affect just one flexor tendon.

The flexor carpi ulnaris

For the flexor carpi ulnaris, the lesion is either proximal or distal to the pisiform bone (*Figure 5.40*); the physician palpates. The cause is normally a single over-strain. Both resisted wrist flexion and resisted ulnar deviation reproduce the familiar symptoms.

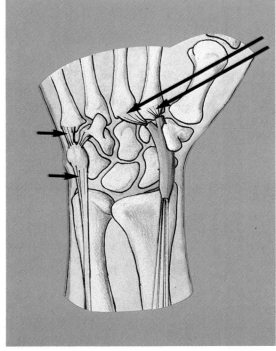

5.40

Fig 5.40 *Right wrist, anterior view. Possible sites of a lesion of the flexor carpi ulnaris (left) and radialis (right).*

Either injection or deep massage work well. Steroid suspension 1ml is injected in droplets into the tendon (*Figures 5.41; 5.42*).

For deep friction the patient's wrist is held in extension (*Figure 5.43*). The massage demands great strength.

The physiotherapist lets the patient's little finger flex in order to relax the hypothenar muscles and counterpressure is supplied at the dorsum of the wrist. The massage is delivered hard at the site of the tear for 20 minutes at a time with a 10-minute rest half-way through; sessions given twice weekly should achieve recovery in about a month. It is tiring work and the physiotherapist may prefer to use the strength of her thumb.

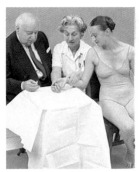
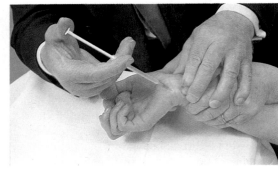

5.41   **5.42**

Figs 5.41, 5.42 *Injection. An assistant positions the patient's hands. Treatment by one or two infiltrations gives lasting quiescence.*

Fig 5.43 *Only an exceptionally strong physiotherapist can give adequate friction. The treatment is ruled out in rheumatoid cases.*

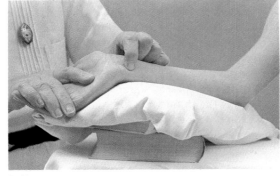

5.43

The flexor carpi radialis

The lesion is often found at the base of the second metacarpal bone (see *Figure 5.40*). The physician palpates. Both injection (steroid suspension 1ml) and massage pay dividends; the wrist is maintained in full extension for either treatment.

The flexor digitorum

The standard indicator for the flexor digitorum is pain on resisted finger flexion. The discomfort is felt either in the palm (see page 72) or in the lower forearm. In the latter case the painful area usually ranges over some 4cm and is due to a tenosynovitis, either of rheumatoid origin or an over-use phenomenon.

Both respond to an injection of steroid suspension 2ml (*Figure 5.44*). The patient sits with her forearm supinated, straightening the wrist and fingers to stretch the tendons. The needle slips in almost horizontally parallel to the tendon, and is pushed along until the tip rests level with the lesion. The entire suspension is deposited there.

Massage must not be contemplated in cases of rheumatoid tenosynovitis, picked out by local warmth and/or nodules along the tendon. In the appropriate circumstances three fingers are placed on the affected tendon with friction imparted by the physiotherapist's drawing her

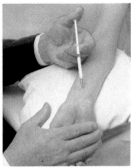
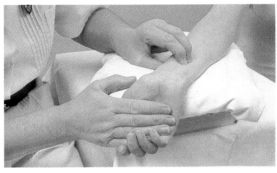

5.44   **5.45**

Fig 5.44 *Injection of steroid suspension is the only treatment if the condition is rheumatoid.*

Fig 5.45 *Massage. Lasting relief is secured in two weeks. The patient's wrist is in extension to stretch the tendons.*

whole forearm to and fro (*Figure 5.45*). The hand is held in extension; treatments last 20 minutes on alternate days and should confer relief in two weeks.

The thumb

Arthritis

The hallmark of arthritis of the trapezio-first-metacarpal joint is pain on a passive backward movement during extension.

Limitation is largely confined to abduction; in the final stage the joint is fixed in adduction. The pain is at the wrist.

Traumatic or rheumatoid arthritis can be relieved by a single injection of steroid suspension 1ml, but in rheumatoid cases the injection is repeated as required. Osteoarthrosis is discernible radiographically and intra-articular injection of silicone 2ml (12 000 centistoke) is often effective.

An assistant distracts the joint surfaces by pulling hard on the thumb and exerting counterpressure with her other hand on the upper forearm (*Figure 5.46*).

The base of the first metacarpal bone is identified dorsally and the needle directed through the gap at a slope of 60° (*Figure 5.47*). If bone is contacted at about 1cm, the needle does not lie inside the joint and the tip must be adjusted until resistance folds at 1.5cm.

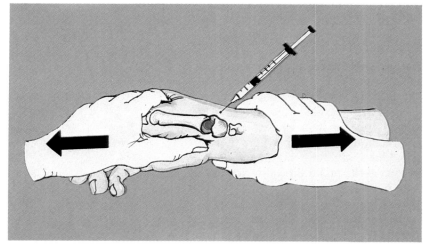

5.46

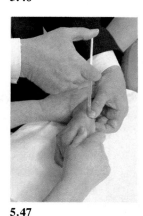

5.47

Fig 5.46 *A physiotherapist opens the joint space for the injection.*

Fig 5.47 *Injection of 1ml steroid suspension. Tenderness is most obvious at the front of the joint.*

Deep massage to the capsule on alternate days can cope with either traumatic arthritis or early osteoarthrosis. One hand hyperabducts the thumb in extension to bring the thenar joint into prominence (*Figure 5.48*).

The thumb of the physiotherapist's other hand on the joint line rubs the capsule—the outer aspect of the joint must also be massaged. Recovery takes two to three weeks.

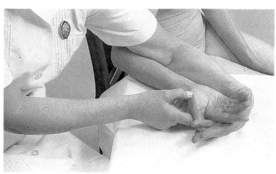

5.48

Fig 5.48 *Massage. Both traumatic arthritis and early osteoarthritis respond well to deep friction delivered by the physiotherapist's thumb.*

Contractile structures

The abductor longus and extensor brevis are often the seat of trouble; in either case, pain will be evoked both by resisted extension and resisted abduction. Because the ache is perceived by the patient to be within the wrist joint, the condition is easy to mistake for a fractured scaphoid unless the resisted thumb movements are tested. The tendinous lesion may lie at the lower forearm, in which case it is some 2 inches in extent, and massage is the treatment of choice. At and below the wrist an injection of steroid suspension 1ml is rapidly effective, rendering both massage and longitudinal slitting of the tendon sheath obsolete. Passive movements may hurt as the inflamed tendon slides through the sheath.

Lesions of the flexor pollicis longus tendon are numerically insignificant.

The abductor longus and extensor brevis pollicis

The cause is over-use or idiopathic. Tenosynovitis results (*Figure 5.49*). Above the wrist all the tendons are affected simultaneously, normally where they curl round the shaft of the radius, and the pain is focused at the radial side of the lower forearm. Crepitus may be present.

At or below the wrist the tendency is towards more diffuse symptoms referred to the thumb. The misleading associated tenderness of the styloid process of the radius should be ignored.

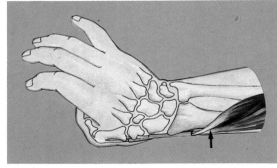

5.49

Fig 5.49 *The arrow marks the musculotendinous site, but often the lesion is an inch or two lower, inside the sheath itself.*

At the lower site, only infiltration avails. For the injection of steroid suspension 0.5–1ml the patient's thumb is fully flexed by an assistant with the wrist in full ulnar deviation and slight extension. This tightens the tendons and leaves the operator with both hands free (*Figure 5.50*).

The needle (2cm) is inserted at the base of the first metacarpal bone and thrust in horizontally.

The tendon is pinched up with the free hand. This enables the point to penetrate the sheath and glide between it and the tendon. As the fluid is injected a little sausage is felt to expand along the tendons as far as the styloid process (*Figure 5.51*).

Rheumatoid tenovaginitis sometimes attacks the carpal extent of the abductor longus and extensor brevis pollicis tendons; it can be relieved by injection of steroid suspension 1ml.

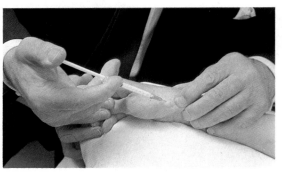

5.50

Fig 5.50 *At the lower site one, or at most two, injections cure. Spontaneous recovery takes three to four years.*

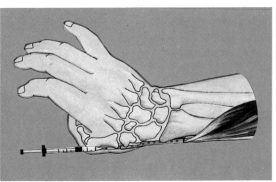

5.51

Fig 5.51 *The only difficulty is to place the injection correctly along the gliding surfaces between tendon and tendon sheath.*

At the upper site, massage is the treatment of choice (*Figure 5.52*). One hand arranges the wrist in flexion. With the operative hand the fingers apply counterpressure while the thumb is laid flat on and parallel to the affected tendons near the lower end of the radius.

The deep friction is imparted by alternate abduction and adduction of the thumb. Sessions last 20 minutes during which the entire extent of the lesion is massaged; treatment is given on alternate days and recovery ensues in about two weeks.

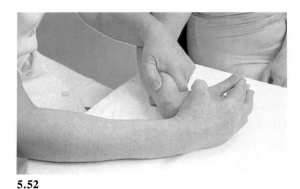

5.52

Fig 5.52 *The thumb delivers the deep friction. Neither crepitus, swelling nor an effusion contraindicate massage.*

The flexor pollicis longus tendon

Two conditions occur; tenosynovitis and a trigger thumb.

Tenosynovitis: strain or over-use will give pain on resisted thumb flexion. There are two sites (*Figure 5.53*). If the lesion lies at the metacarpal extent under the thenar eminence an injection of steroid suspension 1ml is curative but massage usually disappoints. When the lesion is at the wrist, both massage and injection are successful.

Trigger thumb: if the patient cannot voluntarily straighten the thumb following flexion (or *vice versa*) a palpable swelling on the flexor pollicis tendon may be engaged in the tendon sheath. It lies just proximal to the head of the first metacarpal bone.

An injection of steroid suspension 1ml into the swelling is often effective symptomatically (*Figure 5.54*). In the event of failure, the possibility of operation can be investigated.

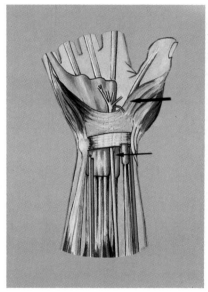

5.53

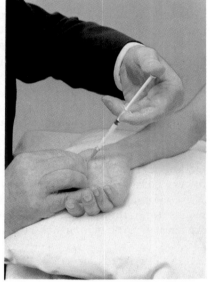

5.54

Fig 5.53 *Tenosynovitis. The two sites.*

Fig 5.54 *Trigger thumb. The injection is made into the nodule.*

Weakness on resisted movements

Consider *inter alia*:

(1) C8 root palsy.
(2) Pressure on the posterior interosseous nerve.
(3) Rupture of a tendon.
(4) Ischaemic contracture.
(5) Cervical rib.

The hand

Capsular lesions

Arthritis may afflict any of the finger joints; the capsular pattern is equal limitation of flexion and extension with the rotations painful at extreme of range rather than limited.

The causes are:

(1) Rheumatoid arthritis—injection of steroid suspension 0.5–1ml (if only a few joints are affected).

(2) Osteoarthrosis—normally symptomless.

(3) Traumatic arthritis—no treatment. Immobilisation is contraindicated.

Local swelling from an unreduced dislocation is sometimes erroneously put down to traumatic arthritis.

Contractile structures

These consist of the dorsal and palmar interosseous muscles and the flexor tendons.

The dorsal interossei are more often to blame than the palmar and give pain on resisted abduction, whereas a lesion of the palmar interossei produces the symptoms on resisted adduction. Tenderness is sought between the metacarpal shafts, normally distally; in both cases the cause may be traumatic or occupational. The bellies and tendons respond to massage imparted by the fingers via rotation of the forearm (*Figure 5.55*) but not to steroid suspension. For the bellies two or three treatments of 15 minutes are enough, even in long-standing cases. The

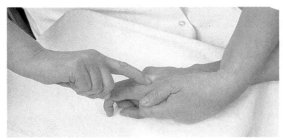

5.55

Fig 5.55 *The dorsal interossei resist every treatment except massage.*

tendons may take a good deal longer.

The long flexor tendons in the palm benefit from steroid suspension 1 ml but not from massage.

The flexor digitorum

Pain on resisted finger flexion incriminates the flexor digitorum. The trouble may be a tenosynovitis at the wrist (see page 68) but if the pain is felt at or below the wrist, either rheumatoid inflammation or a trigger finger is responsible.

For rheumatoid inflammation the injection (1–2ml) is made by a series of droplets along the line of the tendons, about 2 inches in extent. The needle is inserted parallel to the tendon and slides forwards along its surface as the injection proceeds.

A trigger finger may be caused by a swelling on any of the digital flexor tendons. The affected finger, usually the third or fourth, can

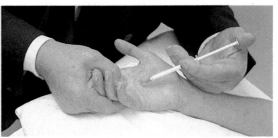

5.56

Fig 5.56 *Injection, trigger finger. Operation is the last recourse.*

no longer be extended voluntarily. In minor cases an injection of steroid suspension 1ml into the swelling abolishes the symptoms (*Figure 5.56*).

Pins and needles

The reader is referred to Appendix II for a summary of the various causes of paraesthesia.

CHAPTER SIX

THE SACROILIAC, BUTTOCK AND HIP

Most pain felt in the buttock is referred from the spine—the sacroiliac joint itself is rarely at fault. However, lesions of the buttock do happen and the serious disorders are readily distinguished from those involving the bursae.

The hip is prey to a number of conditions, including osteoarthrosis, displacements and muscular lesions giving rise to pain in the thigh. These disorders must also be differentiated from symptoms referred from the lumbar spine.

The spine is the most likely cause of pain in the buttock.

Referred pain

Extrasegmental dural reference from a disc lesion may cause pain in the buttock, iliac fossa, groin, thigh or leg (*Figure 6.1*).

A posterolateral disc lesion impinging on the L3, L4, L5, S1 or S2 roots produces pain in the appropriate dermatome (*Figures 6.2; 6.3; 6.4; 6.5; 6.6*). The gluteal bursae are derived from the L4 and L5 segment, and the hip from the L3 segment.

Thus with pain felt in the buttock and thigh, the first issue to settle is whether the symptoms are of lumbar origin and a detailed history (together with examination of the lumbar movements if necessary) is taken to clarify the position. If the spinal joints are exculpated, the examination passes to the sacroiliac, buttock and hip.

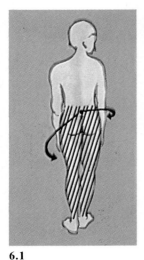

6.1

Fig 6.1 *The dura mater can refer pain anywhere within this region.*

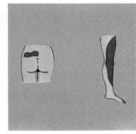

6.2

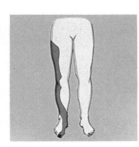

6.3

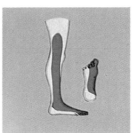

6.4

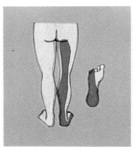

6.5

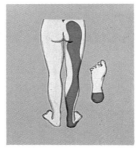
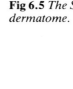

6.6

Fig 6.2 *The hip is an L3 structure.*

Fig 6.3 *The L4 dermatome.*

Fig 6.4 *The L5 dermatome.*

Fig 6.5 *The S1 dermatome.*

Fig 6.6 *The S2 dermatome.*

Examination

Passive movements

The patient lies supine. There are three methods of exerting tension on the sacroiliac joint; for the first, the examiner presses downwards and laterally on the anterior superior spine of each ilium (*Figure 6.7*) thereby stretching the anterior ligaments. As these are unilateral structures, the response to the stretch is positive only if it evokes unilateral gluteal or posterior crural pain.

The posterior ligaments are assessed by putting the patient on her side and forcing the uppermost part of the iliac crest towards the floor (*Figure 6.8*). It is not so delicate a test as the previous measure.

Finally, the patient lies prone and the sacrum is pushed smartly forwards while the pelvis stays motionless supported on the couch (*Figure 6.9*). Again this stretches the anterior ligaments.

Attention now turns to the hip where the state of the capsule is assessed by four passive movements, each of which is repeated on the good side for comparison. But passive hip flexion (*Figure 6.10*) is an ambivalent test as it is also part of 'the sign of the buttock' and will additionally be painful at extreme of range in psoas bursitis.

Passive medial rotation (*Figure 6.11*) of the hip is performed. The capsular pattern is limitation of this and the preceding movement in fixed proportions.

Passive lateral hip rotation (*Figure 6.12*) and passive extension (*Figure 6.13*) are tested. The end-feels are noted; in a healthy joint, flexion is marked by tissue approximation while the other three movements end with elasticity. Arthritis generates a hard end-feel.

Straight-leg raise (*Figure 6.14*) stretches the dura mater via the sciatic nerve, and pain on straight-leg raise alone suggests involvement of the lumbar spine. But if hip flexion with the knee bent is more limited and more painful, this dual finding points to a severe lesion at the buttock ('the sign of the buttock').

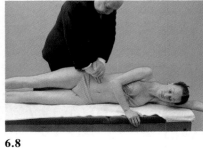

6.7

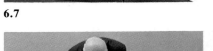

6.8

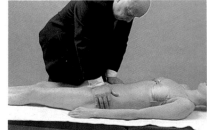

6.9

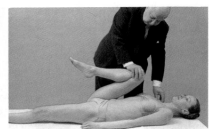

6.10

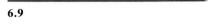

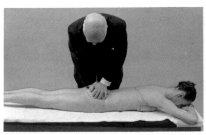

6.11

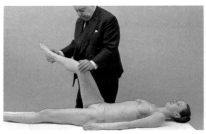

6.12

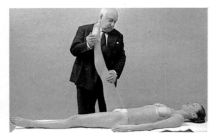

6.13

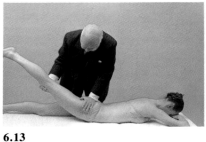

6.14

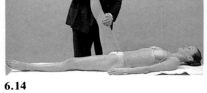

Fig 6.7 *S1J stretch, anterior ligaments. The pelvis is not allowed to rock.*

Fig 6.9 *S1J stretch, anterior ligaments. Attempted forward luxation of the sacrum.*

Fig 6.11 *Passive medial rotation of the hip.*

Fig 6.13 *Passive hip extension.*

Fig 6.8 *S1J stretch, posterior ligaments.*

Fig 6.10 *Passive hip flexion.*

Fig 6.12 *Passive lateral rotation of the hip.*

Fig 6.14 *Straight-leg raise.*

Resisted movements

The examination now proceeds to the resisted movements, but only resisted adduction and resisted flexion are tests for muscular lesions of the hip. The other resisted movements are accessory signs in bursitis when a muscle contracts round or over an inflamed area of bursa.

Resisted hip flexion (*Figure 6.15*) puts strain on the psoas and, to a lesser degree, the quadriceps.

Pain on resisted medial rotation (*Figure 6.16*) or resisted lateral rotation (*Figure 6.17*) or resisted extension are accessory signs in gluteal bursitis. The glutei themselves are practically never the seat of trouble, but they may squeeze the tender extent of bursa.

Resisted abduction (*Figure 6.18*) can compress the gluteal bursa (as may passive abduction), and pain on resisted hip extension (*Figure 6.19*)—the patient presses downwards—is also an accessory sign in bursitis.

However, the next three resisted movements assess contractile structures. Pain on resisted adduction (*Figure 6.20*) suggests a lesion of the adductors, known as rider's sprain. The knees are squeezed together.

Resisted knee extension (*Figure 6.21*) with the patient prone tests the quadriceps. A lesion at the origin of the anterior inferior spine produces pain felt in or about the groin.

Finally, resisted knee flexion (*Figure 6.22*) tests the hamstrings and it is a lesion at the ischial origin which will produce pain around the hip. Lesions at the lower extent of these last two structures are considered as part of the knee (see pages 103–104).

A lesion in a contractile structure will produce pain but not weakness on resisted movement.

Findings may also be made of:

(1) Pain and weakness.
(2) Painless weakness.

These possibilities are set out on page 86.

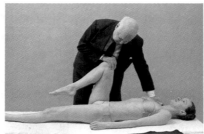

6.15

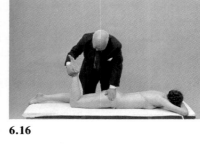

6.16

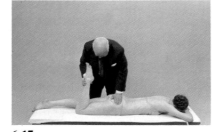

6.17

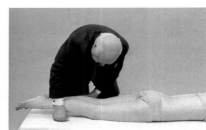

6.18

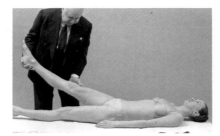

6.19

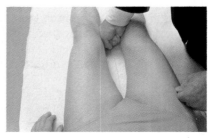

6.20

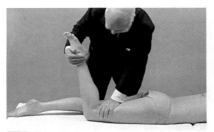

6.21

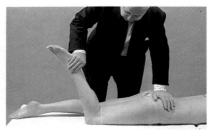

6.22

Fig 6.15 *Resisted hip flexion.*

Fig 6.16 *Resisted medial rotation of the hip.*

Fig 6.17 *Resisted lateral rotation of the hip.*

Fig 6.18 *Resisted hip abduction.*

Fig 6.19 *Resisted hip extension.*

Fig 6.20 *Resisted hip adduction.*

Fig 6.21 *Resisted knee extension.*

Fig 6.22 *Resisted knee flexion.*

The sacroiliac joint

Movement does occur at the sacroiliac joint; at the extreme of trunk flexion and extension, rotation takes place between the sacrum and the ilium, but it is limited to 0.25mm. No muscles span the joint. There is no intra-articular meniscus. All in all, there is little that can go wrong.

The only condition encountered with any frequency is ankylosing spondylitis. Radiography and sedimentation rate may help in diagnosis but are not infallible, nor can local anaesthesia furnish positive confirmation because of the bulk of the posterior ligaments and the inaccessibility of the anterior ones. In difficult cases a lumbar disc lesion may be differentiated by a diagnostic injection of epidural local anaesthetic.

Ankylosing spondylitis starts at any time between the ages of 15 and 39. Its incidence is twice as high in men as in women and the condition is usually symptomless (despite radiographic appearances) until it invades the lumbar spine.

Those who do suffer symptoms of sacroiliac origin normally complain of pain in one buttock radiating to the back of the thigh and calf, because the sacroiliac ligaments are derived from the first and second sacral segments. The pain comes and goes irrespective of exertion and although the symptoms often alternate from one buttock to the other, they never occupy both simultaneously. In four out of five cases the spondylitic invasion progresses to the lumbar spine.

As a rule, some or all of the sacroiliac tests will be positive. The least likely stretch to hurt is the side-lying test for the posterior ligaments. Pain may be felt on walking.

Ankylosing spondylitis can be successfully managed, although none of the treatments prevent recurrence. Both phenylbutazone and indomethacin are highly effective and are continued until the attack passes off.

Osteitis condensans ilii and sacroiliac osteoarthritis are purely radiological findings and sacroiliac strain without spondylitis is practically unknown.

The buttock

Major lesions

It will be remembered that pressure on any nerve root below L3 gives rise to buttock pain.

Major lesions of the buttock are indicated by 'the sign of the buttock', which is:
(1) Slightly limited and painful straight-leg raise (*Figure 6.23*), coupled with
(2) Passive hip flexion with the knee flexed more limited (*Figure 6.24*) and more painful than the straight-leg raise.

These findings show:
(1) The lesion does not involve the dura mater or nerve roots. If it did, straight-leg raise would be painful but passive hip flexion with the knee flexed would be painless.
(2) The lesion has nothing to do with the hip joint since, provided the hip rotations are full and painless, the capsular pattern for the hip is lacking.

The lesion therefore involves structures apart from the joint itself which are stretched by hip flexion. All disorders affecting these structures are serious, for example iliac metastases.

The end-feel is prematurely empty, that is, although the examiner can feel further range is attainable, severe pain makes further movement impracticable.

There is nothing characteristic about the pain which is felt in the buttock and spreads down the back of the thigh to the knee or calf. Sometimes the resisted movements hurt since they alter the tensions in the buttock.

A radiograph is taken without delay. The possibilities include:
Osteomyelitis of the upper femur.
Chronic septic sacroiliac arthritis.
Ischiorectal abscess.
Septic bursitis.
Rheumatic fever with bursitis.
Neoplasm at the upper femur.
Iliac neoplasm.
Fractured sacrum.

Figs 6.23, 6.24 *The sign of the buttock. An arresting combination of signs draws attention to the buttock. Hip flexion is more limited and more painful than straight-leg raise.*

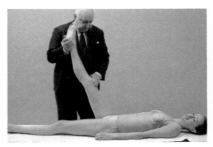

6.23

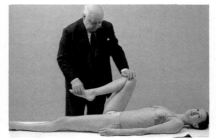

6.24

Minor lesions

A lesion in the buttock itself is suggested when a patient complains of pain in the buttock and the physician draws a blank on testing the lumbar and sacroiliac joints. The main symptom is usually pain brought on or increased by walking.

Diagnosis can be bewildering, not least because the significance of both passive and resisted movements is ambiguous. Thus on full passive hip flexion it is generally the psoas bursa that is being painfully squeezed. Nor is a muscle lesion ordinarily the cause of pain on a resisted movement. For example, contraction of the gluteus medius on resisted abduction squeezes the gluteal bursa and is thus painful in gluteal bursitis. A soft end-feel at the hip is characteristic of bursitis.

In fact muscle lesions in the buttock are almost unknown and the only resisted movements which imply trouble in the muscle itself are:
(1) Flexion—psoas strain.
(2) Lateral rotation—quadratus femoris (very uncommon).

At the hip, resisted adduction tests for rider's sprain.

Psoas bursitis

Psoas bursitis is an uncommon cause of pain at the front of the upper thigh (L2 and L3 dermatomes). It appears gradually for no apparent reason and can go on for years, causing pain near the groin on walking.

Passive adduction in flexion (*Figure 6.25*) is the most painful movement; this compresses the bursa. Passive lateral rotation usually hurts but medial rotation does not, and all the resisted movements are painless.

The symptoms resemble a loose body in the hip (see page 82) which can be distinguished by the sudden twinges of intermittent pain.

The diagnosis is tentative and is pursued simultaneously with treatment. A solution of 0.5% procaine 50ml is injected using an 8cm needle.

The physician palpates for the femoral artery. He then moves his thumb laterally to locate the head of the femur (*Figure 6.26*); the bursa lies anteriorly. The needle is introduced well lateral to the mid-point of the inguinal ligament and 5cm below it (*Figure 6.27*).

This approach gives a wide berth to the femoral artery and nerve. The needle proceeds pointing upwards and medially (*Figure 6.28*) until it strikes bone near the junction of the head and neck of the femur.

It is then withdrawn a few millimetres so it lies extra-articularly. By a series of small withdrawals and reinsertions the area between the hip joint and the psoas muscle is infiltrated; its cubic extent is about the size of a golf ball.

A correctly placed injection often has enduring therapeutic results. If benefit is still manifest at the end of seven days, the injection is repeated two or three times at weekly intervals until the patient is well. If no lasting improvement is afforded, steroid suspension 5ml is substituted.

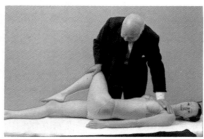

6.25

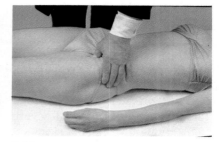

6.26

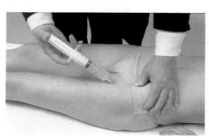

6.27

Fig 6.25 *The most painful movement in psoas bursitis.*

Fig 6.26 *The head of the femur lies immediately deep to the bursa.*

Fig 6.27 *The injection can be both diagnostic and therapeutic.*

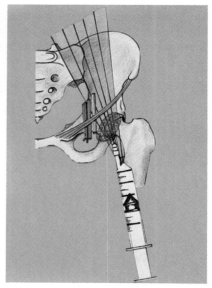

6.28

Fig 6.28 *Local anaesthetic is infiltrated when the needle lies just outside the articular capsule and several centimetres lateral to the artery.*

Gluteal bursitis

Another uncommon cause of pain in this region is gluteal bursitis, but as the bursa is derived from L4 and L5, the symptoms are produced in the buttock and lateral aspect of the thigh. The symptoms come on gradually for no particular reason and once again can persist for years, making walking uncomfortable.

As a rule, full passive hip flexion and full passive lateral hip rotation bring on the pain, although full passive abduction may squeeze the bursa painfully against the blade of the ilium. Resisted abduction can also pinch the lesion between the muscle fibres.

Diagnosis and treatment are identical.

The lateral approach

The patient lies prone. The operator uses his thumb to identify the upper edge of the greater trochanter (*Figure 6.29*) and the injection is delivered to the tender area immediately above its upper surface.

The solution is 0.5% procaine 50ml and the physician inserts the needle horizontally just above the trochanter (*Figure 6.30*).

The likely depth of the lesion is 5–8cm from the skin. By a series of small withdrawals and reinsertions the cubic extent of the area—approaching the size of a tennis ball—is infiltrated.

A well placed injection is often of lasting therapeutic value, although several infiltrations at weekly intervals may be required before the right spot is found. If benefit still persists after a week, the infiltration is repeated two or three times until the patient is well. If the relief does not last, steroid suspension 5ml is substituted.

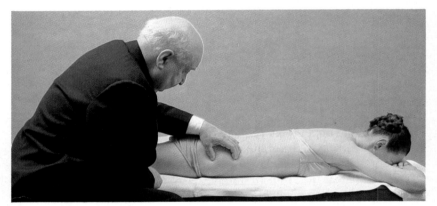

6.29

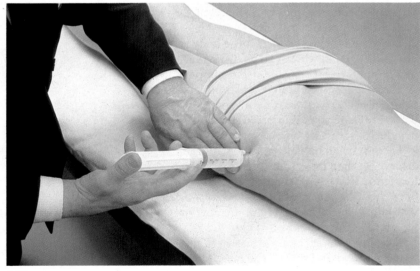

6.30

Fig 6.29 *Tenderness is sought in the area lying between the trochanter and the iliac crest.*

Fig 6.30 *The lesion lies deeply, but within a few minutes of a successful injection the previously painful movements stop hurting.*

The vertical approach

Pain on full passive abduction indicates that the lesion is between the trochanter and the ilium. It thus lies less deeply and may be more accurately located by a vertical approach.

The patient lies prone on a low couch with her leg over the edge so it touches the floor; the upper surface of the greater trochanter can now be seen and felt as a horizontal plateau. The physician palpates deeply for the bone and also for tenderness (*Figure 6.31*).

The needle is inserted almost vertically (*Figure 6.32*) until the tip is felt to touch bone. It is then withdrawn by about 1cm and the injection commences. By a series of small withdrawals and reinsertions, the cubic extent of inflamed tissue is saturated with 0.5% procaine 50ml.

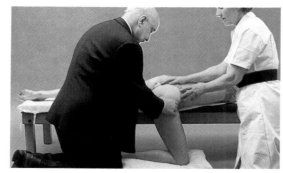

6.31

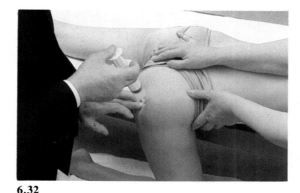

6.32

Figs 6.31, 6.32 *Injection, group and detail. A different position is adopted if the lesion lies close to the trochanter. If local anaesthetic does not give lasting relief, steroid suspension 5ml can be used instead.*

Claudication in the buttock

This is an unusual cause of pain felt at mid-buttock. A severe ache (or sometimes numbness) is produced by walking for 100 yards or so. When the patient stands still the symptoms go, and on examination not one movement is found to hurt.

The condition is diagnosed by raising the patient's fully extended hip (*Figure 6.33*) and asking her to keep the lower limb off the couch for several minutes.

The result of this sustained gluteal contraction is the familiar pain in the buttock. The cause is muscular ischaemia and only operative recanalisation of the artery is effective.

Two other conditions give rise to a similar pain:
(1) The 'mushroom phenomenon' (producing pain when the patient is upright, irrespective of whether he is walking).
(2) Spinal claudication resulting from stenosis (pins and needles in both legs on walking).

Three other rare causes of pain in the region of the buttock and hip are:

(1) Haemorrhagic psoas bursitis—90° limitation of hip flexion; following aspiration, the condition is treated as for psoas bursitis.
(2) Tuberculous abscess—a large, symptomless, fluctuant lump arising from the sacroiliac joint; the condition is treated by anti-tuberculous drugs and rest in bed.
(3) Ischial bursitis—local anaesthesia is induced at the site of tenderness at the tuberosity.

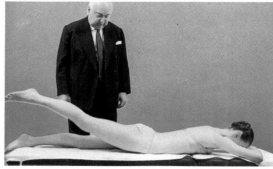

6.33

Fig 6.33 *Pain on prolonged hip extension. This is the only positive finding in claudication of the buttock.*

The hip

The hip is of L3 derivation. Therefore pain originating at the hip may be felt in the upper buttock and the front of the thigh and the knee, on occasions extending as far as the ankle. Pressure on the L3 nerve root causes an identical pain, but often with accompanying pins and needles.

The hip itself is affected by arthritis, displacements and lesions to the contractile structures; bursitis has already been considered. Diagnosis does not present great obstacles.

Disorders of the hip joint in children are nearly all serious.

Capsular lesions

The most marked feature of the capsular pattern is the restriction of medial rotation; this is accompanied by limitation of flexion and abduction linked with slight limitation of extension. The end-feel is hard, most notably on medial rotation which, in advanced cases, is so restricted that the patient walks with the foot turned outwards.

Rheumatoid, spondylitic and traumatic arthritis all benefit from an injection of steroid suspension 5ml (10cm needle). In all three instances, the X-ray of the hip is normal although in spondylitic arthritis the affection of the sacroiliac joint appears radiographically as sclerosis. In rheumatoid arthritis the other hip is the only other joint likely to be involved and traumatic arthritis is distinguished by its history of injury.

For the injection the patient lies on her painfree side and an assistant extends her hip, holding the leg off the couch in slight abduction (*Figure 6.34*).

The edge of the trochanter is identified and the needle introduced just above it (*Figure 6.35*).

The needle is thrust vertically downwards through the resistance of the thick capsule. The tip strikes bone at the neck of the femur close to its junction with the head (*Figure 6.36*).

The injection itself is painful and quite severe discomfort may come back two hours later and continue for several hours. The patient is seen again after two weeks and very often (particularly in rheumatoid cases) does not require a second injection. In cases of ankylosing spondylitis the infiltration should not be repeated more than, say, once every six months to obviate the risk of a steroid arthropathy.

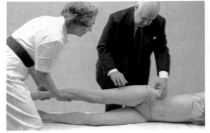

6.34

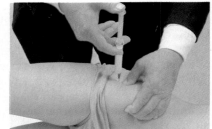

6.35

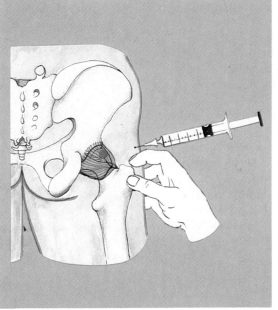

6.36

Fig 6.34 *The lateral approach is simplest, but the leg must be supported in slight abduction.*

Fig 6.35 *Thumb and long finger span the greater trochanter. No large nerves or blood vessels are in the vicinity.*

Fig 6.36 *Posterior view. Reaction to the injection is sufficiently painful to warrant an analgesic.*

Osteoarthrosis

In the early stages, stretching of the capsule is often followed by relief for many months or years but although the pain at night may be abolished, range is not improved. The more elastic the end-feel the better the immediate prognosis. On return of the symptoms following some months' remission the treatment is repeated, probably with diminished success. Sessions are twice weekly for about a month.

The joint is first heated by shortwave diathermy. For stretching, the hip is flexed as far as it will comfortably go and is then forced towards further flexion by slowly increasing pressure applied at the knee (*Figure 6.37*). No jerk is given. This continues with breaks for some 5–10 minutes and then the physiotherapist forces extension.

To do this, she pushes the patient's good hip into fullest possible flexion, thereby raising the bad thigh slightly off the couch. Maintaining the pressure at the good knee, extension is forced by gentle repeated pressure exerted downwards at the lower end of the bad thigh (*Figure 6.38*). With pauses for rest the physiotherapist keeps this up for 5–10 minutes.

If the other way of forcing extension is preferred, the patient must lie prone. The movement has to be confined to the hip joint by preventing any stress reaching the spine, so one hand is used to press the pelvis down. The physiotherapist musters all her strength and gives repeated pulls upwards with her other hand (*Figure 6.39*).

When medial rotation is stretched the pelvis must not be allowed to tilt. The operative hand takes hold of the patient's ankle and repeatedly pushes her leg outwards (*Figure 6.40*).

Forcing of lateral rotation is required only for dancers needing exceptional mobility.

When stretching ceases to benefit, surgery should be considered; the author's results with intra-articular silicone have been disappointing. Cases where the osteoarthritic degeneration is confined to the lateral edge of the femoral head have a relatively hopeful long-term prognosis. A radiotranslucent loose body may form secondary to osteoarthrosis in which case manipulative reduction is the way ahead.

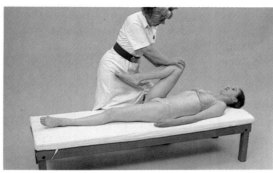

6.37

Fig 6.37 *Forcing hip flexion. Cases that do best with stretching have little erosion of articular cartilage superiorly.*

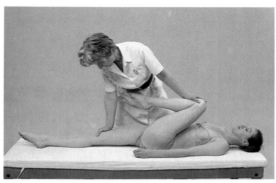

6.38

Fig 6.38 *Forcing extension. Full knee flexion of the good leg lifts the bad thigh off the couch. The physiotherapist has full control and an easier posture.*

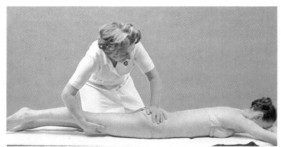

6.39

Fig 6.39 *Forcing extension—the alternative method.*

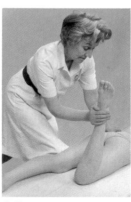

6.40

Fig 6.40 *Forced medial rotation. Too much pressure could fracture the neck of the femur.*

Displacements

The propensity of the hip for loose bodies is not always recognised, the more so since the displacement is usually secondary to osteoarthrosis. The history is diagnostic and consists of sudden twinges of pain shooting down the front of the thigh with the leg giving way, often temporarily immobilising the patient. These attacks punctuate the minor ache from any osteoarthrosis which will be responsible for the capsular pattern.

The attacks of severe pain and inability to bear weight on the affected leg last for, at most, a minute; the lesser symptoms may persist and will be present at the time of the patient's attendance. Generally there is some discomfort on full flexion and full lateral rotation.

The loose body must be shifted to some more favourable part of the joint by manipulative reduction—most cases can be dealt with successfully. Recurrence is common and treated in the same way.

Manipulation—1

The patient lies face upwards on a low couch and an assistant holds the pelvis down to prevent the patient being lifted off by the operator's traction. The operator stands on top of the couch grasping the leg at the ankle (*Figure 6.41*).

The manipulator leans back with all his weight and gradually steps off backwards (*Figures 6.42; 6.43*).

As he does so he extends the patient's leg slowly while repeatedly rotating it, and concludes with a sharp jerk towards one extreme of range (*Figure 6.44*). This final impulse is given in the direction found the most beneficial and thus the manipulation is performed at least three times—once one way, once the other and then in the most favourable direction. Re-examination follows each attempt, and if recovery is incomplete the physician moves on to the next method.

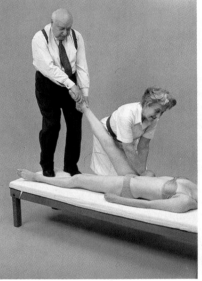

6.41

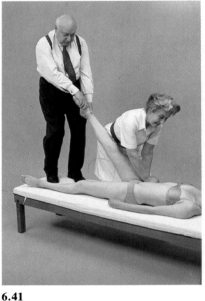

6.42

6.43

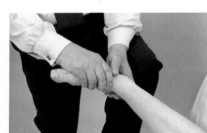

6.44

Fig 6.41 *The starting position, manipulative reduction. Excision is impossible unless the loose body shows radiographically.*
Figs 6.42, 6.43 *Mid-action. The hip is extended during rotation and traction. In Fig 6.43 the operator's right foot is shown suspended in mid-air during his descent.*
Fig 6.44 *The foot is used as a lever.*

Manipulation—2

Usually the last movements to stop hurting are full flexion and full lateral rotation. If they are not rendered painless by the previous manipulation, a stronger rotation strain can be applied (*Figure 6.45*).

The patient lies face upwards on a low couch. Her pelvis is anchored by an assistant, and the operator places the crook of the patient's knee over his. He then plantiflexes his foot and presses down at the patient's ankle over the fulcrum of his thigh, thereby exerting traction on her hip (*Figure 6.46*).

The femur is then smartly rotated (*Figure 6.47*) during continuing traction, with the manipulation first given in the direction previously found to be most beneficial—although the manoeuvre can, of course, be executed in the opposite direction. The patient is re-examined and the process repeated as necessary, say three or four times.

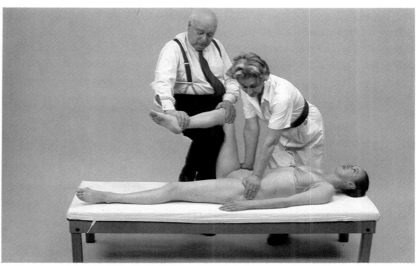

6.45

Fig 6.45 *The starting position. Some two-thirds of loose bodies can be reduced by this and the previous method.*

Fig 6.46 *To assume the starting position, the operator first hooks the patient's knee over his, and then applies traction by raising his heel.*

Fig 6.47 *The finishing position. The patient's lower leg is swung sharply round to push the hip into internal rotation during traction.*

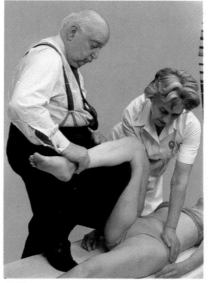

6.46

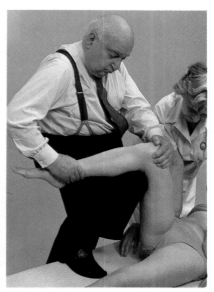

6.47

Lesions of the hip joint in children

Bed-rest and immediate X-ray are crucial if a child is found limping or complaining of even a slight ache in the thigh or knee when coupled with any limitation of movement at the hip joint. The possibilities include:

Congenital dislocation.
Pseudocoxalgia (Perthes' disease).
Tuberculosis of the hip.

Slipped epiphysis.
Transitory arthritis.
Coxa vara.
Haemophilia.
Trapped ligamentum teres.

Nearly all the above produce the capsular pattern. Age and X-ray are, between them, diagnostic.

Contractile structures

Athletes frequently strain the hamstrings; the psoas, adductor longus and rectus femoris do not give trouble so often. When several resisted hip movements hurt the leading possibility is gluteal bursitis (see page 78).

The treatment of choice, whether for the belly or body of a tendon, is massage. Steroids are reserved for the tenoperiosteal junctions.

The psoas

Strain of the psoas is rare and responds well to massage; injection is not employed. The painful movement is resisted flexion with the hip bent to a right angle, a test which excludes involvement of the quadriceps.

It is usually the lower part of the muscle that is injured. The site is below the inguinal ligament just medial to the inner edge of the sartorius (*Figure 6.48*).

Transverse massage with the patient half-lying is administered twice a week and should bring about recovery in a month or so (*Figures 6.49; 6.50*).

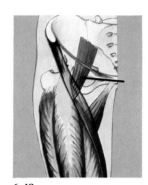

6.48

Fig 6.48 *The usual site.*

Figs 6.49, 6.50 *Massage, group and detail. The lesion responds well to deep friction. In half-lying, the muscle is relaxed.*

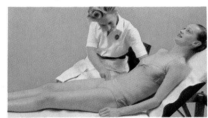

6.49

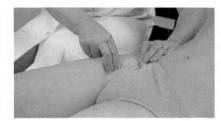

6.50

Adductor longus—rider's sprain

Resisted adduction of the hip is the painful movement, although sometimes full passive abduction hurts as well. The strain is always traumatic and the lesion is more often concealed at the musculotendinous than the tenoperiosteal junction. Treatment differs from site to site (*Figure 6.51*); should the belly be affected (rare) it responds either to massage or local anaesthetic 20ml.

At the tenoperiosteal junction either massage or steroid suspension 2ml is effective. The patient half-lies and for the injection the needle is inserted at the site of tenderness until its point reaches bone (*Figure 6.52*). The entire cubic extent of the tender area is infiltrated with a series of droplets.

Massage is the only effective remedy at the musculotendinous junction. The physiotherapist grasps the affected area between thumb and fingers and the friction is imparted by drawing the hand medially (*Figure 6.53*). Two 20-minute treatments a week are sufficient, with recovery in three to four weeks.

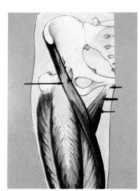

6.51

Fig 6.51 *Possible sites of a lesion of the adductor longus (right) and rectus femoris (left).*

Fig 6.52 *Steroid suspension only works at the tenoperiosteal junction.*

Fig 6.53 *Massage is curative in all recent and most chronic cases.*

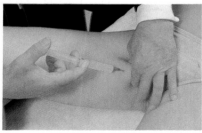

6.52

6.53

Rectus femoris

Athletes sometimes strain the rectus femoris tendon (see *Figure 6.51*). Resisted extension of the knee is the primary painful movement, although full passive flexion or rotation may also pinch or stretch the tissue. Massage is the treatment of choice.

The patient is half-lying so the hip joint is in flexion to relax the overlying tissues. The tendon is about 8cm below the anterior spine of the ilium and two fingers are laid firmly on the lesion with friction applied using the thumb for counterpressure (*Figure 6.54*). Treatments lasting 20 minutes twice a week should ensure recovery in a month or less.

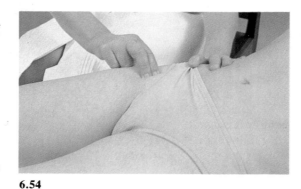

6.54

Fig 6.54 *Results of massage are uniformly good. The overlying sartorius must first be pushed aside.*

The hamstrings

These may be affected at the ischial origin, the belly or the knee (see page 104). Direct trauma or a sudden strain may be responsible and the pain intensifies over 24 hours; the patient—usually an athlete—walks with a limp. Resisted flexion at the knee hurts at the back of the thigh and if a haematoma is present it should be aspirated *stat*.

At the ischial origin, steroid suspension is the treatment of choice. The tendon is identified and the tender area, which usually lies in the upper 5cm, is infiltrated throughout with steroid suspension 5ml delivered in droplets when the tip touches bone (*Figure 6.55*).

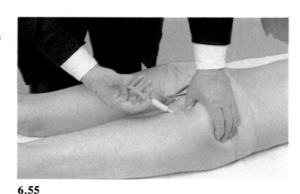

6.55

Fig 6.55 *Ischial origin, injection of steroid suspension.*

Massage is an uphill task because of the size and density of the tendon. To render it palpable, the hip must be supported in flexion (*Figures 6.56; 6.57*). Two or three fingers exert strong transverse friction by flexion and extension of the wrist, emphasised by abduction and adduction of the shoulder.

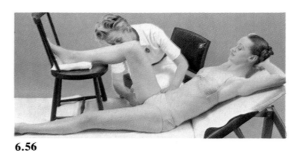

6.56

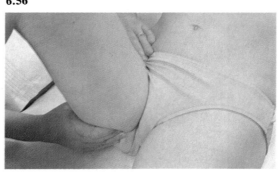

6.57

Figs 6.56, 6.57 *Massage, ischial origin, group and detail. This tendon must be kept taut. In chronic cases relief may take two months.*

If the lesion lies at the belly, local anaesthetic solution 50ml is injected at the first attendance to enable the muscle to move during a period of painlessness. This approach is worthwhile only in the first few days following injury.

On the next attendance massage is administered. The knee is kept flexed to relax the muscle (*Figure 6.58*).

The deep friction is extremely tiring and given for five minutes on, five minutes off, over half an hour. For the first week the sessions are daily, thereafter on alternate days and treatment continues for a week after recovery to forestall recurrence.

The lesion is grasped between thumb and finger of both hands and the fingers are flexed and extended while the hand is drawn upwards (*Figure 6.59*). Each session is concluded by strong Faradism to the affected part of the belly (again with the knee in flexion) to broaden out the muscles without stretching the healing fibres.

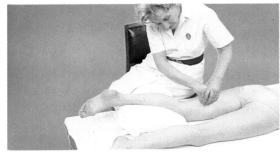

6.58

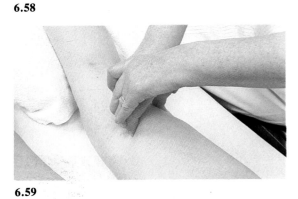

6.59

Figs 6.58, 6.59 *Massage, group and detail. This is the common injury of sprinters and footballers. Note the leg is supported in flexion.*

Other findings on resisted movements

Painful weakness
Flexion—adolescent traction-fracture of the trochanter or the anterior superior spine of the ilium.
Flexion—abdominal neoplasm infiltrating the psoas.
Flexion—metastases at upper femur.

Painless weakness
Lumbar disc lesion if unilateral (common).
Spinal neoplasm.
Abduction—congenital dislocation of the hip.
Hip flexion and knee extension—if bilateral, myopathy or myositis.

CHAPTER SEVEN

THE
KNEE

An exact diagnosis can be made at the knee with greater certainty than at any other joint, and many of the conditions are easily curable. History is of critical diagnostic importance.

Numerically the most important disorders are the ligamentous sprains which are often accompanied by secondary traumatic arthritis; it is, of course, the lesion and not the secondary response that requires treatment. Knee pain is usually well localised and many of the tissues are accessible to palpation. Painless osteoarthrosis should be disregarded.

A straightforward joint.

Referred pain

Pain referred to the knee is characterised by its indefinite extent. The front of the knee is within the territory of the L2 (*Figure 7.1*) and L3 (*Figure 7.2*) dermatomes. Tissues derived from the latter segment provide the more likely cause of referred symptoms, in particular from a disc lesion compressing the L3 root or, more often, osteoarthrosis of the hip.

Disorders of the knee itself very seldom produce posterior pain only. The back of the knee is covered by the S1 (*Figure 7.3*) and S2 (*Figure 7.4*) dermatomes. A fifth lumbar disc displacement exerting pressure on the first or second sacral nerve roots may be responsible for pain in this region, as may a lesion of the lower part of the hamstrings or of the upper part of the gastrocnemius.

It will be borne in mind that extra-segmental referred pain of dural origin may also cause pain in the lower limb (*Figure 7.5*).

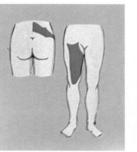
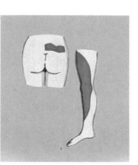

7.1　　　　**7.2**

Figs 7.1, 7.2 *The dermatomes, anterior aspect. L2 (left). L3 (right).*

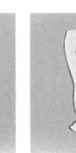
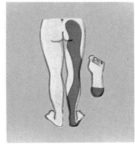
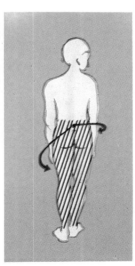

7.3　　　　**7.4**

Figs 7.3, 7.4 *The dermatomes, posterior aspect. S1 (left); S2 (right).*

Fig 7.5 *Pain of dural origin can extend to the knee and beyond.*

7.5

History

Provided the lesion actually lies at the knee, the primary distinction is between disorders of spontaneous origin and those of traumatic origin. In the former case the cause may be, for example, rheumatoid arthritis, ankylosing spondylitis, Reiter's disease, psoriasis, lupus erythematosus.

In the event of injury the most detailed history is needed—for two reasons. First, the physician must assess the exact strain imposed on the joint at the moment of trauma and the exact site of the pain. Thus a valgus strain falls on the medial collateral ligament giving pain on the inner side of the knee.

Second, many disorders can be identified by their typical history and progression. A number of avenues of enquiry should be explored. Did the knee give way? Could the patient get up and walk? Did the joint lock? If so, in flexion or extension? Did it unlock itself? Did the pain and disablement come on suddenly or over some hours? Was the pain momentary? Were there any twinges? Did any swelling come on rapidly? Or slowly?

Each disorder has its idiosyncratic course from which the diagnosis can often be made, being merely confirmed by the physical examination.

Examination

Passive movements

Preliminary examination will, of course, have excluded the lumbar spine and hip as the source of pain.

For examination of the knee the patient lies, and the two primary passive movements of flexion (*Figure 7.6*) and extension (*Figure 7.7*) evaluate the state of the joint capsule.

The capsular pattern is so much limitation of extension, very much more limitation of flexion and no restriction of either rotation (e.g. in the proportion of 5° limitation of extension, 70° limitation of flexion, both rotations full). Gross arthritis with, for example, 90° limitation of flexion may eventually interfere with the rotations.

Fig 7.6 *Passive flexion.*

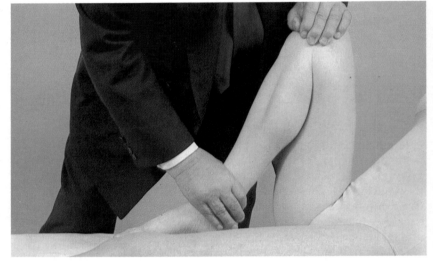

7.6

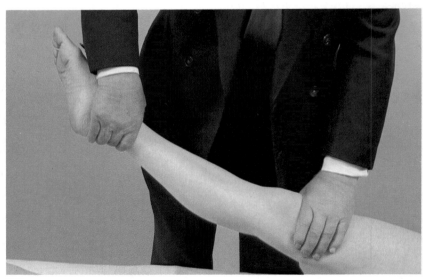

Fig 7.7 *Passive extension.*

7.7

Seven secondary movements follow, testing the ligaments for pain and laxity. Pain indicates a sprain, pain and laxity a severe sprain and laxity alone a past strain.

First valgus strain (*Figure 7.8*) is applied, opening the inner side of the joint. Pain elicited by this test indicates a sprain of the medial collateral ligament, a frequent occurrence.

Varus strain (*Figure 7.9*) opens the outer side of the joint, testing the lateral collateral ligament, infrequently at fault.

Painful passive lateral rotation (*Figure 7.10*) incriminates the medial coronary ligament and is a secondary sign for the medial collateral ligament. Sprain to either coronary ligament is prone to occur in conjunction with damage to the relevant meniscus inflicted by the same injury.

Passive medial rotation (*Figure 7.11*) is tested; pain on this movement suggests a lesion of the lateral coronary ligament.

Pain on forwards shearing implicates the anterior cruciate ligament; the knee is pushed away from, and the lower leg pulled towards, the examiner who sits on the patient's forefoot to stabilise the leg (*Figure 7.12*).

Straining the tibia backwards on the femur (*Figure 7.13*) stretches the posterior cruciate ligament.

The tibia is pushed laterally on the femur (*Figure 7.14*). This is a secondary test for the posterior cruciate although a cracked meniscus may be felt to subluxate momentarily.

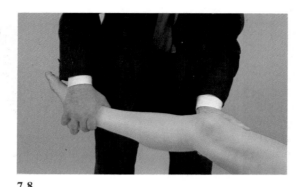

7.8

Fig 7.8 *Valgus strain. Note the knee is in extension.*

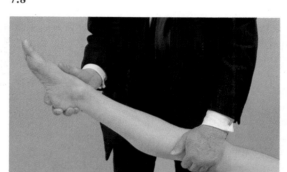

7.9

Fig 7.9 *Varus strain. The operator has reversed his left hand.*

Figs 7.10, 7.11 *Passive lateral and medial rotations. Full rotation is not possible unless the knee is flexed, as extension tautens the ligaments.*

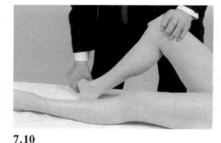

7.10

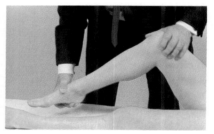

7.11

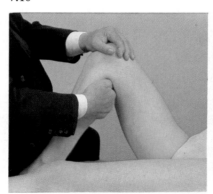

7.12

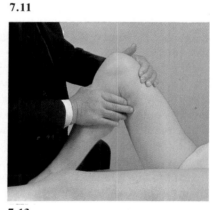

7.13

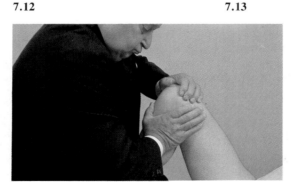

7.14

Fig 7.12 *Forwards shearing.*

Fig 7.13 *Backwards shearing.*

Fig 7.14 *Lateral shearing.*

Resisted movements

The patient lies on her stomach and four resisted movements assess the contractile structures.

Resisted flexion (*Figure 7.15*) tests the hamstrings and so if this movement hurts, the physician must establish from which member of the group the pain originates.

For resisted medial rotation (*Figure 7.16*) the patient attempts to turn her foot inwards. Pain on this movement, if accompanied by painful resisted flexion, suggests a lesion of the semimebranosus (rare), the semitendinosus or popliteus muscles (both very rare). But painful resisted lateral rotation (*Figure 7.17*), together with painful resisted flexion, shows the biceps to be at fault.

Resisted extension with the patient prone (*Figure 7.18*) tensions the quadriceps. If painless weakness is found, a lesion of the nervous system, an L3 tumour, metastases, myopathy or myositis should be considered.

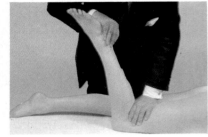

7.15

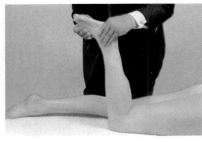

7.16

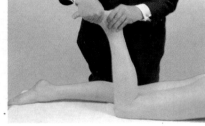

7.17

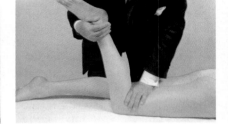

7.18

Fig 7.15 *Resisted flexion.*

Fig 7.16 *Resisted medial rotation.*

Fig 7.17 *Resisted lateral rotation.*

Fig 7.18 *Resisted extension.*

Accessory signs

The physician checks for fluid. The first method is the standard patellar tap (*Figure 7.19*). The more delicate and preferred test is to elicit fluctuation (*Figure 7.20*); with experience, blood and fluid can be distinguished. Blood fluctuates *en bloc* like a jelly whereas fluid runs up and down piecemeal.

One hand is placed flat above the patella and exerts downward pressure. The movement of any fluid thereby induced forces apart the thumb and forefinger positioned on either side of the patella. Blood fills the joint swiftly, fluid in the course of some hours. Blood is an irritant and must be aspirated immediately; that is the therapeutic measure. Aspiration of clear fluid is a waste of time and the treatment is to discover its cause and deal with that.

The examiner searches for heat using the back of the hand, the more sensitive aspect (*Figure 7.21*). Warmth indicates the lesion is still in the active stage and localised heat may pinpoint its exact site. Finally, the physician palpates for the synovial thickening characteristic of the rheumatoid-type arthritises. It may be felt by gently rolling the fingers upwards and downwards (*Figure 7.22*) at the reflexion of the membrane where it overlies each condyle of the femur (*Figure 7.23*). The sound knee is compared.

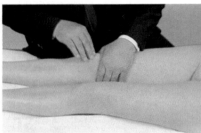

7.19

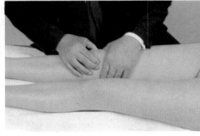

7.20

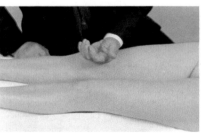

7.21

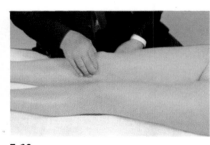

7.22

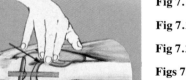

7.23

Fig 7.19 *The patella tap.*

Fig 7.20 *Eliciting fluctuation.*

Fig 7.21 *Feeling for heat.*

Figs 7.22, 7.23 *Palpating for a thickened synovial membrane.*

Findings

Capsular lesions

The commonest capsular lesions—as distinct from secondary traumatic arthritis—are the rheumatoid-type conditions signalled by warmth, fluid, synovial thickening and, in the earliest stages, full range. Later, the capsular pattern supervenes but there is no history of recent trauma.

Osteoarthrosis is visible on the radiograph of nearly all middle-aged patients and of itself is always symptomless. However, the cartilaginous degeneration frequently spawns one or more radiotranslucent loose bodies (see page 99).

It is particularly important to note that if the capsular pattern results from traumatic arthritis, it is the causative lesion and not the secondary response that receives treatment.

Capsular lesions are indicated by markedly more limitation of flexion (*Figure 7.24*)—the patient cannot bend her knee fully—than of extension, when it cannot be fully straightened (*Figure 7.25*).

Except in advanced arthritis, both rotations remain free.

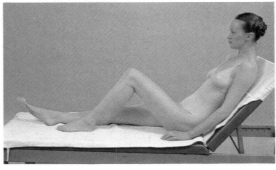

7.24

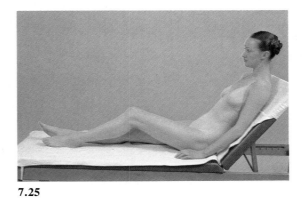

7.25

Figs 7.24, 7.25 *Limitation in the capsular pattern is not necessarily caused by a capsular lesion; almost all traumatic lesions produce a secondary capsulitis.*

Baker's cyst

This produces swelling in the upper calf in the absence of any injury; the patient is found to have long-standing rheumatoid arthritis at the knee. Posterior capsular rupture with extravasation of synovial fluid into the upper calf has taken place and aspiration is the answer (*Figure 7.26*).

Fig 7.26 *A Baker's cyst impedes the venous return. A fluctuant swelling is aspirated via the calf, but if no fluctuation can be detected the fluid is tapped from the joint itself.*

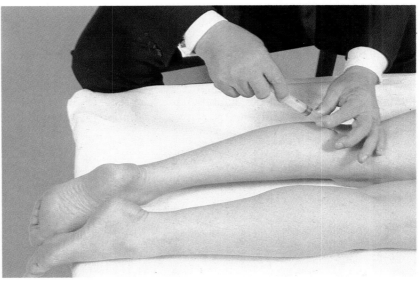

7.26

Primary rheumatoid arthritis

For rheumatoid-type disorders at any stage, the joint is injected. Two or three injections ease or abolish the symptoms but do nothing to eliminate the cause; the treatment must therefore be repeated as the symptoms warrant, but sparingly. Too frequent injection is to be avoided for fear of a steroid arthropathy.

The patient lies with her quadriceps relaxed and steroid suspension 5ml (4cm needle) is injected into the joint. The injection is made at the point where the thumb is placed half-way down the edge of the patella (*Figure 7.27*), lifting it off the condyles.

This allows the needle to slide in parallel to the posterior surface of the patella and the infiltration is made between the two condyles (*Figure 7.28*). Reiter's disease does not benefit from this or any treatment.

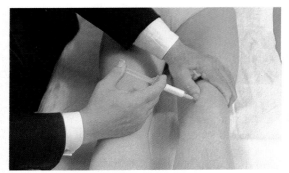

7.27

Figs 7.27, 7.28 *Injection, monarticular rheumatoid arthritis. The patient complains of gradual onset of unprovoked swelling; the injection must not be given more often than once every six months.*

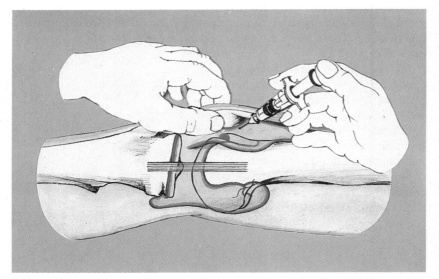

7.28

Haemarthrosis

Internal bleeding may be of either spontaneous or traumatic origin; restriction of movement will in some cases total as much as 45° limitation of extension and 90° limitation of flexion. The blood suddenly fills the capsule, and in a few minutes the joint is distended to near bursting. Aspiration should take place immediately; it may take two attempts to remove all the blood. A haemophiliac needs an injection of globulin prior to the aspiration.

Non-capsular lesions

Ligamentous lesions: general principles

Ligamentous sprains are very common. If untreated, they tend to follow a standard progression best exemplified by the medial collateral ligament. Treatment differs according to the stage reached.

Stage I
A sprain to a ligament (*Figure 7.29*) is accompanied by secondary traumatic arthritis lasting one to two weeks.

Stage II
The traumatic arthritis has subsided. But the lesion must not be allowed to heal in immobility, otherwise adhesions form at the site of tear, binding ligament to bone (*Figure 7.30*).

Stage III
The tear to the ligament has healed but adhesions prevent full painless mobility, unless ruptured (*Figure 7.31*).

Laxity following a sprain is unlikely to be of grave concern to those other than professional athletes. There is no pain and operative suture is the only treatment.

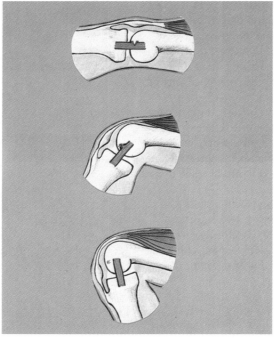

7.29, 7.30, 7.31

Figs 7.29, 7.30, 7.31
After a sprain (top), adhesions may bind the ligament to bone (centre). If untreated, the adhesions will consolidate and must be ruptured (bottom).

Treatment

Stages I and II (except the cruciates)
Massage is given, moving the ligament over bone to inhibit formation of adhesions; any fibrils tethering the tissue to bone are disengaged without interfering with union of scar tissue longitudinally placed. Forcing of the joint towards extension is strongly contraindicated. After the first week or so the massage is given more strenuously and accompanied by gentle encouragement of movement.

Stage III
Manipulative rupture of the adhesions is normally only necessary or feasible at the collateral ligaments, but during this phase—two months plus after injury—it is the sole remedy.

The medial collateral ligament

Sprain of the medial collateral ligament ranks as the commonest ligamentous disorder in the entire body. The history is of a valgus strain with the pain and an acute traumatic arthritis (often making examination impossible) developing rapidly over some hours. The pain is localised to the inner side of the knee and although the lesion may lie at one of three sites (*Figure 7.32*) usually it is at the joint line.

Two weeks after injury the arthritis starts to subside and after three months (if untreated) the symptoms are of an ache following exertion. Except in this chronic stage (see below) the treatment is deep friction. The ligament is never injected with steroid suspension as laxity is apt to ensue.

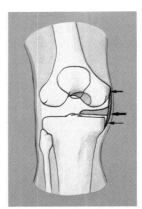

Fig 7.32 *The three sites. Unless the lesion is treated, disability is so severe the patient normally spends some days in bed.*

7.32

First the ligament is massaged in maximum comfortable flexion (*Figure 7.33*). Then massage is given in maximum comfortable extension (*Figure 7.34*). By the end of the session, increased flexion and extension will be attainable and the joint *must* be taken at least once to its new extreme of flexion; extension must not be forced. The starting points for subsequent treatments are the new positions of maximum range.

Massage in flexion is administered to the site of the lesion with strong transverse pressure. The ligament lies roughly in line with the longitudinal axis of the tibia and accordingly the sweep of the fingers is diagonal rather than vertical (*Figure 7.35*).

For massage in extension the ligament lies horizontally; the massage is thus straight up and down (*Figure 7.36*). The reader is referred to *Figures 7.29, 7.30* and *7.31* showing the alignment of the medial collateral ligament for varying knee positions.

The treatments—lasting 20 to 30 minutes—are given daily for the first few days and thereafter are cut back to every other day. In the hyperacute stage the friction must be delivered with a light touch, only penetrating deeply to mobilise the ligament in the last half-minute. Full and painless range should be restored in one to two weeks.

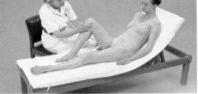

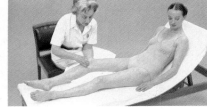

7.33   **7.34**

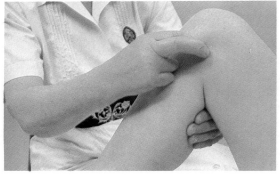

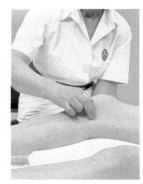

7.35   **7.36**

Figs 7.33, 7.34 *Massage is given for about ten minutes in both flexion and extension.*

Fig 7.35 *Massage in flexion. Note the thrust is slanted diagonally.*

Fig 7.36 *Massage in extension, vertical thrust. With such treatment, most get better in two weeks instead of three months.*

In the final stage, the untreated adhesions must be ruptured by a sharp thrust towards lateral rotation. The patient half-lies with her knee in flexion (*Figure 7.37*) to prevent any rotation taking place at the hip. Lateral rotation of the tibia on the femur is forced using the foot as a lever (*Figure 7.38*); the movement is accentuated by an abrupt adduction of the operator's elbow. If medial rotation is restricted, a thrust is given towards medial rotation (*Figure 7.39*).

If range of movement diminishes rather than increases despite treatment, Stieda–Pellegrini's disease (in which the periosteum has been torn up by the strain) may be to blame. The condition shows clearly on the X-ray after four weeks as a shadow along the whole inner side of the medial femoral condyle. Treatment is useless; recovery takes 6 to 12 months.

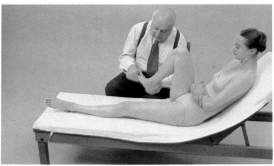

7.37

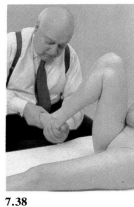

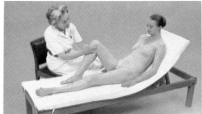

7.38   **7.39**

Fig 7.37 *Untreated adhesions cause pain after strenuous exertion. They must be ruptured.*

Fig 7.38 *The movement is a sharp thrust towards lateral rotation.*

Fig 7.39 *Forcing of medial rotation. The grip corsets the heel to avoid spraining the ankle.*

The coronary ligaments

These fasten the two menisci to the rim of the tibia. Accordingly, a rotation strain may overstretch one of the coronaries with or without accompanying tear of the meniscus (depending on the severity of the stress). As with the meniscus, it is the medial structure (*Figure 7.40*) that is more frequently damaged than the lateral. The appropriate passive rotation (i.e. lateral rotation for the medial ligament) will be uncomfortable as is sometimes passive extension; this shifts the meniscus which bulges out against the ligament. The pain and traumatic arthritis are less pronounced (e.g. 2° limitation of extension, 45°–60° limitation of flexion) than for the medial collateral ligament. It is a common football injury.

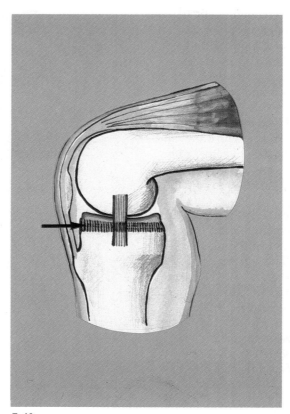

Fig 7.40 *The medial coronary ligament. If untreated, the sprain resolves slowly over a good three months.*

7.40

The medial coronary ligament

The lesion usually straddles the anteromedial quadrant of the joint line but may on occasion reach behind the medial collateral ligament. The physician palpates for tenderness.

Massage is very effective and is the treatment whether the strain is acute, sub-acute or chronic. Sessions last 15–20 minutes daily for the first week and are held on alternate days thereafter. The knee is put into flexion (*Figure 7.41*) to open the joint anteriorly and lateral rotation further exposes the ligament.

The temptation is to press straight inwards towards the femur. This is incorrect; it massages only bone.

The friction must be directed downwards (*Figure 7.42*). The tibial condyle is located from above, the superficial tissues indented and the pressure exerted on to the shelf provided by the tibia. The finger is then pulled to and fro across the site of the sprain, with the index fingernail lying horizontally.

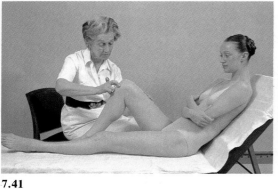

7.41

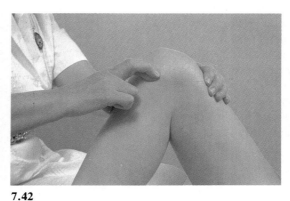

7.42

Figs 7.41, 7.42 *Massage, group and detail. This is the only treatment for the sprain, which is always traumatic. The fingers press downwards on to the ligament.*

The cruciate ligaments

The cruciates (*Figure 7.43*) respond only to injection (2ml steroid suspension). Sprains here often occur as part of a double lesion and—except with a dashboard injury—the causative stress is not in any particular direction. The pain is described as 'right inside the joint'.

The knee is warm and swollen, fluid is present and although full range is possible, all the extremes hurt because the cruciates limit rotation as well as flexion and extension. The collateral and coronary ligaments are palpably normal.

A single correctly placed injection leads to recovery in one to two weeks, but the procedure is difficult because although it is possible to distinguish which ligament is involved, one cannot always tell at which end. The tissues are too deep for palpation, so first one end and later, if need be, the other must be infiltrated.

If one of the ligaments has become permanently elongated after a strain, the history simulates that of a ruptured meniscus.

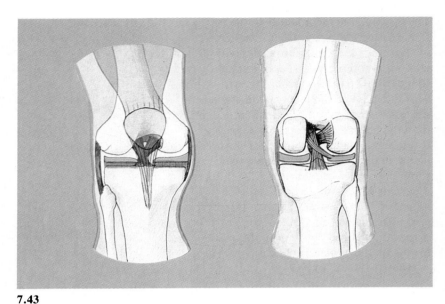

7.43

Fig 7.43 *The anterior ligament runs downwards and forwards from the medial surface of the lateral condyle (left); the posterior runs backwards and downwards from the lateral surface of the medial condyle (right).*

Posterior ligament: posterior end

The posterior ligament is the more commonly injured; the lesion is marked by pain on backwards shearing. Steroid suspension 2ml is injected (*Figure 7.44*) at the site centred across the exact mid-point of the tibia. With experience the physician can judge the optimum point of entry and aim the needle straight at the tibial attachment.

The crux of the matter is to bypass the popliteal vessels which overlie the lesion. The easiest approach is to employ one thumb to locate the apex of the lateral condyle (*Figure 7.45*); the 5cm needle is inserted just there and is inclined at about 60° to the horizontal. It thus passes well under the popliteal vessels and heads distally towards the centre of the posterior aspect of the tibia (*Figure 7.46*).

The angle of entry is then progressively altered until the needle eases into the joint. This is just too far and the tip is returned to the previous position (*Figure 7.47*) and the injection given after the point is felt to penetrate the ligament before hitting bone. A series of tiny insertions and withdrawals is made.

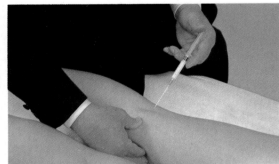

7.44

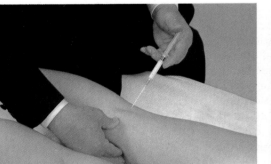

7.45

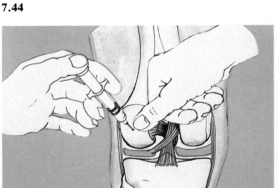

7.46

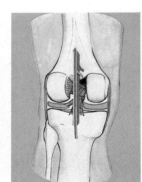

7.47

Fig 7.44 *Injection, left knee. This end is the more often affected.*

Fig 7.45 *One hand locates the lateral condyle.*

Figs 7.46, 7.47 *This lateral approach avoids the popliteals.*

Posterior ligament: anterior end

For injection to the anterior end of the posterior cruciate the patient lies supine with her leg extended. The site of the lesion is masked by the patella (*Figure 7.48*).

One hand tilts the patella, lifting it off the femoral condyle. The 6cm needle is inserted at the patellar margin and enters parallel to the articular surfaces (*Figure 7.49*).

When the needle hits the lateral aspect of the medial femoral condyle, its position is adjusted until the ligamentous resistance is felt. The injection is made by a series of tiny withdrawals and reinsertions.

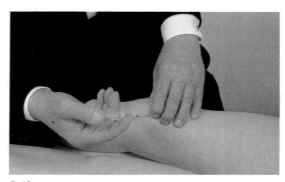

7.48

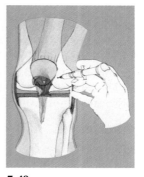

7.49

Fig 7.48 *Injection, right knee. The free hand raises the patella.*

Fig 7.49 *The injection obviates months of traumatic arthritis.*

Anterior ligament: anterior end

Involvement of the anterior cruciate is marked by pain on forwards shearing. The injection to the anterior end of the anterior cruciate is simplicity itself. The patient flexes her knee to a right-angle and the 5cm needle enters immediately below the lower edge of the patella at a slant of about 45° (*Figure 7.50*).

It is aimed for the spine of the tibia; the tip penetrates a resilient tissue—the ligament—before striking bone (*Figure 7.51*). The infiltration is made as before by a series of tiny withdrawals and reinsertions.

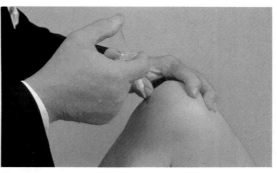

7.50

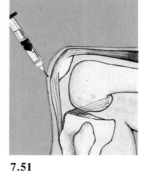

7.51

Fig 7.50 *Injection, left knee. Hyperextension can cause the sprain.*

Fig 7.51 *Injection is effective whether the sprain has lasted days or years.*

Anterior cruciate: posterior end

The techniques mirrors the method for the posterior end of the posterior cruciate, in that the popliteal vessels must be negotiated. But the approach is from the medial side pointing slightly proximally. This time the apex of the medial condyle is identified (*Figure 7.52*) and the needle punctures the skin at an angle about half-way between horizontal and vertical. The tip is directed towards the medial surface of the lateral condyle and ligamentous resistance is encountered before hitting bone (*Figure 7.53; 7.54*). The injection is made by a series of withdrawals and reinsertions.

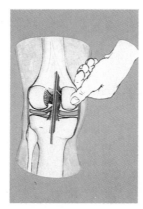

7.52

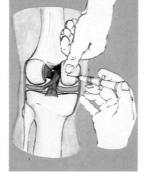

7.53

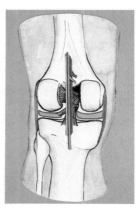

7.54

Fig 7.52 *Again the popliteal vessels mask the lesion. Left leg shown.*

Figs 7.53, 7.54 *The needle passes well posterior to the danger area. The leg is in extension.*

Displacements

The knee has a marked prediliction for displacements, which fall readily into three categories: menisci, loose bodies in the middle-aged and loose bodies in the young.

The latter could result from osteochondrosis dissecans, chondromalacia patellae or a chip fracture. They are insignificant numerically and their common history is of momentary fixation in extension (as opposed to flexion) which is self-unlocking. The loose bodies possess an osseus nucleus and are visible radiographically.

The meniscus

The medial meniscus is the less mobile of the two and consequently more frequently injured. Immediate disabling pain follows a rotation strain and the joint locks in some 10° of flexion so the patient is unable to put her heel to the ground. The knee is warm and full of fluid.

Recurrent dislocation nearly always requires excision; a strain severe enough to tear the meniscus will most likely have sprained the appropriate coronary ligament as well.

A cyst of the lateral meniscus has a history deceptively similar to that of a ruptured meniscus. But then the knee never actually locks and on full extension a small hard bulge is palpable at the joint line. The treatment is to vent the meniscus by puncturing it in a number of different directions with a needle; this liberates the fluid and may result in cure.

The short-term treatment for a torn meniscus is manipulative reduction (*Figure 7.55*) followed by consideration of removal if the condition recurs.

For the medial meniscus the physician opens the inner side of the joint, subjecting it to a valgus strain (*Figure 7.56*) which is maintained while the knee is extended (*Figure 7.57*) during repeated rotation of the tibia; the foot is wielded as a lever. At the last moment a further thrust is given towards both valgus and extension.

The patient is re-examined after each attempt and the process repeated until full range is obtained; reduction is attended by a click. General anaesthesia is sometimes required.

For the lateral meniscus, varus strain is applied. If internal derangement is not present at the time the patient is seen, the examiner may be able to reproduce the tell-tale click by rotating—or applying a shearing strain to—the knee. The history is also suggestive.

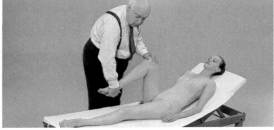

7.55

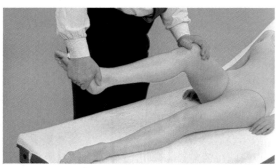

7.56

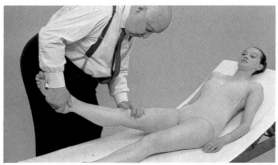

7.57

Figs 7.55, 7.56, 7.57 *Manipulative reduction of a subluxated medial meniscus. The fragment must be shifted medially, since it displaces centrally–hence the valgus strain. Remember the coronary ligament may also require treatment.*

A loose body in the middle-aged or elderly

Initially, rheumatoid arthritis resembles this condition; both show warmth and fluid. However, with a loose body the warmth and pain are localised, the onset is sudden, and the patient complains of twinges and of the knee giving way, especially while walking downstairs. The condition is a frequent product of otherwise symptomless osteoarthritic degeneration.

This pathology should always be taken into account where a middle-aged patient experiences localised pain in the knee with no history of trauma. As well as blocking the joint, the presence of the loose fragment will momentarily strain the medial collateral ligament (which is often tender) from *inside*

the joint. But no *extrinsic* strain will be reflected in the history. Limitation of range and degree of discomfort vary with the size and position of the loose fragment, but often full extension hurts and flexion is limited by 5–10°.

Manipulative reduction abolishes the symptoms. There are four techniques. Each is tried several times and the patient is re-examined after each attempt; if one method does not work, the operator goes on to the next. Following complete reduction, the patient should be warned that recurrence within a year or two is not unlikely. Avoidance of flexion insofar as is possible should help forestall relapse but, if it occurs, the patient must attend again.

Manipulation—1

For the first manipulation the physician hooks the patient's foot over his knee and pulls upwards (*Figure 7.58*) while an assistant presses heavily downwards on the thigh to open the joint (*Figure 7.59*). The distracting force is maintained as the operator removes his foot from the couch and then smartly extends and repeatedly rotates the knee (*Figures 7.60; 7.61*). The patient is re-examined and the procedure repeated as necessary, perhaps a dozen times in a single session.

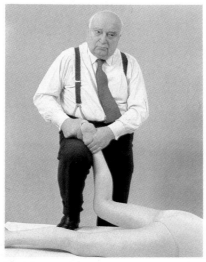

7.58

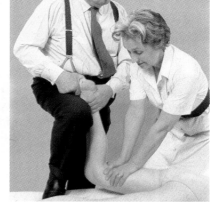

7.59

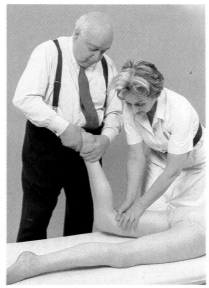

7.60

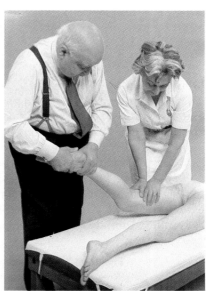

Figs 7.58, 7.59, 7.60, 7.61 *Manipulative reduction, a loose body. The intention is to move the fragment posteriorly from its position between the articulating surfaces. The assistant presses down for some seconds to allow the tibia and femur to come apart. Note how by the final photograph the manipulator has moved right down the couch.*

Manipulation—2

If flexion remains limited, the best method to try next is rocking the tibia on the femur; the movement derives purchase from the fulcrum of an assistant's forearm placed in the popliteal space (*Figure 7.62*).

The anterior movement of the tibia is obtained by jerking the knee strongly towards flexion while simultaneously forcing rotation (*Figure 7.63*); immediately after the overpressure the knee is released to let the tibia snap back.

The patient is re-examined and the manipulation repeated as appropriate. For both this and the succeeding variant, it is vital to check that as flexion eases the range of extension (the more important movement) does not decrease; if so, these techniques are abandoned immediately and, if necessary, the operator resorts to the first manipulation to re-establish the original range.

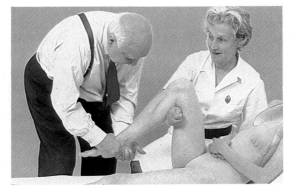

7.62

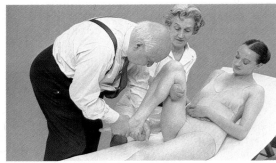

7.63

Figs 7.62, 7.63 *Flexion during rotation, starting and finishing positions. The foot is repeatedly rotated with a final overthrust towards lateral rotation. A click may be felt, flexion suddenly becoming free.*

Manipulation—3

The same manipulation is possible without an assistant (*Figure 7.64*); the manoeuvre is as before but omits the rotation—only flexion is forced (*Figure 7.65*).

Figs 7.64, 7.65 *Rocking the tibia without rotation, starting and finishing positions.*

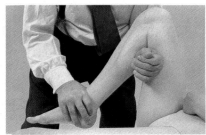

7.64

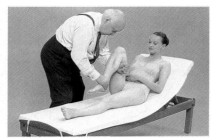

7.65

Manipulation—4

There is another method if pain on full extension persists. The patient half-lies, with her leg in slight flexion, and the operator applies varus pressure (*Figure 7.66*).

While this is maintained, the patient co-operates actively by extending her knee. At the last moment a small jerk encourages full extension (*Figure 7.67*). The patient is re-examined and the procedure repeated as necessary.

Figs 7.66, 7.67 *Full extension can usually be rendered painless provided varus pressure is maintained.*

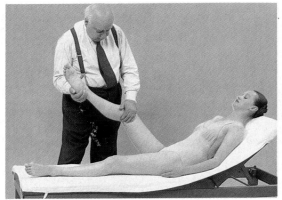

7.66

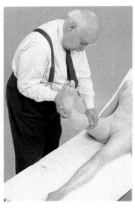

7.67

Contractile structures

The two main groups are the hamstrings at the back of the knee and the quadriceps at the front. Both can be strained at either end.

The extensor mechanism
Painful resisted extension may stem from a lesion of the rectus femoris (at its origin at the anterior inferior spine), the quadriceps belly, the quadriceps expansions, the suprapatellar or the infrapatellar tendon. The last two respond to both massage and injection.

With the exception of the rectus femoris (see page 85) and the quadriceps bellies, they share a history of pain at the front of the knee on walking, with the joint normal. Only resisted extension hurts and palpation reveals the site of the lesion around the patella. In all three tendinous cases the massage is angled so that the supinated fingers reach beneath the patella and catch the affected fibres against the edge of the bone.

The patient is frequently an athlete, dancer or one-legged as amputees put extra strain on the remaining leg.

The quadriceps are most often injured at their origins; for the site at the anterior inferior spine see page 85. At the belly, the patient feels something give way at the front of the thigh.

The suprapatellar tendon
The lesion is found at the insertion of the tendon into the superior border of the patella.

The patient relaxes her quadriceps. For the injection of steroid suspension 2ml (2cm needle) one hand presses downwards on the lower pole of the patella (*Figure 7.68*). This tilts the upper border of the patella upwards, tautening the tendon and bringing the lesion into prominence. The point of entry is through a spot 1.5cm proximal to the lesion (*Figure 7.69*).

The infiltration is not made until the tip of the needle touches bone whereupon the entire affected area is injected by a series of half-withdrawals and reinsertions. For two days there are painful after-effects and the injection may have to be repeated.

The principles of massage are much the same. The web of one hand presses down on the lower edge of the patella while transverse friction is given by the other hand in supination.

The pressure is angled distally and anteriorly to catch the fibres against the upper pole of the patella (*Figure 7.70*). The hand must not be held in pronation pressing downwards only; this rubs the wrong part of the tendon (*Figure 7.71*). The massage is very tiring and is given for 20 minutes on alternate days with recovery in about a month.

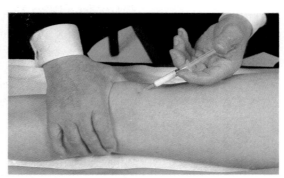

7.68

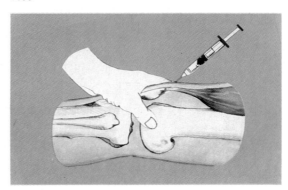

7.69

Figs 7.68, 7.69 *Pressing down on the patella facilitates injection along the tenoperiosteal junction.*

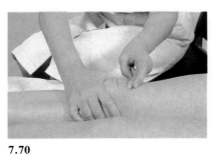

7.70

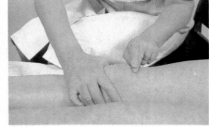

7.71

Fig 7.70 *Massage, correct. Sprain is usually due to sudden over-contraction of the quadriceps.*

Fig 7.71 *Massage, incorrect. The angulation of pressure is wrong.*

The infrapatellar tendon

Strain of the infrapatellar tendon is more common than that of the suprapatellar. The physician palpates at the tenoperiosteal junction (*Figure 7.72*) as the tibial extremity of the tendon is rarely at fault.

The patient relaxes her quadriceps. Altering the angle of the patella is again achieved by downwards pressure of the operator's free hand, but this time it is brought to bear on the upper edge of the patella thus swinging the lower edge upwards. The needle is inserted about 1.5cm inferior to the mid-point of the tender area (*Figure 7.73*).

When the tip touches bone, a series of droplets is distributed fanwise along the tender area—the patient will be sore for two days. Up to three injections may be required since it is easy to leave out a small extent of the lesion.

For massage the free hand tilts the patella while the operative finger, reinforced by its neighbour, presses hard upwards against the tenoperiosteal junction (*Figure 7.74*). The hand is in supination and the whole arm moves to and fro; sessions last about 20 minutes on alternate days and recovery takes anywhere between two and six weeks.

Figs 7.72, 7.73 *Injection. The patella is tilted to tauten the tendon, thus facilitating infiltration of the tender extent.*

Fig 7.74 *Massage. Permanent relief within three weeks is the rule for recent cases.*

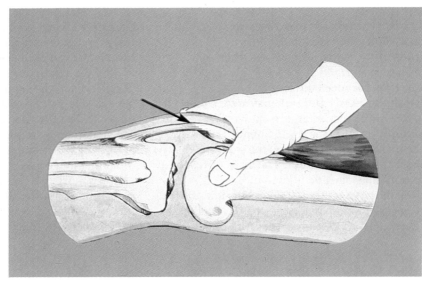

7.72

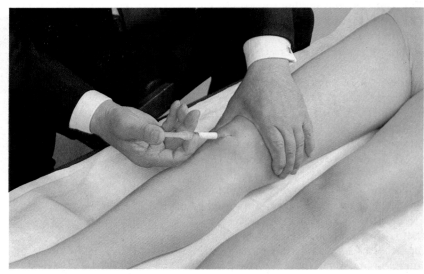

7.73

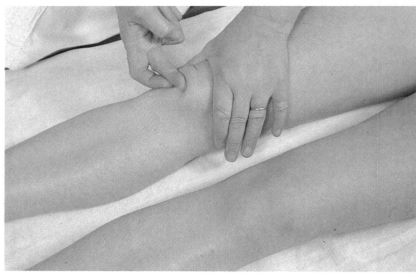

7.74

The quadriceps expansion

The lesion may lie either side of the patella at the junction between the patella and the expansion (*Figure 7.75*).

The only treatment is massage for two to three weeks on alternate days. The first step is to use the thumb of one hand to push the patella towards the affected side. This means that the operative finger can be wedged right under the now projecting edge; the hand is held in supination (*Figure 7.76*). The pressure is directed upwards so that the fibres are massaged against the posterior surface of the patella by drawing the finger back and forth.

The quadriceps mechanism also suffers from a number of surgical conditions. Recurrent dislocation of the patella afflicts children aged eight to 15; the knee gives way suddenly, painfully and repeatedly. Patellar-femoral arthrosis produces an anterior ache coming on after walking, with pronounced crepitus on weight-bearing. In young patients the cause—in the absence of trauma—is chondromalacia patellae. Complete rupture of the belly and fixation of the muscle at the point of fracture at the lower end of the femur also occur.

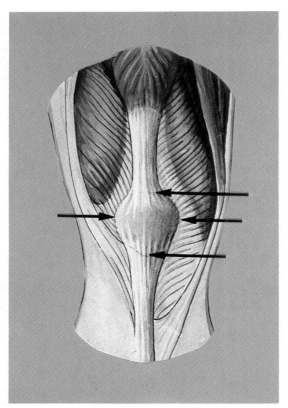

7.75

Fig 7.75 *The sites lie around the periphery of the patella. Sometimes a direct blow rather than overuse is the cause.*

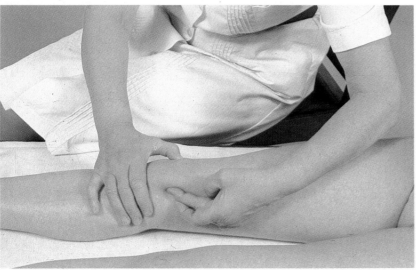

Fig 7.76 *Massage. The pressure is straight upwards against the back of the projecting edge of the patella. Recent cases may be better within the week.*

7.76

The hamstrings

Pain on resisted flexion points to a lesion of the hamstrings which may be injured at any one of a number of sites (*Figure 7.77*); for the ischial origin and bellies, see page 85. A severe lesion in the latter will also limit straight-leg raise.

Occasionally, painful resisted knee flexion is attributable to a lesion of the popliteus tendon or of the posterior cruciate ligament or even of the upper tibiofibular joint.

If lateral rotation hurts in addition to flexion, the sensitive area will be found in the bicipital tendon near its insertion at the head of the fibula. Painful resisted medial rotation probably indicates a lesion of the semimembranosus tendon (rare) as it passes across the head of the tibia. Massage is the treatment of choice in either case.

A lesion of the popliteal muscles (rare) can be cleared up by either massage or infiltration of steroid suspension 1 ml at the tendinous origin, but at the belly only by massage. Both resisted flexion and resisted medial rotation hurt.

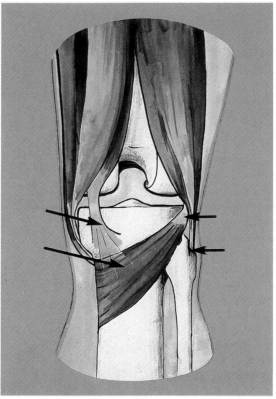

Fig 7.77 *The sites. Palpation may be necessary to differentiate between the popliteus and the semimembranosus, since both hurt on resisted medial rotation. The biceps (bottom right) hurts on resisted lateral rotation.*

7.77

CHAPTER EIGHT

THE LEG

Conditions affecting the leg are simple and diagnosis is easy. Referred pain is rare and the lesions most frequently encountered are muscular.

The usual cause of referred pain in the calf is a fifth lumbar disc lesion compressing the first and/or second sacral nerve root, although pain of dural origin below the knee crops up from time to time; the symptoms are unaltered by resisted movements. It is worthwhile inspecting the calf for signs of bruising and for wasting caused by a disc lesion or ruptured tendon.

The lesions most frequently encountered are muscular.

Examination

Resisted movements

Examination is straightforward. The patient stands on tiptoe, first on one leg, then the other (*Figure 8.1*). This tests both the gastrocnemius and the soleus. The finding may be of painless weakness (an L5 disc lesion) pain and weakness (a ruptured muscle or tendon) or pain alone (a muscular lesion).

The four resisted movements then assess the contractile structures in the leg. Resisted dorsiflexion (*Figure 8.2*) puts strain on the tibialis anterior; the patient pushes her foot upwards.

Resisted plantiflexion (*Figure 8.3*) again tests both the soleus and the gastrocnemius.

Resisted inversion (*Figure 8.4*) puts strain on the tibialis posterior. The patient pushes inwards against the operator's resistance.

Resisted eversion (*Figure 8.5*) tests the peronei.

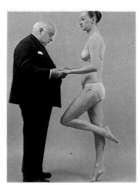

8.1

Fig 8.1 *Rising on tiptoe, the most potent test for plantiflexion.*

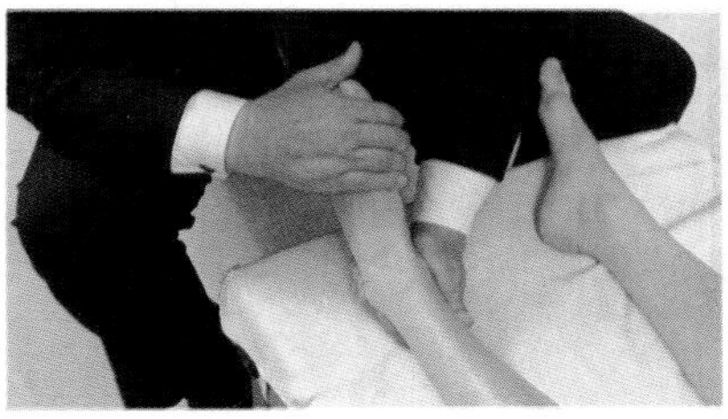

Fig 8.2 *Resisted dorsiflexion.*

Fig 8.3 *Resisted plantiflexion.*

Fig 8.4 *Resisted inversion.*

Fig 8.5 *Resisted eversion.*

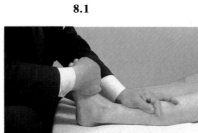

8.2

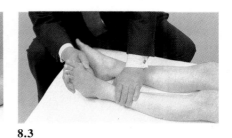

8.3

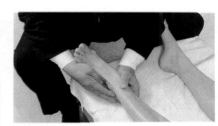

8.4

8.5

Findings

The plantiflexors

'Tennis leg'

A sprain of the gastrocnemius ('tennis leg') is the prevailing muscular lesion in the leg. But pain on resisted plantiflexion is an ambiguous finding as this movement puts strain on both the gastrocnemius and the soleus. But when the knee is flexed the gastrocnemius is relaxed, so pain on resisted plantiflexion which disappears on knee flexion is a sure sign the gastrocnemius is to blame.

The patient reports a sudden severe twinge at mid-calf, with pain on walking ever since. It will emerge that although dorsiflexion is limited by muscular spasm when the knee is extended, full range is attainable merely by flexing the knee to a right angle. The lesion is substantial and normally lies in the muscle about 5cm above the musculotendinous junction; the exact spot is tricky to find, but in severe cases a gap about 1cm wide is palpable. Treatment consists of three co-ordinated measures: local anaesthesia, massage and a raised heel.

Whether the patient is seen on the day of injury or some weeks later, local anaesthesia is immediately induced at the site of rupture (*Figure 8.6*). A solution of 0.5% procaine 50ml is required, and following the injection the patient actively mobilises the muscle for 15 minutes. These active exercises continue daily until recovery.

Meanwhile, a cork support is fitted to the inside of the shoe to compensate for the limitation of dorsiflexion (*Figure 8.7*). The support enables the patient to use the unaffected part of the muscle, without straining the healing breach anew, and is

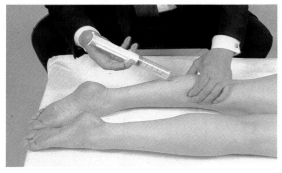

8.6

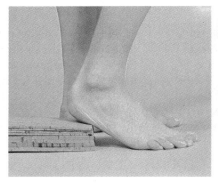

8.7

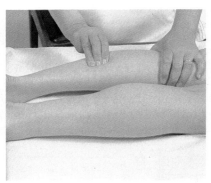

8.8

Fig 8.6 *50 ml local anaesthetic is best, since often the site can only be located approximately.*

Figs 8.7, 8.8 *The muscle is shortened by spasm. So a cork support inside the shoe is needed temporarily. The next day massage is given; in recent cases recovery should take ten days.*

lowered daily as range returns. It can be discarded at the end of a week or 10 days.

Starting the day following the injection the patient receives deep massage, daily for three days, and thereafter on alternate days. Sessions last 20 minutes.

The fingers are placed on the affected area and the friction is imparted by drawing the hand to and fro horizontally (*Figure 8.8*). In chronic cases relief may take up to a month.

The tendo Achillis

The pain is at the back of the heel and standing on tiptoe hurts. Resisted plantiflexion is normally the only other painful movement, but passive dorsiflexion may be uncomfortable. There is no limitation and the condition is often correctly diagnosed by the patient.

The lesion is usually at mid-tendon; the physician must ascertain which aspects are affected. Often both sides as well as the anterior surface are involved—if so all three must be treated. The posterior surface is never at fault (*Figure 8.9*).

Massage is the treatment of choice. Sessions last 20 minutes on alternate days with recovery in about three weeks. For the lateral and medial aspects of the tendon the patient's foot projects over the edge of the couch and dorsiflexion is maintained by the physiotherapist's knee (*Figure 8.10*); this keeps the tendon on the stretch. The tendo Achillis is squeezed firmly between finger and thumb, and the friction is imparted simultaneously to both sides by drawing the hand up and down (*Figure 8.11*). It is hard work and the physiotherapist may wish to change hands mid-session.

For the anterior aspect, the foot lies fully plantiflexed in order to relax the tendon so it can be pushed sideways by the free hand. This brings the anterior surface within reach of the physiotherapist's supinated fingers.

The friction is delivered by supination and pronation of the forearm with upwards pressure maintained by elbow flexion (*Figures 8.12; 8.13*). The finger, hand and forearm are held in line with the patient's lower leg.

An injection of steroid suspension 2ml is effective but relapse often occurs, so massage is to be preferred particularly for athletes or if the lesion is extensive. Infiltrating the anterior aspect of the tendon is difficult if not impossible.

The patient lies prone with her foot dorsiflexed. The needle (5cm) is inserted almost horizontally some 3cm distal to the lesion and the tip is pushed forwards to the proximal edge of the lesion. The needle runs parallel to the tendon along its surface (*Figure 8.14*).

Steroid suspension 0.5ml is infiltrated as the needle is drawn back to the near edge of the lesion. Three or four more lines of fluid are injected in the same way until the entire solution is exhausted (*Figure 8.15*). Rheumatoid tenovaginitis also benefits from this treatment. The substance of the tendon must never be injected because of the risk of rupture, nor is any such approach justified as the lesion lies superficially.

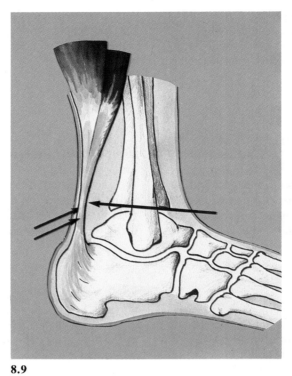

8.9

Fig 8.9 *Any aspect apart from the posterior surface may be involved; treatment must reach every affected portion.*

Figs 8.10, 8.11 *Massage to the lateral and medial aspects. Note the foot is clamped in dorsiflexion. Recovery after friction is nearly always permanent, but the patient should walk as little as possible until well.*

Figs 8.12, 8.13 *Massage to the anterior aspect is only practicable if the tendon is pushed sideways. The forearm is rotated.*

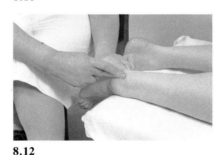

8.10

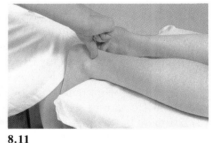

8.11

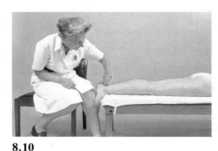

8.12

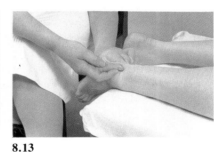

8.13

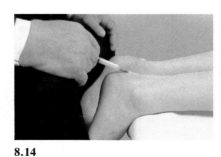

8.14

Figs 8.14, 8.15 *Relapse may follow even successful injection. Steroid is introduced in lines along the tendon's surface.*

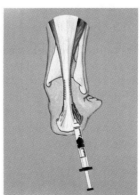

8.15

Plantiflexors: other findings

Rupture of the tendo Achillis is revealed by gross weakness on resisted plantiflexion coupled with excessive range of dorsiflexion. Treatment consists of operative suture and is only fruitful during the first ten days—thereafter spontaneous healing occurs, but only gradually, leaving permanent discomfort.

Intermittent claudication

Owing to the exceptional arrangement of its nutrient arteries, the gastrocnemius muscle is more susceptible than others to ischaemia as the result of arteriosclerosis. The history is characteristic. An elderly patient relates that pain in one calf is brought on by walking a short distance and is relieved by rest; repeated and rapid dorsiflexion and plantiflexion evoke the pain. The condition must not be confused with the 'mushroom phenomenon' (see page 192). Restoration of a patent artery by surgery is the treatment of choice.

Short plantiflexor muscles

Plantiflexor muscles of inadequate length are indicated by painless limitation of dorsiflexion to about 90°. A number of conditions may result.
(1) Excessive range of movement at the mid-tarsal joint (see page 125). Since the ankle itself cannot be fully moved, the patient relies on the adjacent joint instead. Normally, pain results only in middle age and the patient may not be seen until that time. But if the patient is five or under, the calf muscles can be stretched.
(2) Eversion of the tibia. This deformity allows the patient to put his heel to the ground, but the eversion means that with each forward step less distance is covered as the width, not the length, of the foot is employed for forward motion.

Accordingly, the patient is often a very poor runner while at school and has to put up with an awkward gait.

There is no pain. If circumstances warrant, particularly in the young, osteoclasis of the tibia is carried out and the bone is reset with the foot straight. A raised heel may be provided if necessary.
(3) Metatarsalgia. In this condition the patient cannot rest his heel on the ground, so the whole weight of his body is carried on the forefoot. Pain on weight-bearing results. The symptoms generally do not appear until the patient is over 20 and often follow a period of rest in bed sufficiently long for the short flexor muscles to weaken. A permanent support is required.
(4) Plantar fasciitis (see page 123).
(5) Pain/fatigue on standing. As the patient cannot get his heel to the ground, he stands heavily on his forefoot which cannot take the strain for long. A raised heel is required.

The evertor muscles

The peronei

If resisted eversion of the foot hurts, the peroneal muscles are at fault. The site of tenderness defines the position of the lesion which is seldom localised enough for steroid therapy. The cause may be either over-use or a single strain often occurring concurrently with a sprained ankle (see page 114). There are four sites, one at the musculotendinous junction and three on the tendon—above, at and below the malleolus (*Figure 8.16*). Massage is the treatment of choice, with the foot held in inversion to stretch the tendons.

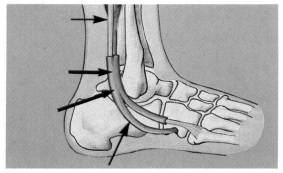

8.16

Fig 8.16 *The four sites. The thick arrows point to the commonest locations. The lesion is seldom localised enough for an injection of steroid.*

The manner of massage is dictated by the size of the lesion. At the upper site only one finger is used, reinforced if need be (*Figure 8.17*). Above the malleolus three digits are required (*Figure 8.18*) and below it two are needed (*Figure 8.19*). The fingers are drawn briskly to and fro across the lesion; recovery in two to three weeks is the norm.

At the malleolus the friction must be imparted by rotation of the digit because the malleolus shields the tendon from direct pressure (*Figure 8.20*).

Spasm of the peroneal muscles results in fixation of the talocalcanean and mid-tarsal joints, produced by arthritis; 'spasmodic pes planus'—see page 124—is a misnomer.

The cause of weak peronei may be a disc protrusion at the fifth lumbar level, an upper motor neurone lesion or peroneal atrophy.

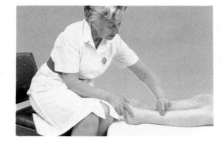

8.17

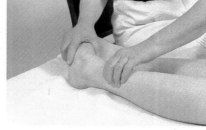

8.18

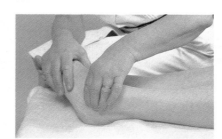

8.19

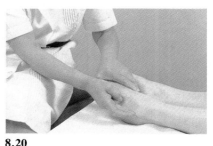

8.20

Fig 8.17 *Massage, upper site. Tenderness is sought from the musculotendinous junction downwards.*

Fig 8.19 *Below the malleolus.*

Fig 8.18 *Above the malleolus. Walking is avoided pending recovery.*

Fig 8.20 *At the malleolus. Massage by rotation.*

The invertor muscles

There are two invertors—the tibialis anterior and the tibialis posterior. However, the anterior tibialis controls dorsiflexion as well and a lesion there will evoke pain not only on resisted inversion but also on resisted dorsiflexion.

The tibialis posterior

If resisted inversion hurts but dorsiflexion does not, the pain is instigated by the tibialis posterior. The underlying factor may be a congenital deformity maintaining the heel in valgus; lateral rotation of the forefoot ('pes planus') is the outcome. This posture imposes constant strain on the posterior tibial tendon and calls for a permanent support; a wedge extending from the front of heel to the metacarpal heads realigns the foot.

The wedge is nearly 1cm higher on the inner side of the foot than on the outer side, with a ridge of additional height under the midtarsal joint. This tips the heel into varus and encourages the forefoot towards medial rotation. As the support is required continuously it is supplied as a removable inner sole.

In the absence of treatment the pain goes on indefinitely, although often it only starts in

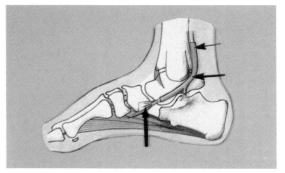

8.21

Fig 8.21 *Possible sites of a lesion to the tibialis posterior. Athletes call the condition at the upper end 'shin-soreness'.*

middle age. Massage is needed as well as support except in cases of non-postural strain, where treatment is confined to deep friction.

There are three sites (*Figure 8.21*) separated by several inches in all. The tendon is put on the stretch; sessions last 20 minutes twice a week for a month or less.

Above the malleolus, massage is angled directly across the tendon (*Figure 8.22*). For the calcanean extent the fingers massage across the tendon using the thumb as a fulcrum (*Figure 8.23*). If the lesion lies at the malleolus, the tibialis posterior is recessed in a groove and is not accessible for transverse pressure; here, transverse friction is achieved by laying the finger flat on the affected sector and rotating the forearm (*Figures 8.24; 8.25*).

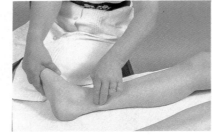
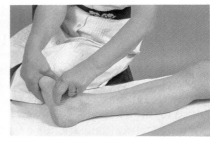

8.22

8.23

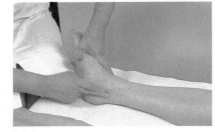
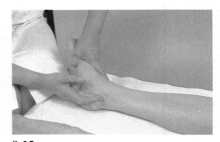

8.24

8.25

Fig 8.22 *Massage, above the malleolus.*

Fig 8.23 *The calcanean extent.*

Figs 8.24, 8.25 *At the malleolus. The fingers rotate in the sulcus between tendo Achillis and tibia.*

The dorsiflexor muscles

The tibialis anterior

Painful resisted dorsiflexion may hurt just above the ankle; resisted inversion should also be painful. These symptoms incriminate the tibialis anterior which boasts a tendon of great length. The lesion is found not at the ankle but a good six inches higher, at the musculotendinous junction next door to the anterior border of the tibia. Crepitus is felt on movement.

The treatment is massage: the thumb is placed on the lesion and the forearm pronated and supinated (*Figure 8.26*). Recovery usually takes two to three weeks.

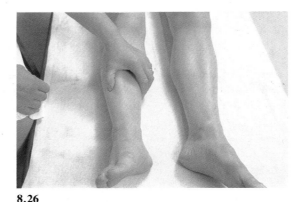

8.26

Fig 8.26 *Massage, tibialis anterior.*

Other findings

Weakness on dorsiflexion is a common finding in lumbar displacements at the fourth level, upper motor neurone lesions and anterior poliomyelitis.

The effects of a tight fascial compartment (rare) superficially resemble intermittent claudication. Voluntary dorsiflexion becomes impossible or difficult after exertion; these symptoms may or may not be accompanied by pins and needles and pain. Treatment by removal of the fascia at the front of the tibial belly is urgent if necrosis is impending.

CHAPTER NINE

THE ANKLE AND FOOT

The ankle joint itself is simple as it permits only two movements in one plane. But a sprained ankle can involve any one of a number of ligaments and tendons at different sites, although these are easy to distinguish. The anterior talofibular ligament is much the most frequently strained.

The foot consists of a highly intricate series of joints which give rise to a multiplicity of possible complaints. Accurate diagnosis is nonetheless practicable and the conditions respond well to treatment. The patient can usually point to the site of the lesion.

In cases of trauma to the foot, a detailed history will ascertain exactly what strains were imposed on the joint.

Dural pain does not extend below the ankles. But root pain, which will not be confined to the foot, and/or paraesthesia from a lumbar disc lesion is common (see page 219).

The intricacy of the joints is no bar to accurate diagnosis.

Examination

After a careful history, the patient's foot is inspected twice, once with the patient standing and once with her supine. This is because the physical examination may reveal nothing, since the momentary stress imposed by manual testing may not be on a scale to evoke the pain caused by sustained weightbearing.

But changes in the foot's contours may be apparent when the patient stands. Any alteration in shape shows where undue strain falls and, by corollary, where it should be diminished. Many conditions can be treated simply by providing a carefully structured support to the foot so alleviating excess strain.

Short plantiflexor muscles may account for a number of disorders and the reader is referred to page 108, minor misalignments of the tibia can cause abnormal stresses in the foot.

The ankle

Two passive movements evaluate the capsule at the ankle joint—passive dorsiflexion (*Figure 9.1*) and passive plantiflexion (*Figure 9.2*). The ligaments stabilising the ankle span the talocalcanean and mid-tarsal joints, which are thus included in the ankle examination.

The talofibular, calcaneofibular and the lateral mid-tarsal ligaments are tested by passive inversion during plantiflexion (*Figure 9.3*).

The deltoid ligament—less frequently strained than the ligaments at the outer side—is assessed by passive eversion, again during plantiflexion (*Figure 9.4*).

Strong varus is applied (*Figure 9.5*). This tests both the tibiofibular ligament and the talocalcanean joint. If the fault lies with the ligament, a click will be felt as the talus overtilts in the enlarged mortice; there is thus pain and excessive range. But if the talocalcanean joint is involved there will be pain and limited range, and the limitation increases as the condition advances. In both cases, valgus strain (*Figure 9.6*) proves full and painless.

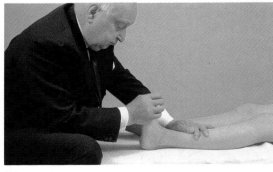

Fig 9.1 *Passive dorsiflexion, ankle.*

9.1

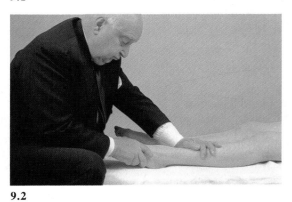

Fig 9.2 *Passive plantiflexion, ankle.*

9.2

Figs 9.3, 9.4 *Passive inversion (Fig 9.3) and eversion (Fig 9.4) during plantiflexion; the ankle ligaments span the mid-tarsal joints.*

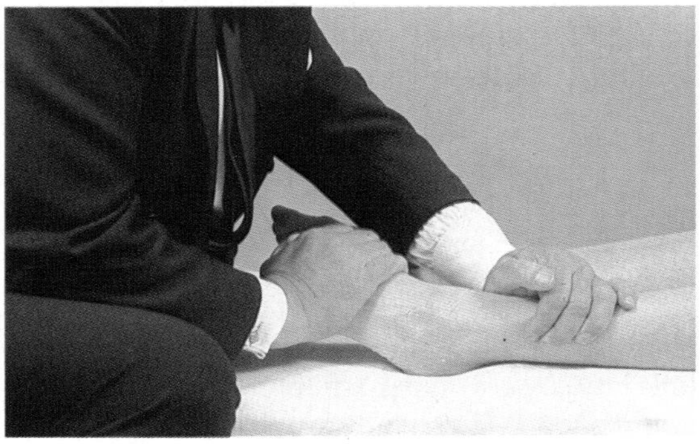

9.3

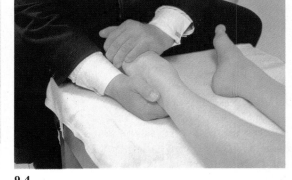

9.4

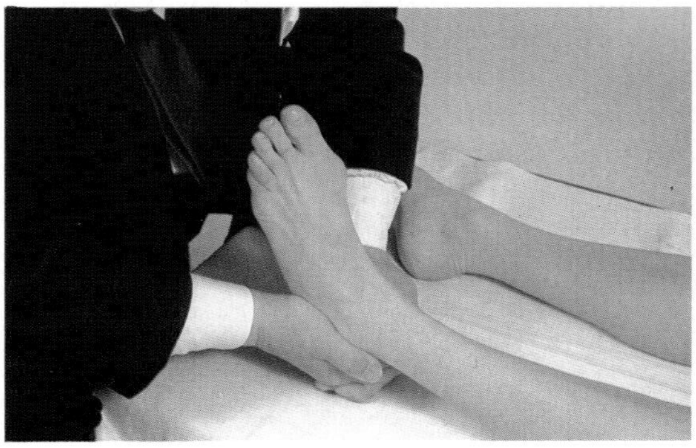

9.5

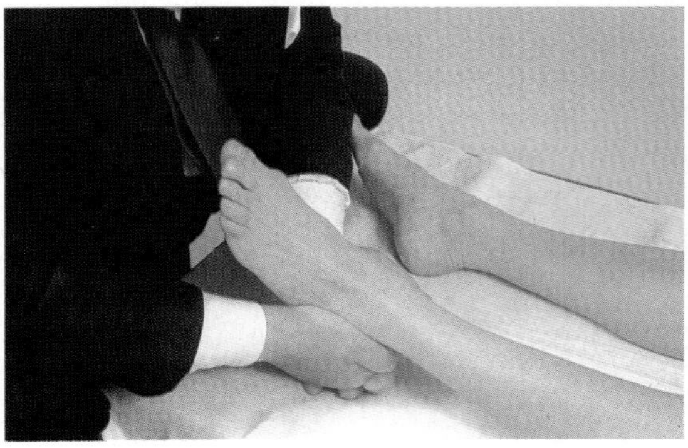

9.6

Fig 9.5 *Varus strain, talocalcanean joint.*

Fig 9.6 *Valgus strain. For these two and the succeeding four movements the heel is grasped in valgus and pulled down towards the examiner to fix the talus. This prevents movement at the ankle joint.*

The mid-tarsal joint

Six movements are now performed for the mid-tarsal joint. They are:

(1) Passive dorsiflexion (*Figure 9.7*).

(2) Passive plantiflexion (*Figure 9.8*).

(3) Passive adduction (*Figure 9.9*).

(4) Passive abduction (*Figure 9.10*).

(5) Passive medial rotation (*Figure 9.11*).

(6) Passive lateral rotation (*Figure 9.12*).

The capsular pattern is announced by limitation of adduction and medial rotation. If necessary, the examination takes in the toes and the resisted movements for the leg may also have to be tested (see page 105).

Finally, the physician feels for the pulsation both of the posterior tibial artery just behind the medial malleolus (*Figure 9.13*) and of the dorsalis pedis on the front of the mid-tarsal joint. If absent, the artery is blocked and the site of obstruction must be established.

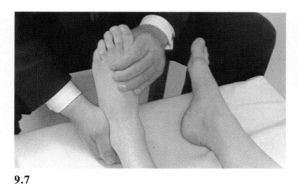

9.7

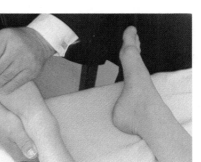

9.8

Fig 9.7 *Passive dorsiflexion.*

Fig 9.8 *Passive plantiflexion.*

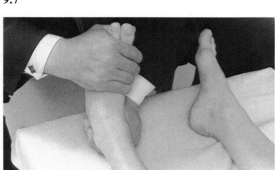

9.9

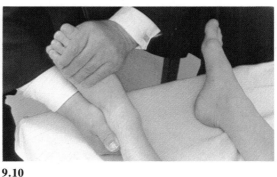

9.10

Fig 9.9 *Passive adduction.*

Fig 9.10 *Passive abduction.*

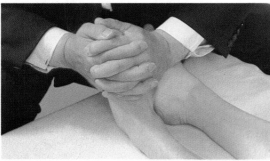

9.11

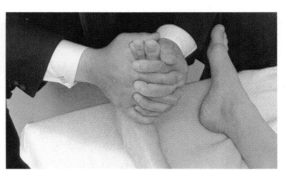

9.12

Fig 9.11 *Passive medial rotation.*

Fig 9.12 *Passive lateral rotation.*

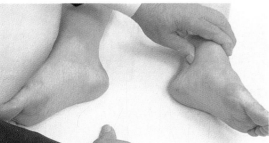

9.13

Fig 9.13 *Feeling for pulsation.*

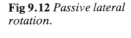

The ankle joint

Capsular lesions

Capsular lesions at the ankle joint are unusual. Rheumatoid arthritis does not occur and in fact the only common condition is osteoarthrosis. Conservative treatment is seldom satisfactory; if the symptoms warrant, arthrodesis is highly effective.

The capsular pattern is some limitation of dorsiflexion and more limitation of plantiflexion, coupled with a hard end-feel. But if short calf muscles restrict dorsiflexion in the normal joint only these last two findings will be apparent.

Ligamentous sprains

Ligamentous sprains are very common and easy to differentiate. Following examination by selective tension, the physician palpates for tenderness of the affected structure. If gross oedema renders this impossible, the swelling is first reduced by effleurage.

Valgus sprains do not often happen and are considered at page 118. It is the varus sprains that are routinely encountered and the sites (*Figure 9.14*) are listed in order of descending frequency:

(1) The anterior talofibular ligament at the fibular origin.
(2) The calcaneofibular ligament at the fibular origin.
(3) The anterior talofibular ligament at the talar insertion.
(4) The calcaneocuboid ligament.
(5) The peronei (see page 108).
(6) The tibiofibular ligament.
(7) The extensor longus digitorum (very rare).
(8) The anterior talotibial ligament (very rare).

The lesion most frequently met with is a combined sprain of the anterior talofibular ligament and the calcaneocuboid ligament.

With the exception of the rare valgus injuries, most sprained ankles clear up of themselves in due course. But full painless mobility can be greatly expedited by proper treatment, which varies according to the period elapsed since the tissue damage.

Acute stage
During the first 24 hours, steroid suspension 2ml is injected into the ligament—the sooner after the injury the better the results. Deep effleurage may be needed first to diminish oedema, and massage follows the next day, continuing daily until recovery.

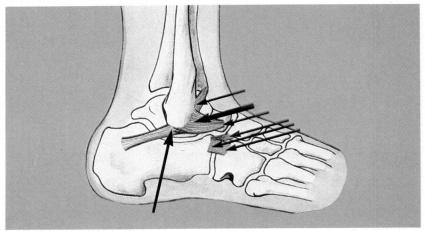

9.14

Subacute stage
Deep massage moves the ligament in imitation of its normal behaviour, preventing the formation of adhesions both in the ligament and between it and bone. The massage is given to the site of the tear, at first for a few minutes but for longer at later treatments. After each session the joint is encouraged towards its new extreme of range by gentle passive movements.

Chronic stage
Pain on prolonged exertion persisting some months later is disposed of by manipulative rupture of the adhesions. Peroneal tendinitis following a sprained ankle is often mistaken for adhesions and is manipulated in vain; resisted eversion must be tested to avoid committing this error.

None of the foregoing procedures have any bearing on the tibiofibular ligament. Sprain here results in elongation and consequent instability of the mortice joint and frequent recurrent strains (see page 117).

Fig 9.14 *Possible sites of a sprained ankle. The calcaneofibular (left), anterior talotibial (top), anterior talofibular (centre, thick arrow), calcaneocuboid or bifurcate ligament (right). The fibular origins of the two main ligaments are far and away the commonest sites of tear. Note the lesion may lie at various sites within individual ligaments. The peronei and the extensor digitorum can also suffer.*

Varus sprain

The anterior talofibular ligament

The anterior talofibular ligament may be
strained at either the fibular origin or the talar
insertion (see *Figure 9.14*). Passive inversion
during plantiflexion is the most painful
movement and at both sites the treatment is
the same.

First effleurage is applied.

If the injury occurred within the last 24 hours
steroid suspension 2ml (3cm needle) is
injected. The foot is held in the maximum
possible plantiflexion and inversion and the
insertion made about 2cm distal to the
lesion—most often at the fibular origin. The
needle is thrust in almost horizontally (*Figure
9.15*) until it meets bone and a series of
droplets are distributed fanwise. The pain is
quite considerable for 48 hours but then the
symptoms start to resolve rapidly until the
patient is well in a couple of days. Most
probably massage will not be necessary.

Massage is the only treatment if the time for
injection has passed, or if the patient proposes
to do without the discomfort caused by the
injection. The foot is held in the same position
with the digit lodged against the lower tip of
the malleolus. The hand is in supination and
the fingers press medially and proximally to
rub the ligamentous fibres against their origin
from the bone (*Figure 9.16*).

The principles of treatment are unchanged at
the talar site. For the injection the needle is
thrust directly into the tear (*Figure 9.17*). For
the massage the pressure is directed medially
only, while the fingers travel in a straight line
across the fibres (*Figure 9.18*). At neither site
is massage vigorous in the acute stage; more
than two weeks' treatment is a rarity.

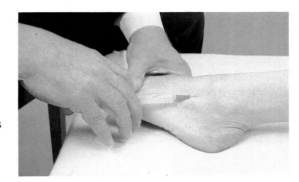
9.15

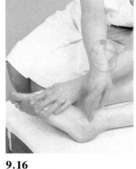
9.16

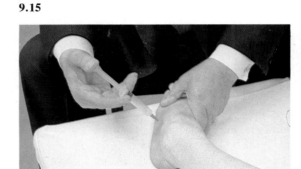
9.17

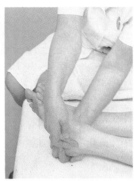
9.18

Fig 9.15 *Injection, fibular origin. The sooner the infiltration the better.*

Fig 9.16 *Massage, fibular origin. In recent cases, deepish friction is only necessary or tolerable for a few minutes. Treatment may have to be preceeded by effleurage.*

Fig 9.17 *Injection, talar insertion. The two sites are hardly more than 1cm apart.*

Fig 9.18 *Massage, talar insertion. Whatever the site, the treatment must include instruction on normal heel-and-toe gait to ensure mobility of the ligament.*

The calcaneofibular ligament

As the ligament spans the talocalcanean joint
but not the mid-tarsal joint, the only painful
movement is varus and the tenderness is found
just below the lower edge of the fibula (see
Figure 9.14). The treatment is infiltration
(*Figure 9.19*) with steroid suspension 1–2ml
during the first few days and massage
thereafter (*Figure 9.20*).

Sometimes the ligament is totally or partially
ruptured, producing instability and pain on
movement. The foot must be kept in full valgus
by fixing an adhesive strapping to the inner
aspect of the heel and tightly drawing it up the
outer aspect of the leg (*Figure 9.21*). After
three weeks the ligament should have healed.

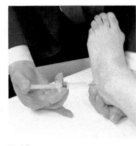
9.19

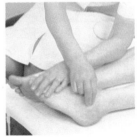
9.20

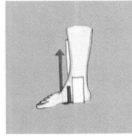
9.21

Fig 9.19 *Injection is the treatment immediately following injury.*

Fig 9.20 *Massage may be needed a few days after the injection, or by itself as the treatment of choice.*

Fig 9.21 *If the ligament is ruptured, firm strapping prevents varus movement.*

The calcaneocuboid ligament

The tear is usually found at the outer side of the joint (*Figure 9.22*). Often the talofibular ligament is sprained at the same time, but the calcaneocuboid can be tested in isolation by holding the foot in both dorsiflexion and valgus via the heel, which is maintained stationary while the forefoot is medially rotated. Pain arising from the calcaneocuboid joint is at the outer side of the mid-foot.

In a recent sprain, after the effleurage the patient is injected with steroid suspension 2ml (2cm needle). The needle punctures the skin just above the lowest palpable extent of the joint line and slants upwards into the joint (*Figure 9.23*). A series of droplets is injected as the needle proceeds. The resultant pain is enough to make walking difficult for one or two days; then the symptoms rapidly abate.

Massage is given the next day or as the only treatment (*Figure 9.24*). The foot is held in adduction, bringing the joint into prominence; the digit is placed on the joint line and friction is imparted by a movement of the whole forearm. Treatment on alternate days for a week should result in recovery.

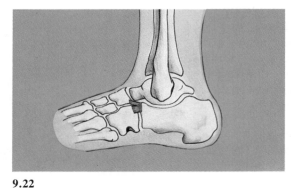

9.22

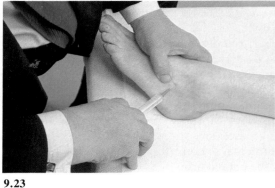

9.23

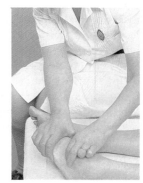

9.24

Fig 9.22 *The ligament binds the calcaneus, cuboid and navicular bones.*

Fig 9.23 *Injection is painful but the results uniformly good.*

Fig 9.24 *Massage is given by vertical movements.*

Rupture of adhesions

Adhesions may develop following an untreated sprain of the talofibular or calcaneocuboid ligament. The consequence is pain and slight swelling persisting for some days after extended exertion. The treatment is manipulative rupture of the adhesions.

One hand grasps the heel, forcing it into full varus and keeping it there throughout the manipulation (*Figure 9.25*).

The other hand puts the patient's foot into the starting position, consisting of fullest possible plantiflexion, adduction and medial rotation (*Figure 9.26*). The operator then gives a sharp thrust to accentuate this position by crisply bringing his elbow in towards his side (*Figure 9.27*).

The manipulation is done only once each session. If re-examination shows no—or incomplete—improvement, the patient attends again the next day.

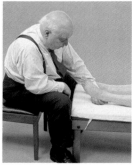

9.25   9.26

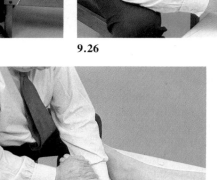

9.27

Fig 9.25 *Manipulative rupture: starting position, anchoring hand. Despite the adhesions, the foot is adequate for ordinary purposes and only aches after vigorous use.*
Figs 9.26, 9.27 *The degree of movement is most apparent by comparison of the right forearm's positions on the knee.*

The anterior tibiofibular ligament

Sprain of the anterior tibiofibular ligament (*Figure 9.28*) is almost invariably part of a composite varus sprain. It is treated by massage; the foot is held in full plantiflexion to tauten the ligament (*Figure 9.29*). A late effect of an untreated sprain is elongation of the tibiofibular ligament. An unstable mortice joint results, provoking momentary pain within the ankle which turns over easily with a click. The two malleoli can be felt to move apart, and a history of tibiofibular sprain some years previously is suggestive.

Sclerosis may be attempted, the bones wired together or a floated heel fitted (*Figure 9.30*).

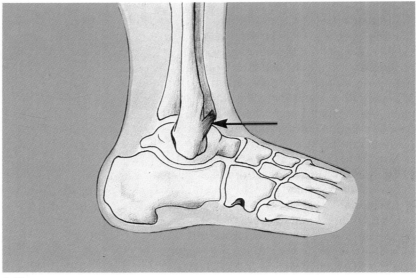

9.28

Fig 9.28 *Pain from the anterior tibiofibular ligament is never severe but may last for years.*

Fig 9.29 *Massage is extremely effective.*

Fig 9.30 *Unstable mortice joint. A false heel can be floated on the outer side of the shoe to prevent recurrent strain.*

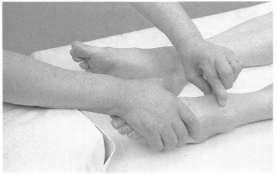

9.29

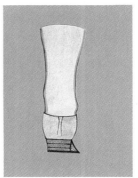

9.30

Recurrent sprain

The occasional individual complains of recurrent minor sprain during ordinary usage. There are two main explanations. The first is an untreated tibiofibular sprain (see above) giving attacks of pain lasting a day or two. Alternatively, a sluggish reflex arc between the lateral ligaments and the peroneal muscles leads to delayed contraction of the peronei. The muscles therefore fail to prevent varus strain during walking.

The condition is managed by a floated heel at the outer side of the foot combined with proprioceptive training of the peronei (on a wobble board) to speed up the reflex arc.

Valgus strain

The deltoid ligament

It is unusual for a valgus strain to end in a sprain of the deltoid ligament (*Figure 9.31*). More often the lesion—which is long lasting—is brought on by chronic strain in patients with a valgus foot. Massage is useless, manipulation and stretching are harmful. Full passive eversion during plantiflexion is the painful movement.

As soon as the patient is seen, a support 1–2cm thick is fitted under the mid-tarsal area to obviate the repeated stretch at every step. It is worn for months.

In addition, steroid suspension 2ml is injected to allay the persistent traumatic inflammation which lies at the tibial origin. The foot is held in eversion and the 3cm needle enters 2cm below and in front of the ligament (*Figure 9.32*). The tip heads towards the inferior aspect of the tibia and a series of droplets are deposited fanwise along the affected extent of the ligamento-osseous junction. The ankle is painful for a day.

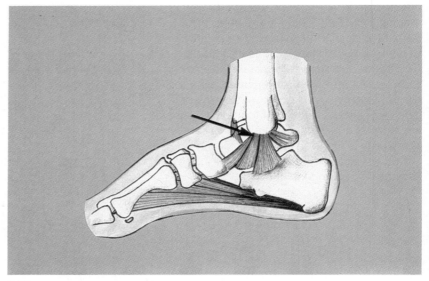

9.31

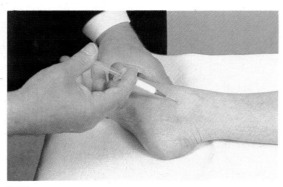

9.32

Fig 9.31 *Tenderness is found along the tibial origin.*

Fig 9.32 *Injection. Beads of fluid are delivered all along the affected extent.*

The anterior tibiotalar ligament

An uncommon result of a pure plantiflexion stress is sprain of the anterior tibiotalar ligament. The pain may linger on for years but is never severe; the symptoms are felt at the front of the ankle on full plantiflexion. To palpate, the extensor tendons must first be pushed aside.

Massage is the invariable treatment of choice (*Figure 9.33*).

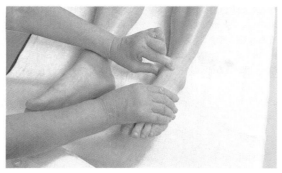

9.33

Fig 9.33 *Massage. The ligament is too thin for steroid infiltration; it is just visible to the left of the head of the arrow in Fig 9.31.*

A loose body

After a sprain, a small fragment of cartilage may become detached within the ankle joint. The patient complains of sudden erratic twinges on plantiflexion of the foot, often when walking downstairs.

The pain is momentary and the displacement self-reducing. Thus the patient is well at the time of attendance and treatment must be conducted without the framework of symptoms and signs that normally guide the manipulator; the patient cannot immediately report whether or not the loose body has been shifted to a better position.

The patient therefore returns a week after treatment stating whether attacks are now spaced at wider intervals. If no improvement has been registered the method given for the talocalcanean joint should be tried; as an alternative an anterior wedge may be affixed to the heel of the shoe.

For the manipulation, the patient lies on a high couch, her heel level with its edge (*Figure 9.34*). An assistant at the other end supplies traction.

The operator's lower hand does not move. Instead it acts as a fulcrum, protected from the hard edge of the couch by a foam rubber pad.

The upper hand grasps the dorsum and the physician leans back, pulling hard to distract the talus from its mortice. A strong circumduction movement is then carried out several times while the traction is maintained (*Figure 9.35*).

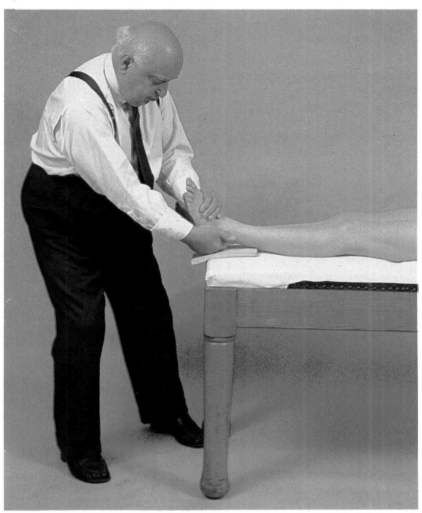

9.34

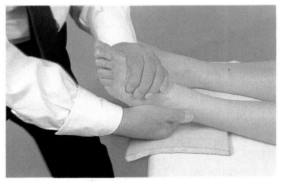

9.35

Fig 9.34 *Reduction, a loose body. The manipulator leans back and distracts the joint; an assistant at the other end supplies countertraction.*

Fig 9.35 *The foot is used as a lever to distract talus from mortice during a circular movement in plantiflexion. About half the cases are relieved.*

The talocalcanean joint and heel

Capsular lesions

The disorders habitually encountered are monarticular rheumatoid arthritis and osteoarthrosis. Sub-acute traumatic arthritis retards recovery after a sprained ankle; it can be readily distinguished from ligamentous adhesions following the sprain by the limitation of movement at the talocalcanean joint.

Rheumatoid arthritis is often bilateral and is given away by local heat and palpable synovial thickening. There is no history of sprain.

Osteoarthrosis follows fractures involving the articular surface of the calcaneus. Persistent pain is apt to result which is curable only by arthrodesis.

A normal joint has a full range of varus. As the capsular pattern encroaches, varus becomes increasingly limited and in due course fixation in full valgus (*Figure 9.36*) results.

Rheumatoid arthritis and sub-acute traumatic arthritis respond well to one or two injections of steroid suspension 2ml. Since the heel is in valgus, the simpler approach is at the inner side.

The physician identifies the sustentaculum taili. The 2cm needle is thrust in parallel to the joint surface (*Figures 9.37; 9.38*) and usually strikes bone at 1cm. The tip is manoeuvred until it slips in further without resistance and steroid suspension 1ml is injected into the anterior joint, the needle partly withdrawn, reinserted 45° posteriorly and a further 1ml discharged into the posterior compartment. Failure after two infiltrations is the exception, and indicates several months' immobilisation in plaster.

Post-traumatic osteoporosis ('Sudeck's atrophy') may trouble the talocalcanean joint but then the capsular pattern amounts to fixation in the mid-position rather than in full valgus. The condition is visible radiographically, the whole foot hurts, the nails stop growing and when the leg is dependent the foot turns black. No treatment avails but the patient recovers within two years.

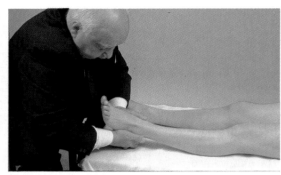

9.36

Fig 9.36 *Arthritis. The foot cannot be persuaded into varus.*

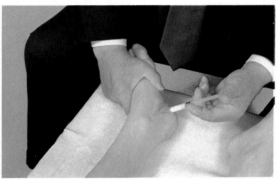

9.37

Fig 9.37 *In advanced rheumatoid cases the injection cannot restore range but still abolishes pain.*

Fig 9.38 *The suspension is delivered into the entire length of the joint.*

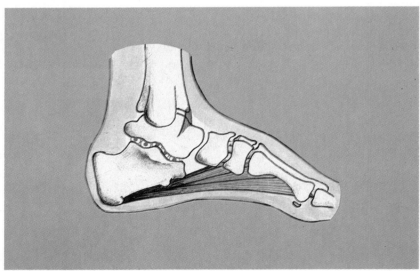

9.38

Non-capsular lesions

Dancer's heel

Dancers can provoke a traumatic periostitis at the posterior articular margin of the tibia (*Figure 9.39*) precipitated by pressure on the upper surface of the calcaneus by the posterior aspect of the tibia. Full passive plantiflexion of the foot sets up pain at the back of the heel but rising on tiptoe does not hurt, thus exculpating the tendo Achillis.

The cause is over-pointing (i.e. plantiflexion beyond the 180° position) when the dancer is *sur les pointes*. The physician palpates for tenderness along the length of the articular margin. For the injection of steroid suspension 2ml (4cm needle) the patient lies prone. The posterior articular margin of the tibia is identified about 2cm superior to a line joining the tips of the malleoli, and the needle enters to one side of the tendo Achillis (*Figure 9.40*).

The tip is adjusted until it rests on the tibial edge (*Figure 9.41*). This is about 1mm above the point at which the bone gives way to the articular cartilage and when the tip contacts the periosteum a number of droplets are delivered along this horizontal line (*Figure 9.42*).

The patient must not rise *sur les pointes* for a week and should cease over-pointing.

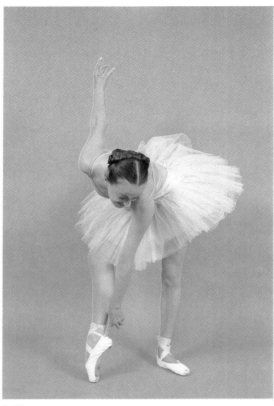

9.39

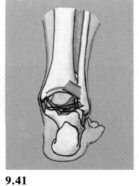

9.40

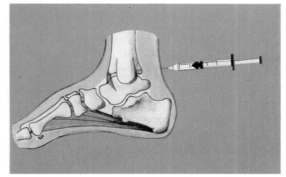

9.41   **9.42**

Fig 9.39 *Site of dancer's heel. Sometimes the pain is mistakenly ascribed to the tendo Achillis.*

Fig 9.40 *Injection. The foot is plantiflexed so that the tendo Achillis can be pushed aside.*

Figs 9.41, 9.42 *The injection is made all along the bruised edge.*

Immobilisation limitation

Immobilisation in plaster for several months following a tibiofibular fracture may result in permanent limitation; the joint becomes fixed in the mid-position (*cf.* arthritis). The capsule has to be stretched out but the treatment is difficult because it is hard to get much leverage. But if only half the normal range can be restored, the lesion ceases to trouble the patient.

The heel is clasped as strongly as possible between the two palms. By alternately swinging one elbow away from, and the other towards, herself the physiotherapist imparts a varus and valgus movement (*Figures 9.43; 9.44*). This forcing is repeated with the utmost vigour a great number of times. Sessions take place twice a week for up to several months; after some range has been regained, the symptoms may well abate of themselves.

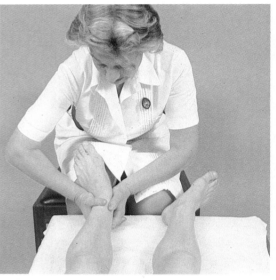

9.43

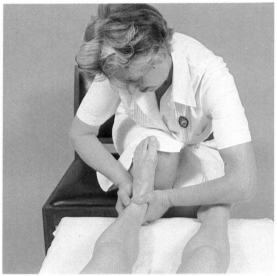

9.44

Figs 9.43, 9.44 *Capsular stretching. The physiotherapist grips the heel firmly below the malleoli and swings her trunk and arms from side to side. Note the patient's foot is maintained in comfortable dorsiflexion against her knee.*

Subcutaneous nodules

A nodule about the size of a small pea may form spontaneously in the subcutaneous fascia. It engenders severe momentary pain but only when pinched by the back of the shoe.

Division by subcutaneous tenotomy (*Figure 9.45*) under local anaesthesia pays good dividends. Shoes with a gap posteriorly are an excellent alternative.

The calcaneofibular ligament is discussed as part of the sprained ankle (see page 115).

Fig 9.45 *Tenotomy gives results as good as excision.*

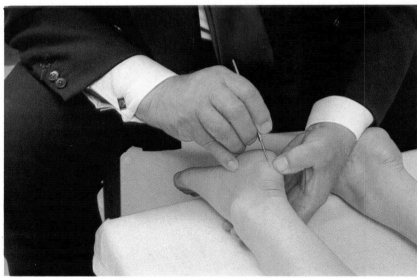

9.45

Plantar fasciitis

Chronic strain is the only common cause of pain arising from the plantar fascia. It normally stems from prolonged strain during standing by patients with an over-arched foot or short calf muscles. The most distinctive symptom is severe pain at the heel on first getting up to walk after sitting.

On examination, the movements of the foot are found normal and painless: all findings are negative. The tender spot is palpable and always at the inner aspect, just distal to the origin from the calcaneus (*Figure 9.46*).

Continued overstrain may pull the periosteum away at its origin from the calcaneus. A bony spur results which of itself is symptomless and has no influence on treatment.

The fascia must be relaxed by dropping the forefoot. This is accomplished by raising the heel of the shoe while keeping horizontal the platform on which the patient's heel rests (*Figure 9.47*). Permanent support can be achieved by a wedge applied to the heel, the thick end lying anteriorly (*Figure 9.48*). This should afford immediate relief.

However, in obdurate cases the patient is injected with steroid suspension 2ml. The foot is dorsiflexed to tauten the plantar fascia. The skin must be sterilised and the point of entry is through thin skin some 3–4cm anterior to the lesion. The approach is oblique (*Figure 9.49*).

As the needle advances it traverses fascia before touching bone and the affected area is infiltrated all over by a series of minor withdrawals and reinsertions (*Figures 9.50; 9.51*). Severe discomfort is provoked lasting two days, making walking painful, and a strong analgesic is prescribed.

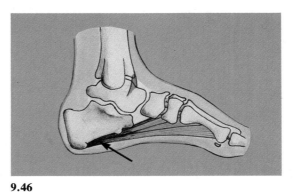

9.46

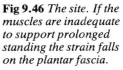

Fig 9.46 *The site. If the muscles are inadequate to support prolonged standing the strain falls on the plantar fascia.*

Figs 9.47, 9.48 *Most cases are dealt with by a modified heel. An internal or external wedge raises the front edge of the heel so the platform is horizontal.*

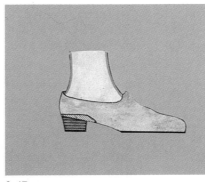 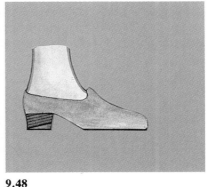

9.47   9.48

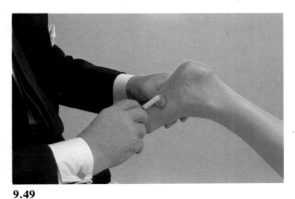

9.49

Fig 9.49 *Injection. The patient lies prone with her knee flexed.*

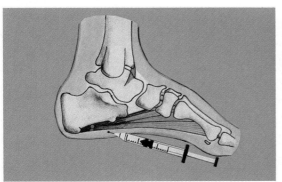

9.50

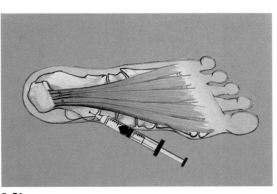

9.51

Figs 9.50, 9.51 *The point of entry is some distance from the lesion, as the plantar skin overlying the site is too thick for sterilisation.*

The mid-tarsal joint

The mid-tarsal joint is constituted by the talonavicular and calcaneocuboid joints.

Between them they run the full width of the foot and permit movement in six directions.

Capsular lesions

Several types of arthritis afflict the mid-tarsal joint. Osteoarthrosis—unless gross—causes no symptoms.

Monarticular rheumatoid arthritis is recognisable by the oedema and synovial swelling at the dorsum of the foot: immobilisation in a plaster cast is required at once. The pain ceases in a few days but the cast must be worn for a full year to prevent relapse.

Sub-acute arthritis in middle age and adolescence are dealt with below.

The capsular pattern is limitation of adduction and medial rotation with the other movements full.

Sub-acute arthritis in middle age

Over-use far outweighs an isolated strain as the cause; usually the patients are stout women. An inversion movement at the talocalcanean and mid-tarsal joints is partially restricted by muscular spasm.

If—as sometimes happens—only one joint is affected, it can be infiltrated with steroid suspension 2ml delivered in droplets over the entire extent of the tender area (*Figures 9.52; 9.53*). One injection should suffice.

But if the lesion is diffuse, treatment is by rest which entails tilting the heel towards varus and maintaining it there by a figure-of-eight adhesive strapping (*Figure 9.54*).

The foot is held at right angles to the leg. The plaster starts off at the inner side of the leg; it then crosses the front of the ankle and goes under the foot. Strong traction is applied as the strapping passes upwards across the inner side of the mid-tarsus and the front of the ankle to achieve maximum inversion of the forefoot. At least two layers of strapping are required. The patient is seen every few days to have the bandage—which is worn for some months—renewed to keep up tension.

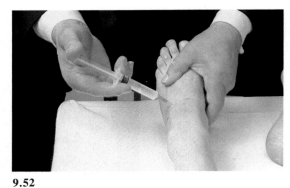

9.52

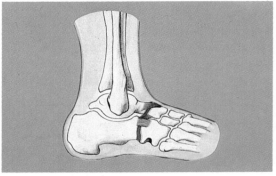

9.53

9.54

Fig 9.52 *Injection, calcaneocuboid joint; the likeliest site.*

Fig 9.53 *The lesion can lie anywhere on the joint line, marked in blue.*

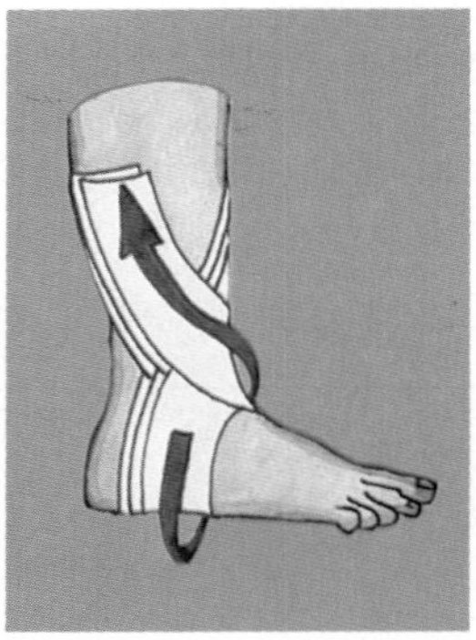

Fig 9.54 *Strapping is the alternative.*

Sub-acute arthritis in adolescence

This condition presents as a painless deformity: the foot is fixed in valgus at the heel and in lateral rotation and abduction of the forefoot. It is often called spasmodic pes planus because of the secondary spasm of the peroneal muscles which accompanies the arthritis. The condition is brought on by prolonged standing and is rarer than formerly; the raising of the school leaving age has deferred employment in jobs involving much standing. The essence of treatment is support for the joint and relief from weight-bearing. The patient needs a sedentary job, a bicycle, a wedge on the heel of his shoes, and strapping (see above).

The mid-tarsal ligaments

The mid-tarsal ligaments (see *Figure 9.57*) are susceptible to two contrasting disorders. Strain may lead to pain with excessive range, and contracture to pain and limitation.

Mid-tarsal strain

This should be anticipated in patients with an over-arched foot or an equinus deformity caused by short calf muscles. In such cases, weight-bearing dorsiflexes and therefore abducts the foot at the mid-tarsal joint. First the foot becomes wobbly. Later, an ache appears at the extremes of passive range, especially rotation, and finally increasing abduction of the forefoot puts undue strain on the calcaneonavicular ligament.

Treatment is made up by a combination of four measures. First, the heel of the shoe is raised to allow the forefoot to adopt a more plantigrade position. Second, the short flexor muscles are given resisted exercises so they become adequate to take the strain of weight-bearing. Third, the joint is mobilised (see below); this is the only example of manipulation at a joint already possessing excessive range. Fourth, sprain of the calcaneonavicular ligament is tackled by infiltration of steroid suspension.

The aim of mobilisation is to attain full painless range. Repeated strains during healing of minor ligamentous ruptures will have led to the formation of adhesions which now must themselves be ruptured.

The operator clasps his hands about the outer aspect of the forefoot; great strength is required. The heel of the dorsally placed hand presses chiefly on the first metatarsal bone, the heel of the other hand acts mostly against the plantar surface of the fifth metatarsal bone and the rotation is imparted by the operator forcibly swinging his elbows, one towards and the other away from himself (*Figures 9.55; 9.56*). This movement is repeated scores of times each session for three or four treatments.

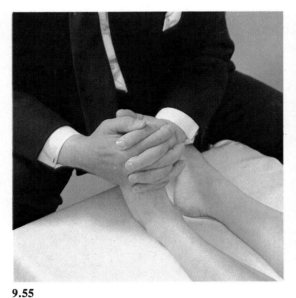

9.55

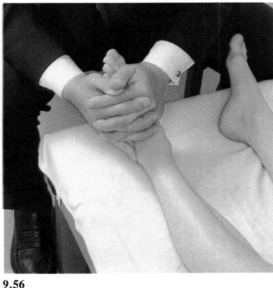

9.56

Figs 9.55, 9.56 *Forcing lateral rotation. A surprising degree of vigour is necessary; the operator's widely spread legs give him a stable platform. Note the swing of his elbows.*

Mid-tarsal ligamentous contracture

Limitation of movement at the mid-tarsal joint
may arise from ligamentous contracture
following some months in a plaster cast for
fractures of the lower leg. The shortened
ligaments on the dorsum of the foot are tender
and although walking is painless, more
pronounced exertion provokes immediate
symptoms.

Mobilisation does not work. Instead, the
affected ligaments are infiltrated with steroid
suspension 2–5ml. The solution is injected into
the ligaments along their length wherever they
are tender (*Figure 9.57*).

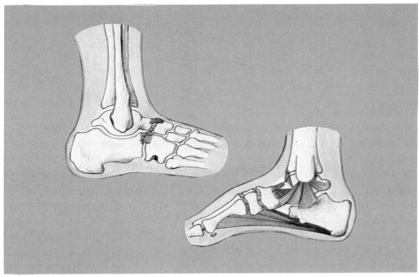

Fig 9.57 *The tender area
lies anywhere on the
joint line across the
dorsum.*

9.57

The cuneo-first-metatarsal joint

The cuneo-first-metatarsal joint suffers from
only one condition—osteoarthrosis of insidious
onset, usually bilateral, probably the legacy of
a previous adolescent osteochondrosis. Pain
for some months may result from osteophytes
pinching the skin when cramped by the uppers
of a tight shoe. The osteophyte is palpable as a
small projection at the dorsum of the foot.

The pain is localised and produced by the
shoes; the problem can normally be solved by
wearing footwear no part of which touches the
joint. At the worst the osteophyte might have
to be chiselled away, but in any case recovery
from the pain is a certainty.

The metatarsal shafts

A marching fracture

A short first metatarsal bone visible
radiographically is compatible with full
painless function; the common cause of pain in
the forefoot is a marching fracture.

The marching fracture is characterised by
unilateral localised warmth and oedema lying
in a circular patch. There is no history of injury
or even of over-use. The condition is a stress
fracture, most often at the neck of the second
or fourth metatarsal bone, and it is only after
the first two weeks that the break shows on the
X-ray. Spontaneous recovery within six weeks
is facilitated by strapping the foot so that the
intact bones splint the fracture.

Differential diagnosis

Localised warmth, swelling and tenderness at
the dorsum of the distal part of the foot are
also features of a number of other conditions,
all relatively rare, which are listed together
with their treatment:

(1) Strained interosseus muscles secondary to a
    marching fracture—massage.
(2) Gout—phenylbutazone.
(3) Gonorrhoea—penicillin.
(4) Rheumatoid arthritis of the
    metatarsophalangeal joint—steroid
    suspension.
(5) Freiburg's arthritis.
(6) Sarcoidosis and Reiter's disease—systemic
    treatment.
(7) Ringworm.
(8) Morton's metatarsalgia—see page 129.

The toe joints

Capsular lesions

The first metatarsophalangeal joint

Gout, adolescent arthritis or osteoarthrosis may attack the first metatarsophalangeal joint. The joint is normally capable of 30° of flexion and 90° of extension—the latter movement is the one that matters. The capsular pattern is gross limitation of extension and some limitation of flexion. Fixation in the neutral position (hallux rigidus) eventually results.

Arthritis in adolescence may follow osteochondrosis dissecans. The patient is normally male, aged 15–20. Conservative treatment consists of the prescription of a rocker to the sole of the shoe, thus exonerating the big toe from the necessity of extension during walking.

Osteoarthrosis in middle age produces no symptoms until extension is limited by 45° or so, whereupon the joint is forced beyond its painfree range by each step the patient takes. In minor cases the disorder is really a superimposed traumatic arthritis.

Rheumatoid arthritis is frequently met and is treated by an injection of steroids.

Whatever the cause, the pain is accurately localised and the joint tender. Resisted flexion proves painless, thereby excluding sesamoiditis as a cause of pain.

Steroid suspension 1ml is injected into the joint. The patient lies on a couch while an assistant grasps the big toe and pulls hard to distract the joint surfaces (*Figure 9.58*).

Rotation of the toe facilitates identification of the proximal phalanx. The needle is passed into the space between the two bones and the injection given there (*Figure 9.59*); considerable pain results for 12 hours, but both rheumatoid arthritis and osteoarthrosis are normally relieved for a year or longer.

Typically gout affects the big toe in elderly men. The attacks are unprovoked, recurrent and switch from one foot to the other; often the joint is normal for some years at a stretch. Phenylbutazone or indomethacin are both effective in resolving the symptoms within a day or two. In periods of respite, the excretion of urates is enhanced by aspirin, probenecid, sulphinpyrazone or allopurinal.

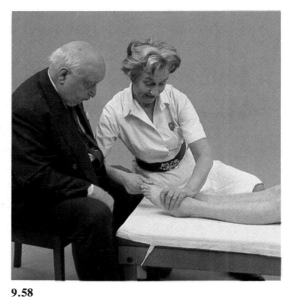

9.58

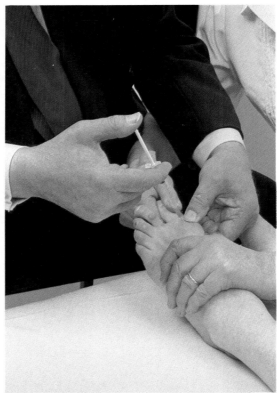

9.59

Figs 9.58, 9.59 *Injection, group and detail. The physiotherapist opens the joint space to facilitate entry of the needle.*

Sesamoiditis

Over-use may set up a traumatic arthritis at the sesamo-first-metatarsal joint. This is particularly likely in a patient with short calf muscles fixing the foot in plantiflexion so that he comes down too hard on the forefoot. Resisted flexion of the hallux is painful and, contrary to expectation, the position of the tender spot does not change with flexion and extension of the big toe.

The treatment is injection of steroid suspension 1ml. Recurrence is prevented both by fitting a metarsal support and by raising the heel of the shoe, keeping its upper surface horizontal the while.

An ingrowing toenail

An ingrowing toenail is aggravated by cutting away the sides of the nail; this stimulates further lateral growth of the flesh. But if the centre of the convex surface of the nail is pared away with a knife, the nail loses its rigidity and can no longer slice painfully into the skin. Thinning is maintained until a nail of full width has grown and from then on the patient makes a practice of cutting the nail straight across.

The other joints

Rheumatoid and traumatic arthritis

The capsular pattern is restricted flexion but little limitation of extension (*cf.* the first metatarsophalangeal joint). Rheumatoid and traumatic arthritis are both rare and an injection of steroid suspension 1ml is curative, although the infiltration provokes severe pain for 12 hours. In advanced cases of rheumatoid arthritis the toes become fixed in the clawed position; at this stage it is too late to inject and the only effective measure is a support relieving the metatarsal heads from weight-bearing.

Freiburg's arthritis

This is normally confined to the second metatarsophalangeal joint. It is a late result of osteochondrosis dissecans starting in adolescence and continuing intractable indefinitely. A support may be fitted to prevent the joint from touching the ground during walking; alternatively the head of the bone can be removed.

Metatarsalgia

Pain at the plantar aspect of the forefoot is called metatarsalgia. Acute metatarsalgia has a standard history of agonising pain felt at the outer border of the forefoot on walking. The attack is brief, lasting for a minute or so during which the patient stands still on the other foot. After some minutes the twinges cease but the foot becomes warm and remains so for several hours. Incidents are normally separated by intervals of several months.

The cause is a fibrous swelling of the fourth digital nerve proximal to its point of division. This is nipped between the heads of the fourth and fifth metatarsal bones (*Figure 9.60*).

Examination between attacks is wholly negative. Conservative treatment consists merely of a small support under the toe to alter the alignment of the metatarsal heads (*Figure 9.61*). If this fails the nerve with its neuroma should be excised.

Chronic metatarsalgia affects the middle three toes; it arises in conditions in which an excessive proportion of the body-weight falls on the forefoot. The pain is brought on by standing or walking and relieved by rest. The causes are:

(1) Short calf muscles.
(2) Pes cavus.
(3) Weak flexor muscles.

Treatment is a combination of two measures—a support and exercises. For the former, the thickness of the support lies just behind the heads of the second, third and fourth metatarsal bones. This makes the shaft bear more weight.

The exercises are directed at strengthening the flexor muscles. This ensures the toes flex properly at every step and carry weight on their tips, thus taking load off the capsule of the joint.

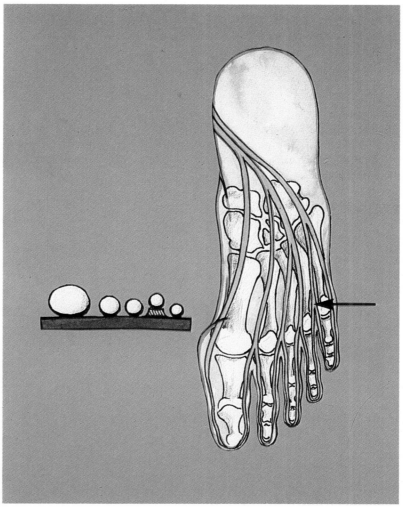

9.60, 9.61

Dancer's metatarsalgia is confined to those who do much tiptoe work (not *sur les pointes*); a bruised pad of fibrous tissue is found in the sole lying anterior to the second, third and fourth metatarsophalangeal joints. The ballet shoes are fitted with a small semi-lunar pad so the proximal phalanges bear more weight.

Figs 9.60, 9.61 *Morton's metatarsalgia. A small fibrous tumour on the digital nerve causes severe twinges at the outer toes. A support under the head of the fourth toe keeps the bones slightly out of line and prevents the nerve from being squeezed.*

Arteriosclerosis

In advanced arteriosclerosis, the circulatory defect may show itself at the sole rather than in the calf muscles; it is provoked by walking. The dorsalis pedis and posterior tibial pulses are both absent, and the X-ray may show the arteries to be calcified.

Paraesthesia

The cause of pins and needles in the feet normally lies in the spine (see Appendix II):

    Cervical disc lesions—Cord sign
    Thoracic disc lesion—Cord sign
    Lumbar disc lesion—Root pressure
    Spondylolisthesis—Root pressure
    Spinal claudication—Lack of arterial blood
       supply.

PART THREE

THE
SPINE

CHAPTER TEN

PRINCIPLES OF EXAMINATION

As at other joints, diagnosis at the spine is dependent on assessment of function. At all spinal levels—cervical, thoracic and lumbar—a number of general anatomical considerations hold sway which together dictate the format of the examination. In practice, the physician will consider only one level at a time and thus subsequent chapters have been organised to reflect this. In order to cover the basic theory the present chapter treats the spine in its entirety.

Because disc lesions are common and generally responsive to treatment, the examination sets out to differentiate between disc lesions and the other sources of pain as well as establishing the particular treatment that will benefit any given displacement. As elsewhere in the body, displacements give rise to certain characteristic symptoms and signs.

First, the history is indicative.

Second, any loose fragment in the joint restricts spinal movement in some but not all directions, producing the non-capsular pattern characteristic of internal derangement.

Third, a displacement protruding posteriorly interferes with the dura mater; apart from pain, this adversely affects the dura's normal painless mobility.

Fourth, a displacement protruding laterally connects with the appropriate nerve root emerging from the dura mater. Where the pressure is only mild the external aspect of the nerve root suffers, engendering pain in the dermatome and hindering the nerve root's mobility. But if pressure is severe, conduction suffers as well, making for weakness in the relevant muscle groups.

Examination for a disc lesion is thus conducted for each of the above. However, in many cases the dural signs, nerve root symptoms and nerve root signs are absent, leaving the diagnosis to be made on history and joint signs alone.

Finally, compression of the spinal cord strongly contraindicates manipulation, the primary treatment for cartilaginous displacements. Accordingly, the physician checks for cord signs.

The basic clinical principles do not differ greatly from one spinal level to another and repay close study. Lesions of the spine account for somewhere in the region of half the orthopaedic physician's cases; moreover, symptoms of spinal origin often affect the upper or lower limb and thus a sound grasp of peripheral pain is founded on an understanding of the spine.

The various structures involved are analysed in detail and the inferences drawn are progressively tabulated under the appropriate headings. Discussion commences with the dura mater as its role is paramount; it provides the mechanism of spinal pain.

The role of the dura mater.

EXAMINATION FOR A SPINAL DISPLACEMENT: SUMMARY I

History	Joint Signs	Dural Signs	Nerve Root Signs		Cord Signs
			Mobility	Weakness	
Always characteristic.	Always characteristic.	Sometimes present.	Sometimes present.	Sometimes present.	Rare.

The dura mater

This tough membranous tube extends from the foramen magnum of the skull down to the caudal edge of the first or second sacral vertebra (*Figures 10.1; 10.2*). It houses the spinal cord surrounded by cerebrospinal fluid.

Figs 10.1, 10.2 *The dura mater. This membrane runs the length of the spine and is sensitive anteriorly, where it is vulnerable to pressure from intervertebral displacements.*

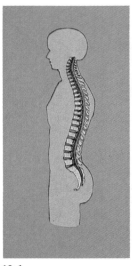
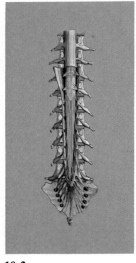

10.1   10.2

Two important characteristics of the dura mater are not always appreciated:

(1) It is sensitive, being innervated from the sinuvertebral nerve by three separate routes[1]. However, these fibres all run to the ventral aspect of the dura and no nerves have been traced to or discovered at the dorsal surface of the membrane. This partial innervation, confined to the anterior aspect of the dura, explains why no pain is felt at lumbar puncture.

At its anterior aspect the dura is sensitive to two stimuli: stretching and compression. In addition, pain may be provoked by a vascular jolt (e.g. coughing) which momentarily enlarges the intradural veins and starts an impulse transmitted throughout the cerebrospinal fluid.

(2) It moves slightly in relation to the vertebrae it traverses. Thus neck flexion lifts the dural tube upwards by an average of 3cm and draws the thoracic extent with it. The dura can, of course, be stretched from below (e.g. by straight-leg raising via the sciatic nerve).

The dura mater is thus an inert, mobile, sensitive structure. Accordingly, its function can be examined by stretching and any compression limiting mobility will result in pain and limitation on passive movements.

As noted previously, dural pain is not subject to the rules of segmental reference. At the cervical level (*Figure 10.3*) pain of dural origin may be felt running up the neck and through the forehead—C2 and C3 dermatomes—or down towards the mid-scapular area—T3, T4, T5 and T6. Thus in the stages of central and posterolateral dural pressure, the pain is usually felt in areas derived from a segment quite other than that in due course found to contain the lesion. A small area of tenderness within the painful area may be identified by the patient as the source of his troubles; this tenderness is, like the pain, referred.

Interference with the dura mater at thoracic levels may give rise to posterior pain spreading to the base of the neck or down to the mid-lumbar region (*Figure 10.4*).

Extrasegmental reference is also common in the lumbar region (*Figure 10.5*). The pain often radiates to the abdomen or up to the back of the chest. In acute lumbago, the symptoms are frequently referred to one or both groins or to one or both iliac fossae, thus encroaching on the lower thoracic segments. Pain the the buttock or one or both legs often results from interference with the dura mater.

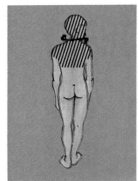

Figs 10.3, 10.4, 10.5 *Dural pain and extrasegmental reference. The figures show the extensive areas to which pain can be referred from cervical, thoracic and lumbar displacements respectively.*

10.3

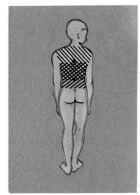
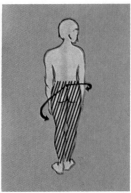

10.4   10.5

1. Edgar, M.A. and Nundy, S. (1966). Innervation of the spinal dura mater. *Neurol. Neurosurg. Psychiat.*, **29**, 530

EXAMINATION FOR A SPINAL DISPLACEMENT: SUMMARY II

Spinal level	CERVICAL	THORACIC	LUMBAR
History *Always characteristic.*	Usually unilateral scapular pain, almost always referred extrasegmentally.	Posterior trunk pain, often referred extrasegmentally.	Pain in lumbar region, buttocks, legs, often referred extrasegmentally.
Joint Signs			
Dural Signs *Sometimes present.*	Painful neck flexion (ambiguous; stretches thoracic extent of dura).	Painful neck flexion (ambiguous, see across). Check for pain on moving shoulder girdle backwards, forwards and upwards. Ask if deep breath or coughing painful.	Test for bilateral limitation on SLR. Ask if deep breath or coughing painful.
Nerve Root Signs			
Cord Signs			

Dural signs

Dural involvement may give rise to any of the following signs:

At cervical levels

Painful neck flexion. This tugs the dura mater upwards; if mobility is restricted pain will result, but it is an ambiguous finding as dural mobility could be impaired at thoracic rather than cervical levels.

At thoracic levels

Painful neck flexion (see above).

Scapular approximation pulls on the first and second nerve roots and thereby raises the whole thoracic extent of the dura mater upwards. Bringing the shoulder girdle forwards or upwards may also (although less often) have the same effect. If mobility is impeded pain will result.

Pain on a deep breath or (less often) coughing.

At lumbar levels

Painful straight-leg raise. This stretches the dura mater via the sciatic nerve. A central protrusion limiting dural mobility would thus produce pain on bilateral straight-leg raise.

Pain on coughing or (less distinctly) on a deep breath.

Each of these signs can be specifically examined for as set out in Table 2.

The nerve roots

Thirty pairs of nerve roots project from the dura mater. Each nerve root draws out with it an investment of the dura mater[2] that extends, judging by clinical data, for at least 2cm (see *Figure 10.2*).

Compression of the dural sheath causes pain distributed on an accurate segmental basis, for example, from the C8 root to the third, fourth and fifth fingers, and from the L4 root down the leg to the big toe.

Mobility

In addition, the dural sheath is mobile at the lumbar levels and any interference with mobility may be detected by unilateral pain on stretching by passive movements—straight-leg raise and prone-lying knee flexion. These are the tests for nerve root mobility.

Each root also possesses an internal aspect—the parenchyma—which serves conduction only. Mild pressure on the dural sheath may not be great enough to hamper the conduction of the parenchyma. In such a case the tests will show:

(1) Interference with mobility of the dural sheath (i.e. pain increased by stretching).
(2) No impedence of conduction (i.e. neither paraesthesia nor weakness on resisted movements nor absence or sluggishness of jerks).

2. Frykholm, R. (1951). Lower cervical nerve-roots and their investments. *Acta chir. scand.*, **101**, 457.

Conduction

Greater pressure disrupts mobility and conduction, giving positive results for both tests.

Interference with sensory conduction produces pins and needles or numbness generally located at the distal end of the dermatome. The weakness (motor conduction) will be detectable in the appropriate muscle groups and the reflexes absent or sluggish. Accordingly, at cervical levels the upper limb is examined against resistance; at lumbar levels the lower limb is similarly tested. These are the tests for motor nerve root conduction.

Extreme pressure may result in ischaemic root atrophy.

Mobility and conduction

However, the clinical picture at the different spinal levels is not so straightforward as invariably to permit examination for both mobility and conduction. At the cervical spine the nerve roots are tethered to the transverse processes and therefore no movement of the arm can stretch the nerve roots: they are immobile. Consequently, examination of the nerve roots at cervical levels is limited to the parenchyma. Any weakness detected by the resisted arm movements should be monoradicular (see below).

At the thoracic spine, root pain is not uncommon and is a particularly deceptive symptom as the pain is only felt anteriorly. However, no practicable way exists of testing the nerve roots for mobility although neck flexion provides an occasional indicator. Conduction is very rarely interfered with.

At the lumbar levels, a disc lesion could, theoretically, affect any nerve root(s) between L1 and S4. In fact displacements at L1 and L2 are extremely rare, L3 is relatively uncommon and a protrusion here attacks only the third lumbar nerve root. Fourth or fifth lumbar disc lesions are run of the mill and may give rise to monoradicular or polyradicular root signs as discussed below. So the parenchyma is examined by resisted movements for weakness; the mobility of the nerve root at L3 is tested by prone-lying knee flexion and at L4, L5, S1 and S2 by straight-leg raise.

Polyradicular and monoradicular symptoms

Fig 10.6 *Lumbar nerve roots, posterior view. The exact site of a displacement determines the root(s) compressed. An L4 protrusion (left) can affect either the L4 or the L5 root, or both simultaneously. L5 disc lesions (right) have an even wider choice.*

At cervical levels, the nerve roots are aligned horizontally. Hence any symptoms emanating from impingement on a nerve root by a cervical displacement of disc material will be monoradicular. Theoretically, any root between C3 and T2 is at risk from a disc lesion. In practice, the physician is most often concerned with the roots at C5, C6, C7 and C8.

At lumbar levels, the nerve roots project obliquely. This downward slope has an important practical bearing: it enables a displacement of disc material to compress two nerve roots simultaneously (*Figure 10.6*). Furthermore, a displacement at a particular level will not necessarily be paired with one particular root. Thus it is possible for a protrusion lying almost centrally at the fourth level to pinch the fifth root or, by inclining a little more to one side, compress only the fourth root. A larger protrusion can, of course, squeeze both roots. Thus the symptoms may be polyradicular.

These findings are consolidated overleaf.

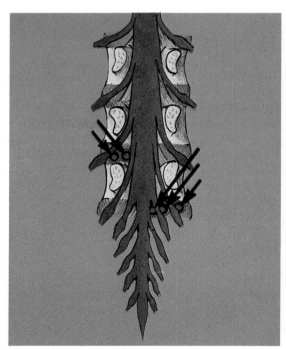

10.6

EXAMINATION FOR A SPINAL DISPLACEMENT: SUMMARY III

Spinal level	CERVICAL	THORACIC	LUMBAR
History *Always characteristic.*	Usually unilateral scapular pain, almost always referred extrasegmentally. Any nerve root pain felt in appropriate dermatome.	Posterior trunk pain, often referred extrasegmentally. Any nerve root pain felt anteriorly (sometimes the only symptom).	Pain in lumbar region, buttocks, legs, often referred extrasegmentally. Nerve root pain felt in lower limb in appropriate dermatome(s).
Joint Signs			
Dural Signs *Sometimes present.*	Painful neck flexion (ambiguous; stretches thoracic extent of dura).	Painful neck flexion (ambiguous, see across). Check for pain on moving shoulder girdle backwards, forwards and upwards. Ask if deep breath or coughing painful.	Test for bilateral limitation on SLR. Ask if deep breath or coughing painful.
Nerve Root Signs: Mobility *Sometimes present.*	No test—nerve roots tethered to transverse processes (but see across for T1 and T2).	Mobility of T1 and T2 roots tested by scapular approximation during cervical examination. No test for other thoracic roots.	Test for unilateral limitation on SLR (L4, L5, S1 and S2 roots). Test for unilateral pain on prone knee flexion (L3 root).
Nerve Root Signs: Weakness *Sometimes present.*	Any signs monoradicular. Test upper limb for muscle weakness (revealed on resisted movements) and absent or sluggish jerks. T1 and T2 included in this examination.	No test for T3–T12; weakness not detectable. For T1 and T2, see across.	Signs may be polyradicular. Test lower limb for weakness (revealed on resisted movements) and absent or sluggish jerks.
Cord Signs			

The posterior longitudinal ligament

The posterior longitudinal ligament runs from one vertebra to the next and protects the dura mater from the intervertebral disc. It occupies the midline but is deficient at each side; it does not span the full width of the vertebrae.

Hence a displacement of disc material initially protruding centrally runs into the barrier of a tough ligament (*Figure 10.7; 10.8*). The ligament may bulge out enough to compress the dura mater, resulting in extrasegmental pain. But the resistance of the ligament tends to push the displacement back again anteriorly, and accounts for the regular occurrence of spontaneous reduction in lumbago.

After repeated attacks, the protrusion is apt to shift towards the lightly defended zone to one side of the ligament. There it contacts the nerve roots (*Figure 10.9*), and this means that as a protrusion enlarges it usually becomes unilateral. As a result central pain in the back is replaced by root pain in the lower limb; and unilateral scapular pain is exchanged for brachial symptoms. This is echoed in the history.

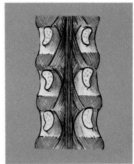

10.7

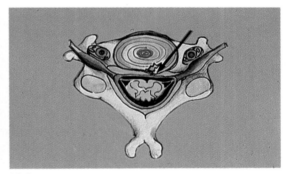

10.8

Figs 10.7, 10.8, 10.9 *The posterior ligament is strong centrally (Fig 10.7) but can be bulged backwards by a central displacement (Fig 10.8). Its absence at the sides allows direct access to the nerve roots (Fig 10.9).*

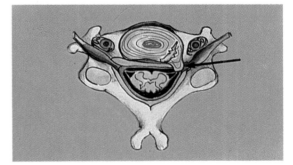

10.9

The disc

Between the bodies of each two vertebrae—except C1 and C2—lies a disc, the largest avascular structure in the whole body. Each is separated from the anterior aspect of the dura mater by the posterior longitudinal ligament.

Being of cartilage the disc:

(1) Has no nerves[3].
(2) Is radiotranslucent.
(3) Cannot heal once cracked.

A wide capsule of fibrocartilage (*annulus fibrosus*) composed of various criss-crossing layers encases a soft water–absorbent *nucleus pulposus* which distributes pressure hydrostatically. The nucleus consists of a softish gelatinous polysaccharide. In the young it is quite distinct from the annulus, less so in adults and by middle age has disappeared completely, degenerating into fibrils of cartilage.

When time and the multiple traumata of ordinary active life have initiated damage, the cartilage becomes slightly, and then more, cracked. In the end, a fragment forms that is either completely detached within the joint or lies hinged.

The nucleus sometimes pushes past the annulus. If so, pure herniation of pulp with an intact annulus results. Alternatively, a cartilaginous displacement of sufficient size

EXAMINATION FOR A SPINAL DISPLACEMENT: SUMMARY IV

Spinal level	CERVICAL	THORACIC	LUMBAR

History
Always
characteristic.
	Usually unilateral scapular pain, almost always referred extrasegmentally. Any nerve root pain felt in appropriate dermatome.
	    Brachial symptoms may follow scapular pain. Pain in upper limb recovers spontaneously within four months from onset.
	    Discs radiotranslucent. History of recurrent attacks.
		Posterior trunk pain, often referred extrasegmentally. Any nerve root pain felt anteriorly (sometimes the only symptom).
		    No spontaneous recovery from root pain.
		    Discs radiotranslucent.
		History of recurrent attacks.
			Pain in lumbar region, buttocks, legs, often referred extrasegmentally. Nerve root pain felt in lower limb in appropriate dermatome(s).
			    Root pain in leg comes on as pain in back fades. Spontaneous recovery from pain in lower limb within one year from onset.
			    Discs radiotranslucent. Cartilaginous displacements characterised by rapid onset; nuclear displacements (confined to those under 60) by slow onset. History of recurrent attacks.

Joint Signs			

Dural Signs
Sometimes
present.
	Painful neck flexion (ambiguous; stretches thoracic extent of dura).	Painful neck flexion (ambiguous, see across).
		    Check for pain on moving shoulder girdle backwards, forwards and upwards.
		    Ask if deep breath or coughing painful.
			Test for bilateral limitation on SLR.
			    Ask if deep breath or coughing painful.

Nerve Root Signs: Mobility *Sometimes* *present.*	No test—nerve roots tethered to transverse processes (but see across for T1 and T2).	Mobility of T1 and T2 roots tested by scapular approximation during cervical examination. No test for other thoracic roots.	Test for unilateral limitation on SLR (L4, L5, S1 and S2 roots). Test for unilateral pain on prone knee flexion (L3 root).
Nerve Root Signs: Weakness *Sometimes* *present.*	Any signs monoradicular. Test upper limb for muscle weakness (revealed on resisted movements) and absent or sluggish jerks. T1 and T2 included in this examination.	No test for T3–T12; weakness not detectable. For T1 and T2, see across.	Signs may be polyradicular. Test lower limb for weakness (revealed on resisted movements) and absent or sluggish jerks.
Cord Signs			

3. Jung, A. and Brunschwig, A. (1932). Recherches histologiques sur l'innervation des corps vertebraux. *Presse med.*, **17**, 136.

may become aggravated by secondary herniation of nuclear material.

Thus a displacement of disc material may consist either of a cartilaginous loose fragment or of nuclear material. Either may move posteriorly to compress the dura mater centrally via the posterior longitudinal ligament or laterally to impinge on the nerve roots. Pain will result.

Cartilage is hard and such a displacement is often susceptible to manipulative reduction. Nuclear material is soft and cannot be jerked back into place. Sustained heavy traction is the treatment of choice.

A lateral protrusion of disc material indenting the nerve roots lies outside the joint, and its extra-articular position deprives the fragment of its nutrient synovial fluid. Hence the protrusion slowly shrivels. At the neck, spontaneous recovery from nerve root impingement giving brachial pain may be expected four months after the pain went down the arm. For some unknown reason such spontaneous recovery does not occur at thoracic levels. But at the lumbar spine the corresponding period is recovery within a year.

However, this mechanism is not brought into play when the displacement reposes centrally, causing pain chiefly in the back. Thus backache or neckache may persist or recur indefinitely.

The onset of backache from a cartilaginous displacement is rapid and often immediate. The pain from a nuclear displacement tends to come on over some hours or overnight, intensifying bit by bit as the pulp seeps out and the bulge enlarges. At the neck nuclear displacements are rare; at the thoracic spine they are even more unusual but at the lumbar spine they contribute about one case in three in patients under 60. Patients over 60 can no longer boast a nucleus.

Displacements at the spine, as elsewhere, give rise to the characteristic history of sporadic attacks; cartilage is an avascular structure and hence cannot heal after it has been damaged.

In common with other structures, cartilage degenerates with the passage of time but this causes no pain of itself. In old age the discs crumble away, an individual sometimes losing two inches or more in height. Disc trouble then ceases and although spinal mobility is often minimal the limitation is nearly always painless. In fact, the highest incidence of back trouble is in the age group 40 to 49, tailing off thereafter (Leavitt *et al.* 1972)[4]. It must therefore be abundantly clear that degeneration of any tissue in the spine cannot provide the explanation for back trouble.

These findings are tabulated on page 138.

The joints

In principle, the joints at the spine are examined by the normal routine of resisted and passive movements. However, in practice, resisted movements are not found to be painful at the spine and hence are often omitted. At the thoracic and lumbar spine active movements are substituted for the passive ones, as the body weight ensures that the active movements are largely passive in their diagnostic import; the active movements are only instigated by muscular action, thereafter the body weight takes over.

As at other joints the findings may be of:

(1) The capsular pattern (uncommon).
(2) The non-capsular pattern, nearly always of the kind characteristic of internal derangement (common).

Movement about the joint will painfully force any protrusion against the dura mater; the pain will then be present on some, but not all, movements. Additionally, a displacement will obstruct free movement at the joint giving rise to limitation. So any displacement will produce pain and limitation in the non-capsular pattern characteristic of internal derangement. This is in addition to the dural signs (previously discussed) where the dura mater is stretched by traction exerted from a distance by, for example, straight-leg raising.

In fact, often a disc lesion will be evident only from its history and the limitation of the spinal movements in the pattern of internal derangement. Examination of the dura mater, nerve root sheath and parenchyma often prove negative.

4. Leavitt, S.S., Johnson, T.L. and Beyer, R.D. (1971). Patterns in industrial back injury. *Industry Med. Surg.*, **40**, 8.

The spine: intervertebral pressure

Fig 10.10 *Lordosis of the lumbar spine subjects the disc to anterior pressure, directing it away from sensitive structures.*

The spine is constructed in curves. The neck and lumbar concavities are compensated for by thoracic kyphosis. Both neck flexion and lumbar flexion open the posterior aspect of the joint and close the anterior. So the tilt of the surfaces of the vertebra during flexion subjects the disc, by the parallelogram of forces, to pressure directed posteriorly towards the dura mater. By contrast, a healthy degree of lordosis generates anterior pressure (*Figure 10.10*). Moreover, the experimental findings of Nachemson (1960)[5] show it is during flexion that intervertebral pressure reaches its peak. If the pressure within the disc while an individual is standing is taken to be 100, then on lying supine it is 25, while lying on the side it is 75 and while sitting it is 140. While standing slightly bent forwards it is 150; sitting slightly bent forwards, 180; standing bent well forwards, 210 and sitting bent well forwards, 270.

Flexion of the spine thus:

(1) Exerts strong pressure on the disc.
(2) Exerts pressure directed posteriorly.

Not surprisingly, many attacks of disc trouble are triggered off by bending and lifting.

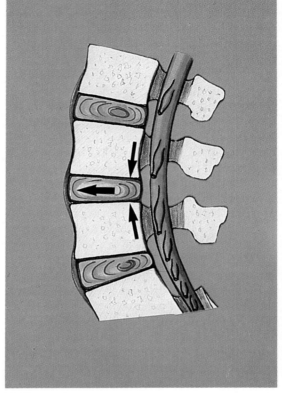

10.10

The spinal cord

A major disc lesion may jeopardise the integrity of the spinal cord. Whether at cervical, thoracic or first lumbar levels this affords the strongest possible bar to manipulation. The physician always examines for cord signs.

Compression of the spinal cord is not painful. At the cervical spine pins and needles (unaccompanied by pain) in both upper limbs or all four limbs may result. These symptoms may possibly be elicited only by neck flexion.

Encroachment on the spinal cord at thoracic or the first lumbar levels may give rise to a tingling sensation in both lower limbs.

The physician tests the plantar response for all levels.

Summary

Examination

Espousal of the mode of examination described in the previous sections will:

(1) show disc lesions constitute by far the largest category of spinal disorders; most symptoms are referable to this condition alone. A condensation of additional clinical support for this hypothesis is on page 15.

(2) facilitate differentiation of other spinal disorders, as they do not conform to the known characteristics of a disc lesion.

Treatment

Examination, diagnosis and treatment at each spinal level will be elaborated in the ensuing chapters.

5. Nachemson, A. (1960). Measurement of intradiscal pressure. *Acta orthop. scand.*, Suppl. **43**, 1.

EXAMINATION FOR A SPINAL DISPLACEMENT: SUMMARY V

Spinal level	CERVICAL	THORACIC	LUMBAR

History
Always characteristic.
	Usually unilateral scapular pain, almost always referred extrasegmentally. Any nerve root pain felt in appropriate dermatome.
	    Brachial symptoms may follow scapular pain. Pain in upper limb recovers spontaneously within four months from onset.
	    Discs radiotranslucent.
	History of recurrent attacks limiting spinal mobility.
		Posterior trunk pain, often referred extrasegmentally. Any nerve root pain felt anteriorly (sometimes the only symptom).
		    No spontaneous recovery from root pain.
		    Discs radiotranslucent.
		History of recurrent attacks limiting spinal mobility. Onset of pain often during bending/lifting.
			Pain in lumbar region, buttocks, legs, often referred extrasegmentally. Nerve root pain felt in lower limb in appropriate dermatome(s).
			    Root pain in leg comes on as pain in back fades. Spontaneous recovery from pain in lower limb within one year from onset.
			    Discs radiotranslucent. Cartilaginous displacements characterised by rapid onset; nuclear displacements (confined to those under 60) by slow onset.
			History of recurrent attacks limiting lumbar mobility. Onset often during bending and/or lifting.

Joint Signs *Always characteristic.*	Test for pain and limitation on passive cervical movements in some but not all directions.	Test for pain and limitation on thoracic movements in some but not all directions.	Test for pain and limitation on lumbar movements in some but not all directions (except lumbago, where all movements asymmetrically limited).

Dural Signs
Sometimes present.
	Painful neck flexion (ambiguous; stretches thoracic extent of dura).	Painful neck flexion (ambiguous, see across).
		    Check for pain on moving shoulder girdle backwards, forwards and upwards.
		    Ask if deep breath or coughing painful.
			Test for bilateral limitation on SLR.
			    Ask if deep breath or coughing painful.

Nerve Root Signs: Mobility *Sometimes present.*	No test—nerve roots tethered to transverse processes (but see across for T1 and T2).	Mobility of T1 and T2 roots tested by scapular approximation during cervical examination. No test for other thoracic roots.	Test for unilateral limitation on SLR (L4, L5, S1 and S2 roots). Test for unilateral pain on prone knee flexion (L3 root).
Nerve Root Signs: Weakness *Sometimes present.*	Any signs monoradicular. Test upper limb for muscle weakness (revealed on resisted movements) and absent or sluggish jerks. T1 and T2 included in this examination.	No test for T3–T12; weakness not detectable. For T1 and T2, see across.	Signs may be polyradicular. Test lower limb for weakness (revealed on resisted movements) and absent or sluggish jerks.
Cord Signs *Rare.*	Check plantar response. Never manipulate if cord signs present.	Check plantar response. Never manipulate if cord signs present.	Check plantar response (L1 only). Never manipulate if cord signs present.

NB Although this mode of examination is specifically geared towards detection and classification of a displacement, it also serves to differentiate other causes of spinal pain.

At cervical levels nearly all displacements are cartilaginous and respond to manipulation.

At thoracic levels the pattern is similar but with a greater tendency to relapse—countered by injections of sclerosant material.

At lumbar levels, nuclear displacements can be dealt with by sustained traction[6] and cartilaginous displacements by manipulation. Sclerosants diminish the tendency to relapse and epidural local anaesthesia may abolish the pain[7] from an otherwise irreducible displacement. Laminectomy is only very seldom required.

6. Mathews, J.A. (1968). Dynamic discography: a study of lumbar traction. *Ann. phys. Med.*, **7**, 275.

7. Coomes, E.N. (1963). Comparison between epidural local anaesthesia and bed rest in sciatica. *Br. med. J.*, **i**, 20.

Spinal manipulation

At joints containing a meniscus it has long been accepted that manipulation acts to abolish symptoms caused by a displacement.

However, the same logic is not always extended to intra-articular displacements at the spine. Spinal manipulation is sometimes denigrated as an unorthodox procedure.

The principal reason appears to be diagnostic. Pain from a spinal disc lesion is often misascribed to strained back muscles, osteoarthrosis, and so on, through, for example, failure to test the patient's movements against resistance or excessive reliance on the X-ray. Many such cases nevertheless respond readily to manipulation because the original diagnosis was incorrect and the relief is brought about by reduction of the undiagnosed displacement.

But in theory many complications arise. Doctors are understandably reluctant to concede that twisting the vertebrae has healed a sprained muscle or abolished osteophytes still visible radiographically. The picture is further complicated by the claims of laymen.

But the facts are simple. At the spine as elsewhere, manipulation reduces displacements. Clinically both its *modus operandi* and effect are clear: a loose body is identified, the joints are twisted, the displacement shifts, the pain eases and mobility returns. That this is what happens has now been objectively confirmed. In 1978 three Hungarian doctors conducted a trial on a sequence of 50 patients with the 'one-sided sciatic syndrome'. Forty-six of these had disc lesions visible on the epidurogram. The entire group of 46 was manipulated with epidurograms taken immediately before and after treatment. Eighteen patients were rendered pain-free immediately and in 12 of those patients the second epidurogram showed reduced or negative disc herniation (Szechery, F., Csispo, L., Kiss, E., 1978)[8].

Manipulation: technique

Reappraisal is an integral part of each manipulative manoeuvre. The physician's clinical judgement, based on reassessment of the patient, will tell him what to do next— whether to abandon the session or repeat the same method as before with equal strength, greater strength or in the opposite direction, or whether to try some different manipulation altogether. At lumbar and thoracic levels there are two basic manoeuvres—extension strains and rotation strains. On the whole the manipulator will start a session with the weaker methods before progressing to those deploying greater purchase.

At the cervical spine a variety of different approaches are viable; as well as extension and rotation, the neck can undergo side flexion and lateral or antero-posterior gliding. Each yields a slightly different effect and generally each is suitable for a particular purpose. But even so it is not possible to be categoric about which manipulations must be tried in which order. During the original examination the physician will have noted which movements were limited and which were painful; guided by his findings on re-examination he must make up his own mind as to the next step, and the fundamental principle is that if something has improved the patient it is worth repeating.

By trial and error and relying on a growing body of experience, the physician strives to achieve full reduction. He need not regard himself as bound by the sequences set out in the ensuing pages—which are nonetheless tried and tested; the most effective technique is the best. It is this continual recourse to reappraisal that makes spinal manipulation both productive and safe.

Occasionally re-examination will show manipulation has made the patient not better but worse. In such cases, normally the first resort is to perform the same manoeuvre but in the opposite direction.

TREATMENT OF AN INTERVERTEBRAL DISC LESION: SUMMARY

Cervical displacement	Thoracic displacement	Lumbar displacement

Manipulative reduction.	Manipulative reduction.
	
	To forestall relapse: Sclerosants.
		Manipulative reduction if cartilaginous.
		
		Traction if nuclear.
		
		Epidural local anaesthesia if irreducible.
		
		To forestall relapse:
		   1. Posture.
		   2. Corset.
		   3. Sclerosants
		
		Only a tiny proportion of cases go to operation.

Note that signs or symptoms may strongly contraindicate manipulation or traction.		

8. Szechery, F., Csispo, L. and Kiss, E. (1978). *Psychopathology, Szentes; Psychiatric Theory*, **31**, 436–440.

Misleading phenomena

X-ray

The disc is cartilaginous and does not show on the X-ray. As elsewhere with soft tissue trouble, a number of misleading conclusions may be deduced from radiographic appearances.

(1) Osteoarthrosis/osteophytosis are both symptomless. Radiological surveys have shown that, by the age of 50, lumbar osteophytosis is present in 90% of normal men. Osteophytes (with very rare exceptions) protrude anteriorly away from the dura mater.

(2) A narrowed joint space is immaterial of itself; it merely proves the disc to be thinned. But many discs atrophy with advancing age without becoming displaced, and a normal disc space by no means excludes gross displacement of disc material. By discography, Collis (1963)[9] showed that 56% of herniations arose at intervertebral spaces of normal thickness.

(3) Osteoporosis is normally symptomless[10]. Elderly patients, usually women, with marked generalised rarefraction of the spine may sustain a pathological fracture of one or more vertebrae. It is more frequent in the thoracic than the lumbar region.

The wedging may evolve slowly. It is then painless (unless a secondary disc lesion develops on account of the upper lumbar kyphosis at the joints to either side of the collapse).

However, if the wedging comes on suddenly, bone pain results. It may be severe for a week or two but fades in two to three months. The kyphosis is visible and palpable. Osteoporosis does not appear to cause aching unless fracture supervenes, but frequent bouts of lesser pain may well be caused by repeated micro-fractures.

Symptomless osteoporosis visible on the radiograph may thus occur simultaneously with a disc lesion.

(4) Spondylolisthesis—particularly if posterior—does not necessarily cause symptoms[11]. It may result in no more than instability of the lateral joints (see page 218).

(5) Scoliosis and lordosis are the names of shapes and do not contribute any pain of themselves. Schmorl's nodes produce no symptoms.

Myelography

When a neuroma is suspected, contrast myelography is obviously indicated. For disc lesions it is a highly unreliable diagnostic aid.

If the disc protrusion passes laterally, the dural tube is not indented and the displacement is not disclosed. Gurdjian and Thomas's (1970) findings[12] for the invisibility of disc lesions are 11.9% at the fourth lumbar level and 23.8% at the fifth. Hence a negative finding does not exclude herniation. Nor, for that matter, is a positive finding necessarily relevant. Both cervical and lumbar filling defects may be entirely inconsequential, as Hitselberger and Whitten found in 1968[13] when investigating patients with suspected acoustic tumour. They extended their observations to the spinal canal. Even when all patients with a past history of back troubles were excluded, they detected myelographic defects indicating disc abnormality in no less than 37%. Clinical judgement is a surer arbiter of a displacement's presence or severity.

9. Collis, J.S. (1963). *Lumbar discography.* Springfield, Ill.: Charles C. Thomas.

10. Ross, E. (1962). Ergebnisse einer Reihenröntgenuntersuchung der Wirbelsäule bei 5000 Jugendlichen. *Fortschr. Rontgenstr.*, **97**, 734.

11. Key, J.A. (1945). Intervertebral disc lesions are the commonest cause of low back pain with or without sciatica. *Ann. Surg.*, **121**, 534.

12. Gurdjian, E.S. and Thomas, L.M. (1970). *Neckache and Backache.* Springfield, Ill.: Charles C Thomas.

13. Hitselberger, W.E. and Whitten, R.M. (1968). Abnormal myelograms in asymptomatic patients. *J. Neurosurg.*, **28**, 204.

General observations

Muscle spasm is a symptomless secondary phenomenon brought into play to guard the joint and does not require treatment. Attention should instead be brought to bear on the causative lesion, on reduction of which the muscle spasm will be abolished.

Resisted movements will be found painless in nearly all cases of spinal trouble, with occasional exceptions at the thoracic level—hence the exculpation of muscle spasm and muscles as a cause of pain. Treatment to muscles is not justified, whether in the form of heat, massage, relaxants or exercises. Bulging muscles do not diminish the liability to a disc displacement[14].

The spinal ligaments are capable of causing pain but in fact do not appear to do so. No clinical evidence supports—and the bulk of clinical evidence conflicts with—their involvement or that of the sacroiliac and facet joints. Lumbago and sciatica are of course not diagnoses but names of pain.

Spinal stenosis does not produce backache of itself, but patients with too small a spinal canal are apt to suffer more from encroachment on its space by, for example, a disc lesion, than those whose dura mater can avoid compression by retreating backwards. This explains the higher incidence of backache reported in recent surveys in those with spinal stenosis.

14. Nachemson, A. and Lind, (1969). Measurement of abdominal and back muscle strength with and without low back pain. *Scand. J. rehab. Med.*, **1**, 60.

CHAPTER ELEVEN

THE CERVICAL SPINE

The great majority of soft-tissue symptoms at the neck originate from different stages of the same disorder and respond to the same treatment: manipulative reduction of the disc displacement.

The examination is nonetheless thorough because a number of alternative causes of pain (some serious and/or strongly contraindicating manipulation) must be recognised. In particular, the arm is examined for weakness to ascertain if any neurological deficit detected is consistent with a disc lesion.

Disc lesions and cervico/brachial pain

The dura mater

A central disc lesion impinges on the dura mater via the posterior longitudinal ligament, most often giving rise to unilateral scapular pain or less frequently pain in the head and neck (*Figures 11.1; 11.2*). Displacements are common at the C4, C5, C6 and C7 levels.

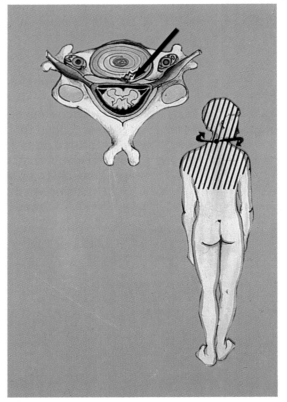

Figs 11.1, 11.2 *Possible areas to which pain can be referred by pressure on the dura mater at cervical levels. Normally the symptoms are unilateral.*

11.1, 11.2

The nerve roots

A posterolateral disc protrusion may compress the dural sleeve and nerve root within it (*Figure 11.3*). Pressure slight enough to affect the sleeve alone engenders pain in the relevant dermatome (*Figure 11.4*). Greater pressure hinders conduction along the nerve root, making for weakness in the appropriate muscles, absent or sluggish jerks and paraesthesia in the distal end of the dermatome.

The symptoms of a disc lesion may thus be dual. First, the displacement may block the joint, leading to pain and limitation of movement in the non-capsular pattern of internal derangement. Second, the loose fragment may produce root signs.

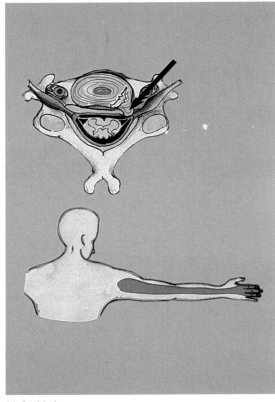

11.3, 11.4

Figs 11.3, 11.4 *A lateral displacement affecting a nerve root gives pain down the arm. C7 dermatome illustrated.*

History

Displacements

A displacement has a characteristic history. The attacks are usually recurrent, sometimes accompanied by sudden fixation of the joint and severe pain; milder symptoms accompany less limitation. The condition may abate over a week or continue on and off for years, and the patient complains of a stiff neck.

Root pain and weakness from a displacement are highly unusual in those under 35 and recovery follows within four months of the pain commencing in the arm.

The slightest jolt may be sufficient to account for onset, but many displacements occur through no more than maintenance of postural asymmetry at night. Whiplash injuries are a common cause of disc displacement but evoke central pain; they are tackled by a special manipulation (see page 161).

Examination

Joint signs

The neck can move in six directions. If all movements prove full and painless, the lesion must be sought elsewhere. First the active movements are performed, starting with active extension (*Figure 11.5*).

The two active side flexions follow (*Figures 11.6; 11.7*).

The patient then rotates her head first in one direction (*Figure 11.8*) and then the other (*Figure 11.9*).

Finally, active flexion is tested (*Figure 11.10*). This stretches both the cervical and the thoracic extents of the dura mater, so pain on this cervical movement alone may stem from a thoracic disc lesion. Pain and limitation on each active movement are noted for correlation later with the symptoms elicited by passive movements, which immediately ensue.

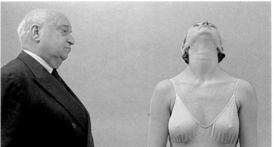
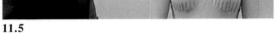

11.5

Fig 11.5 *Pain on active cervical movements suggests a cervical lesion. Active extension.*

Figs 11.6, 11.7 *Active side flexions.*

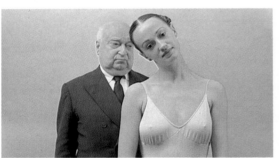

11.6

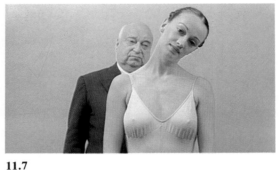

11.7

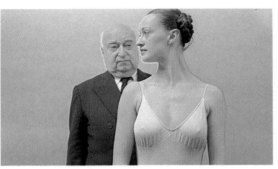

11.8

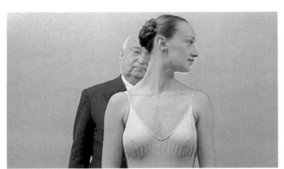

11.9

Figs 11.8, 11.9 *Active rotations.*

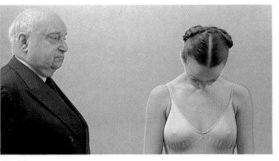

11.10

Fig 11.10 *Active flexion. Usually the patient finds this the most uncomfortable and worrying movement, so it is tested last.*

The first passive movement is extension (*Figure 11.11*). For the passive side flexions (*Figures 11.12; 11.13*), care must be taken to limit the movement to the neck by counterpressure to the thorax, otherwise trunk movements will complicate the clinical picture.

When the passive rotations (*Figures 11.14; 11.15*) are tested, rotation of the patient's trunk is precluded by the examiner's elbows, one placed in front of the shoulder and the other behind, against the opposite scapula.

Passive flexion is normally passed over as any disc lesion may be exacerbated. The end-feel should be noted throughout, particularly on passive rotation: vertebral metastases are signalled by the sudden twang of muscle spasm. The passive movements should hurt in the same pattern as the active ones but slightly more so because the joint is taken slightly further by the operator towards painful limitation.

The capsular pattern at the neck is marked by limitation of all movements except flexion, which remains relatively full. The non-capsular pattern of internal derangement is pain and limitation of two, three or four movements.

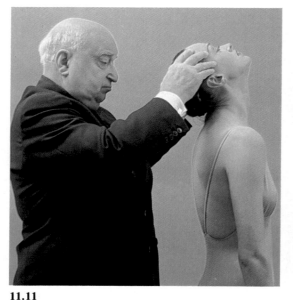

11.11

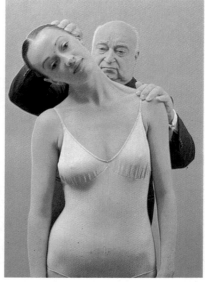

11.12

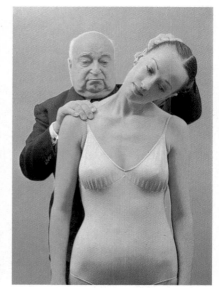

11.13

Fig 11.11 *The same movements are performed passively, for correlation with the active movements. Passive extension.*

Figs 11.12, 11.13 *Passive side flexions.*

Figs 11.14, 11.15 *Passive rotations. Since it is never safe to force flexion, it is not even tested passively.*

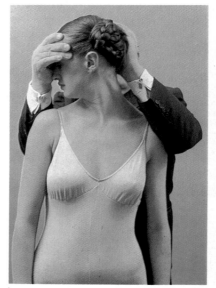

11.14

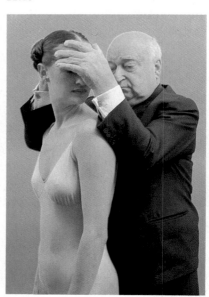

11.15

The next step is the six resisted movements. First, the physician resists extension, preventing all movement at the joint so that only the neck muscles are brought into play (*Figure 11.16*).

If the patient is not adequately restrained by counterpressure, the extensors of the entire trunk will be used (*Figure 11.17*).

Both side flexions are tried against resistance with counterpressure again afforded at the opposing shoulder (*Figures 11.18; 11.19*). Muscular lesions at the neck are extremely rare so the resisted movements normally prove painless; however, acute torticollis is occasionally aggravated by movement against resistance.

Both resisted rotations (*Figures 11.20; 11.21*) are tested. If strength is below par (rare) a C1 root palsy, probably the result of serious disease, may be present with limitation in the capsular pattern. The elbows are employed to prevent trunk movement.

Flexion is resisted (*Figure 11.22*) with the free hand applying counterpressure to the thorax. Other causes of pain on resisted movement are fracture of the first rib, anginal glandular fever, vertebral metastases or neurosis.

Fig 11.16 *The same movements are tested against resistance, sticking to the same order. Pain from genuine cervical lesions is rarely aggravated. Resisted extension, correct.*

Fig 11.17 *Resisted extension, incorrect.*

Figs 11.18, 11.19 *Resisted side flexions.*

Figs 11.20, 11.21 *Resisted rotations.*

Fig 11.22 *Resisted flexion.*

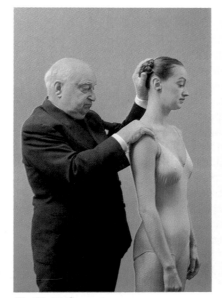

Fig 11.16 *Correct*

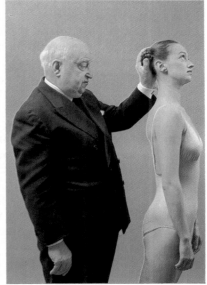

Fig 11.17 *Incorrect*

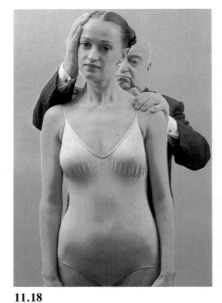

11.18

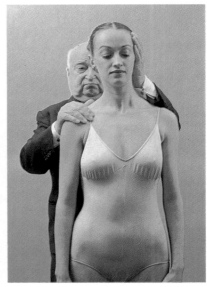

11.19

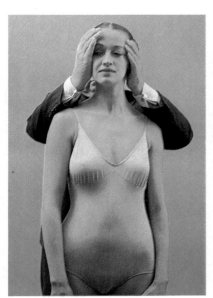

11.20

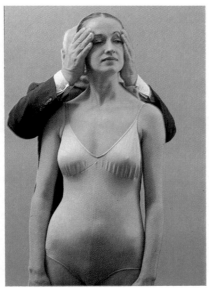

11.21

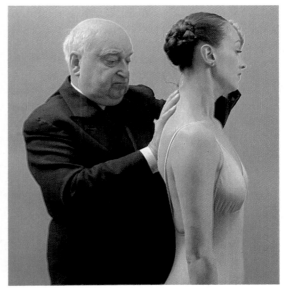

11.22

The thorax and scapula:
dural and nerve root signs

The examination now turns to the thorax, scapula and arm. No tests exist for mobility of the nerve roots as each adheres to a transverse process (*Figure 11.23*). However, any weakness of the upper limb from interference with conduction can be detected by painless weakness on resisted brachial movements.

Brachial symptoms fall broadly into three categories and the first is monoradicular signs consistent with a disc lesion. Second, there may be polyradicular signs (rare) inconsistent with a disc lesion and this suggests serious disease. Third, a finding of pain on resisted arm movements incriminates a contractile structure at the shoulder as an alternative source of brachial symptoms.

It may well be that examination of the arm draws a blank. In that case the diagnosis is based on the neck movements and history alone.

Shoulder girdle elevation (*Figure 11.24*) demonstrates whether the scapula—as is the almost invariable case—possesses normal mobility in relation to the thorax. Pulmonary neoplasm, contracture of the costocoracoid fascia, secondary malignant deposits or advanced ankylosing spondylitis in the acromioclavicular joint may limit range.

The trapezius and levator scapulae muscles are tested against resistance (*Figure 11.25*). A root palsy at C2 (never a disc) or C3 or C4—both unlikely to be a disc—would produce weakness.

Active scapular approximation (*Figure 11.26*) tugs on the first and second thoracic nerve roots, thereby lifting the whole thoracic (but not the cervical) extent of the dura upwards.

Moving the shoulder girdle forwards (*Figure 11.27*) similarly shifts the thoracic extent of the dura. Pain on both or either of these motions suggests a thoracic dural lesion. The examination now passes to the shoulder.

The patient elevates both arms (*Figure 11.28*). Full elevation through 180° is to be expected and would exclude a capsular lesion of the shoulder. Limitation unaccompanied by subsequent pathological findings is attributable to neurosis—the reader is referred to page 31 for the mechanism of arm elevation.

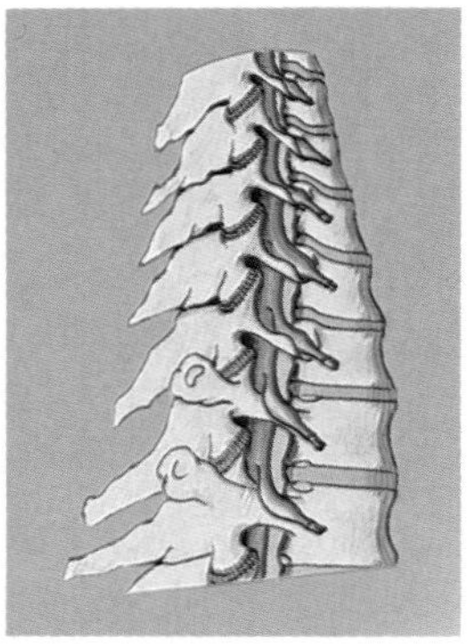

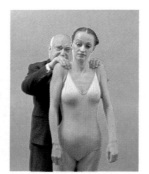

11.23

Fig 11.23 *The cervical nerve roots. A disc lesion compresses the root one higher in number. Thus the C6 disc impinges on the C7 root. The roots are immobile, cradled in the transverse processes.*

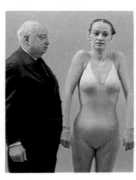

11.24

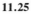

11.25

Fig 11.24 *Active shoulder girdle elevation. Immobility of the scapula or ostensible weakness of the trapezius suggests either neurosis or serious disease.*

Fig 11.25 *Resisted shoulder girdle elevation.*

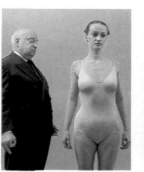

11.26

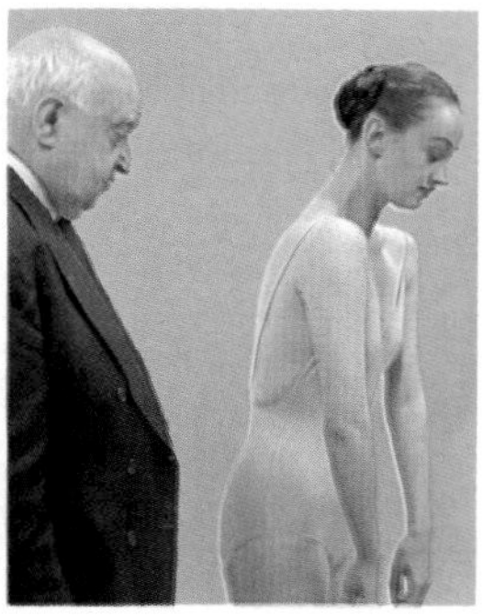

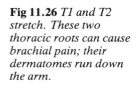

11.27

Fig 11.26 *T1 and T2 stretch. These two thoracic roots can cause brachial pain; their dermatomes run down the arm.*

Fig 11.27 *Dural stretch.*

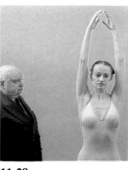

11.28

Fig 11.28 *Active arm elevation. If full and painless, this rules out capsular lesions of the shoulder; muscular lesions are cleared during examination of the nerve roots—see next page.*

Nerve root signs

The physician now runs through a series of resisted movements, primarily to check for weakness caused by nerve root pressure. A protrusion large enough to hinder conduction is too large to be shifted by manipulation and thus contraindicates successful treatment, although the condition will get better spontaneously. If weakness is found, the good side is compared. Pain on resisted movement suggests a lesion of the appropriate contractile structure.

Abduction is resisted (*Figure 11.29*). Pain indicates a defect of the deltoid or supraspinatus muscle and painless weakness a C5 root palsy. To detect weakness here and elsewhere the physician must dispose himself correctly, applying counterpressure to the far side of the patient's body. Incorrect positioning (*Figure 11.35*) will activate other groups of muscles.

If resisted adduction (*Figure 11.30*) proves weak and painless, a C7 palsy is present.

Painless weakness on resisted medial rotation (*Figure 11.31*) is rare and normally attributable to a partial rupture of the subscapular tendon.

Painless weakness on resisted lateral rotation (*Figure 11.32*) incriminates the C5 root although suprascapular neuritis should also be considered. Pain suggests a lesion of the infraspinatus (common) or the teres minor (rare). The patient pushes her arm outwards with counterpressure applied at the opposite shoulder.

Elbow flexion is tried against resistance (*Figure 11.33*). Painless weakness points to the C5 or the C6 root; pain indicates a lesion of the biceps or brachialis.

If resisted elbow extension (*Figure 11.34*) is weak, the C7 root is at fault and in fact the great majority of nerve root palsies caused by cervical disc lesions favour this root. If the movement is painful, a lesion of the triceps (rare) is suggested.

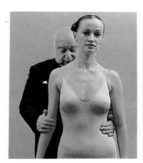

11.29

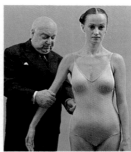

11.30

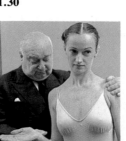

11.31

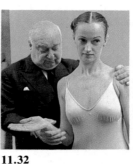

11.32

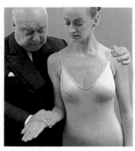

11.33

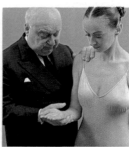

11.34

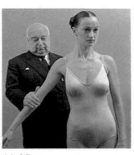

11.35

Fig 11.29 *Resisted brachial movements are primarily tests for nerve root signs, but also serve to pick out any muscular lesion. Resisted abduction, correct: C5 root.*

Fig 11.30 *Resisted adduction: C7 root.*

Fig 11.31 *Resisted medial rotation.*

Fig 11.32 *Resisted lateral rotation: C5 root.*

Fig 11.33 *Resisted elbow flexion: C5 or C6 roots.*

Fig 11.34 *Resisted elbow extension: C7 root.*

Fig 11.35 *Resisted abduction, incorrect.*

If resisted wrist extension (*Figure 11.36*) proves weak, the C6 root is at fault. If the movement is painful, the extensores carpi radialis longus and brevis are incriminated.

If resisted wrist flexion (*Figure 11.37*) is below strength, the C7 root is implicated. If it is painful, the common flexor tendons are responsible.

Painless weakness on resisted ulnar deviation (*Figure 11.38*) denotes involvement of the C8 root but pain shows the ulnar deviators are to blame.

For resisted thumb adduction (*Figure 11.39*) the patient presses her thumb inwards; painless weakness is attributable to a palsy of the C8 root as is weakness on resisted thumb extension (*Figure 11.40*).

The patient pushes her thumb outwards—abduction is resisted (*Figure 11.41*). Theoretically any weakness is attributable to the C8 root but in practice the cause is far more often a cervical rib.

The fingers are squeezed together for resisted finger adduction (*Figure 11.42*). Painless weakness suggests a lesion of the T1 root but in fact a disc lesion is never responsible; serious disease is more probable.

Next the reflexes are tested. A sluggish

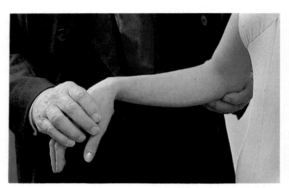

11.36

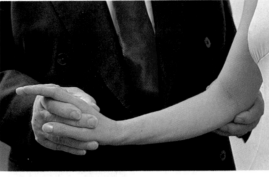
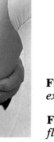

11.37

Fig 11.36 *Resisted wrist extension: C6 root.*

Fig 11.37 *Resisted wrist flexion: C7 root.*

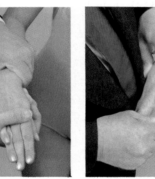

11.38

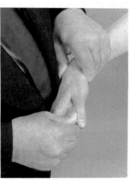

11.39

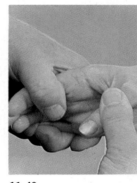

11.40

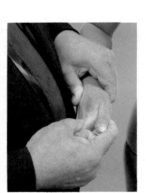

11.41

Fig 11.38 *Resisted ulnar deviation: C8 root.*

Fig 11.39 *Resisted thumb adduction: C8 root.*

Fig 11.40 *Resisted thumb extension: C8 root.*

Fig 11.41 *Resisted thumb abduction: cervical rib, C8 root.*

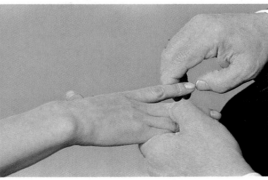

11.42

Fig 11.42 *Resisted finger adduction.*

brachioradialis jerk (*Figure 11.43*) points to a defect of the C5 root.

A sluggish or absent biceps jerk (*Figure 11.44*) incriminates the C5 or C6 root.

A sluggish or absent triceps jerk (*Figure 11.45*) incriminates the C7 root.

Cutaneous analgesia is sought at the hand.

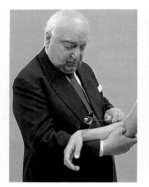 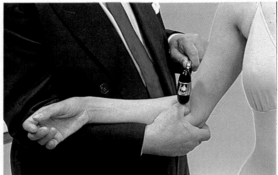 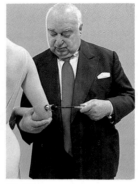

11.43   11.44   11.45

Fig 11.43 *Brachioradialis jerk: C5 root.*

Fig 11.44 *Biceps jerk: C5 or C6 root.*

Fig 11.45 *Triceps jerk: C7 root.*

Cord signs

Finally, evidence of an upper motor neurone lesion is checked by assessing the patient's plantar response (*Figure 11.46*).

A spastic gait and inco-ordination of the lower limbs are also diagnostic; all the above are cord signs. A central posterior protrusion at cervical (or thoracic) levels may compress the spinal cord and is an absolute bar to manipulation.

Paraesthesia in hands and/or feet is a cord symptom calling for circumspection.

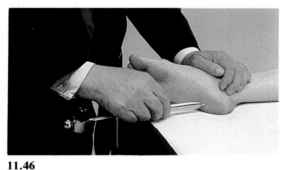

11.46

Fig 11.46 *Plantar response: cord sign.*

Root signs

The roots emerge from the cervical spine horizontally so any palsy from a cervical protrusion would be monoradicular. The root indented by a disc lesion is one greater in number than the disc; thus the C2 disc impinges on the C3 root, and so on, with nine out of ten disc lesions concentrated at the sixth cervical level compressing the C7 root (although C4, C5 and C7 lesions are encountered).

Root signs (i.e. weakness) indicate that treatment by manipulation will fail whereas root symptoms (i.e. pain without weakness) indicate that manipulation may fail.

The discovery of brachial symptoms is a prime diagnostic consideration, and before progressing to treatment for a disc lesion the physician must be assured his diagnosis is correct and that history and joint signs tally. Although disc lesions far outnumber other disorders at the cervical spine, differential diagnosis is of paramount importance and error could prove dangerous.

During the examination, the root signs are tested for in a logical order, working down the arm for the patient's convenience. On pages 164–166 the maximum root signs are grouped together root by root. It should be recalled that in addition to pain in the dermatome, the symptoms may be preceded or accompanied by scapular pain brought on by pressure on the dura mater.

Alternative causes of cervical or brachial symptoms will be found on page 163.

Findings

Capsular lesions

The capsular pattern is recognisable by pain and equal limitation of all movements apart from flexion, which is scarcely restricted. The end-feel on all the other movements is liable to be hard, except in early rheumatoid arthritis where it is soggy or empty, that is, the movement ceases at a point the examiner can tell is far short of its structural limit.

Possible explanations of the capsular pattern include fracture, ankylosing spondylitis, cervical myeloma, chordoma and rheumatoid arthritis. Secondary neoplasm is characterised by rapid onset with polyradicular signs if the invasion is at the fourth to seventh level; at the upper vertebrae detection is more difficult, but resisted movements will be both painful and

weak. All these disorders fall outside the orthopaedic physician's scope and rarely come his way. The commonest cause of capsular limitation is painless loss of mobility attendant on ageing.

Osteoarthrosis does not account for any symptoms except in advanced cases where painless limitation in the capsular pattern is apparent. So a disc lesion at an osteoarthritic joint will superimpose painful non-capsular limitation on the painless capsular limitation and should be treated as for a disc lesion at a non-osteoarthritic joint. This means that anterior osteophytes can be safely disregarded as they are themselves painless and do not interfere with sentient structures.

Displacements

A disc lesion is signalled by pain and limitation of two, three or four movements, the others retaining full painless range. The limitation is asymmetric (*cf.* the capsular pattern) and the pain is usually unilateral, felt anywhere in the neck or scapular area. Very occasionally a central displacement—often a whiplash injury—will cause pain and/or paraesthesia in both upper limbs.

Brachial pain from a cervical disc lesion hardly ever occurs before the age of 35 and

disappears (although scapular pain may remain) within four months. Nor—with rare exceptions—will the neck movements either cause or accentuate pain down the arm.

If only one movement is painfully limited by a disc lesion, it is nearly always rotation towards the painful side.

A finding of no painful movements except side flexion *away* from the painful side usually means a cancerous tumour in the upper lung.

Treatment

The treatment for a disc lesion is immediate manipulative reduction. Cervical manipulation is thus contraindicated where the diagnosis is not of a cervical displacement.

Absolute bars to manipulation

There are a number of outright bars to cervical manipulation. One should never manipulate in the presence of a displacement causing cord signs and serious consequences may also ensue in cases of rheumatoid arthritis, basilar ischaemia and patients suffering from drop attacks. It should be borne in mind that patients with these last three conditions may also have a disc lesion which must be left well alone, although a special manipulative

technique may be tried when cord symptoms only are disclosed.

The manipulations which rely on rotation during traction are dangerous in any postero-central disc protrusion, often marked by central pain and/or postural vertigo. The rotation may bruise the vertebral artery by pressing it against the body of the atlas; if spasm results in a patient with basilar ischaemia, the consequence may be cerebral ischaemia leading to death.

A comprehensive history and examination will readily sift out the conditions where manipulation could prove dangerous. For further information on differential diagnosis see page 163.

Caution

Manipulation should cease immediately if it brings on or increases brachial pain. Patients with gross cervical deformity (e.g. with chin on the chest or the ear on the shoulder) must first be given half a session of repeated pulls of manual traction in the line of deformity until this has been overcome. If standard manipulations are resorted to first, damage to the spinal cord may result. Acute torticollis in young patients should be treated by the special method noted on page 162. Manipulation is ill-advised if a patient is on anticoagulants.

Contraindications

Cervical manipulation will hardly ever succeed in the following cases; the rationale is that the protrusion is too large to be readily shifted.

(1) Root palsy. Minor pins and needles do not count. Await spontaneous recovery (four months from onset of pain in the arm).
(2) Cervical movements cause or increase brachial pain. Await spontaneous recovery as above.
(3) Brachial pain (without a root palsy) of more than two months' standing. Await spontaneous recovery as above.
(4) Primary posterolateral protrusion, that is, where the symptoms arrive in the reverse of the usual order commencing with paraesthetic digits, and brachial and scapular pain appearing subsequently. Await spontaneous recovery as above.

Other conditions benefited by manipulation

For reasons that remain obscure, manipulation occasionally helps disorders other than displacements. These conditions are tinnitus, migraine, and old man's matutinal headache set up by ligamentous contracture at the upper two joints. In the last-named case, the patient wakes with a headache that passes off normally by lunchtime and is lastingly relieved by stretching out the contracted ligaments.

Summary

Nearly all pain of cervical origin is caused by disc displacements. Nearly all the displacements can be manipulated.

In the long term the consequences of *not* reducing a cervical disc lesion can be drastic. A displacement may draw out the intervertebral ligaments, and because bone grows until it meets its lining membrane, over the years posterior osteophytes form. Eventually the spinal cord is menaced and paraplegia may ultimately ensue; this train of events could have been aborted decades previously by manipulative reduction.

Manipulation

Manipulation is set about at once in an endeavour to produce immediate recovery by shifting the loose fragment to a position where it no longer compresses sensitive structures. Further general information is set out in Chapters 2 and 10.

The sessions may last some 20 minutes. Using only one manoeuvre can occasionally secure complete reduction, but more likely a sequence of techniques will be employed during each treatment. Most relief is obtained during the first two sessions and a fourth is a great rarity. The principles are simple:

(1) Manual traction is applied throughout. Neglect of this injunction may lead to aggravation.
(2) The over-pressure is then administered during continued traction.
(3) The patient is then re-examined.

The importance of really strong manual traction cannot be overestimated. It distracts the joint surfaces, tautens the ligaments and creates a negative pressure within the joint. These factors do not merely facilitate reduction; by ensuring that if the loose fragment moves it moves centrally they make manipulation safe.

A high couch is required and an assistant holds on to the patient's feet to supply counterpressure to the operator's traction. Audible clicks during the manipulation are insignificant. The neck should never be manipulated in flexion; the head must be held either in the neutral position or in slight extension.

Before the manipulative attempt starts, the neck movements are memorised so the operator knows which movements hurt and which do not and the approximate degree of limitation—this allows progress to be monitored by re-examination. If one method results in improvement, it is repeated; if not, another is tried. The rotary manipulations (*cf.* side flexion) are first carried out in the direction in which movement is painless, irrespective of which side the pain is felt.

The first manoeuvre may be no more than traction accompanied by slow rotary movements (not approaching full range) for some seconds to win the patient's confidence. Nonetheless, improvement may result and the patient should be re-examined; treatment then passes to the first manipulation proper.

Rotation during traction—1

The head is rotated in the direction that does not hurt while an assistant grasps the patient's ankles, bracing her thighs against the couch (*Figure 11.47*).

The operator's grip makes strong traction easy to maintain. One hand supports the occiput, while the other is hooked under the patient's jaw with the little finger keeping clear of the trachea (*Figure 11.48*).

The operator steps up the traction by leaning back heavily until his arms are straight, and stays pulling for a second or two (*Figure 11.49*). Then, during continued traction, he turns the head smoothly until the resistance that heralds the approach of full range (*Figure 11.50*).

Finally, a quick thrust of tiny amplitude forces another degree or two of rotation by pulling downwards with the hand at the jaw.

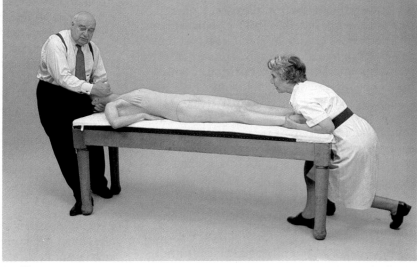

11.47

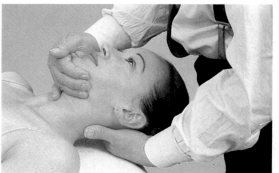

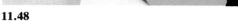

11.48

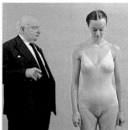

11.49

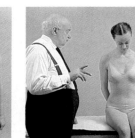

11.50

Fig 11.47 *Starting position. Traction is a vital safety factor.*

Fig 11.48 *The grip (seen from the other side).*

Figs 11.49, 11.50 *Manipulation to the right. The operator leans back, rotates the head and gives the overpressure.*

Re-examination: an example

The examiner checks that the movements previously found to have full painless range—say extension, both side flexions and one rotation—are normal. But whereas flexion was previously limited (*Figure 11.51*) it may now be found to have improved (*Figure 11.52*) and the previous restriction of rotation (*Figure 11.53*) may likewise have diminished (*Figure 11.54*). On this basis there has been some improvement, and subject always to the provisos on page 142, the manipulation merits another go with re-examination after each attempt. A sound rule-of-thumb is that the harder the end-feel, the less likely that repetition will do any good. When maximum benefit is manifest after a couple of attempts, then—unless the patient is well—rotation during traction in the direction that causes the pain (i.e. the other way) is tried, gently at first. The patient is re-examined.

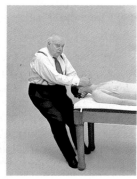

11.51

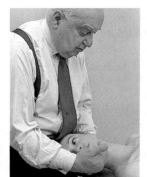

11.52

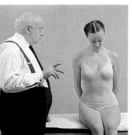

11.53

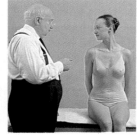

11.54

Figs 11.51, 11.52 *Re-examination. Flexion before the manipulation (left) and after (right). Any improvement is clearly detectable.*

Figs 11.53, 11.54 *Rotation, before and after. The operator is guided by his findings on re-examination.*

Rotation during traction—2

When the previous manipulation ceases to benefit, the second rotation follows (*Figure 11.55*). It resembles the first, but a new grip gives greater power at the extreme of rotary range because it is the uppermost hand that thrusts downwards. Again an assistant anchors the feet.

The operator's motive hand is applied to the patient's cheek, pressing on her maxilla with his thenar eminence while the other hand supports the occiput. A solid grip of the head is thus secured (*Figure 11.56*).

The operator leans back (*Figure 11.57*) and during considerable traction turns the head in the painless direction until he feels the gathering tissue resistance (*Figure 11.58*).

A further thrust is now given (*Figure 11.59*). The patient is re-examined and, if there has been additional improvement, the manoeuvre is repeated and followed by reappraisal. If not, rotation may be attempted in the direction that hurts.

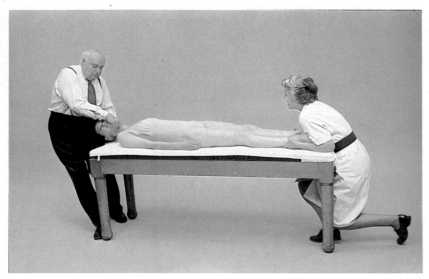

11.55

Figs 11.55, 11.56 *The starting position. The method differs from its predecessor in that reversal of the operator's hands gives stronger purchase. Fig 11.56 demonstrates the grip in detail, seen from the other side.*

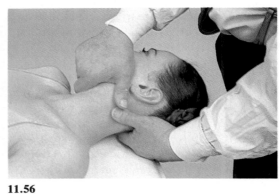

11.56

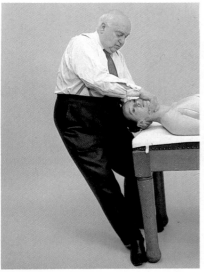

11.57

11.58

Figs 11.57, 11.58 *Manipulation to the right. The patient's head is taken smoothly to the extreme of comfortable range. Note flexion is avoided throughout.*

11.59

Fig 11.59 *The final thrust.*

Side flexion during traction

If full reduction has not been accomplished by the previous manipulations, side flexion during traction is the next measure (*Figure 11.60*). The assistant stops the patient from slipping sideways by placing her abdomen against the patient's arm, and from riding up the couch by bracing her forearm against the patient's shoulder. The operator will pivot on his left leg through a right-angle, thereby achieving side flexion of the cervical spine.

Side flexion is always performed *away* from the side on which the pain is felt; it is immaterial which side flexion produced that pain. The operator's forearm, pressing against the skull just above the ear, will be used to force side flexion at the last moment.

The operator braces his left leg against the couch and leans back to apply traction. He kicks backwards and to the left with his right leg using the momentum to swivel his body on the left leg (*Figure 11.61*). As he swings round, the patient's head is side-flexed until the approach of tissue resistance.

The overthrust is set in motion by the operator drawing his elbow—which has been allowed to lag behind—crisply into his side (*Figure 11.62*). The patient is re-examined and, if improvement is noted, the manoeuvre is re-enacted. Should side flexion towards the painful side be the only movement which remains uncomfortable, manipulation in this direction may be cautiously attempted.

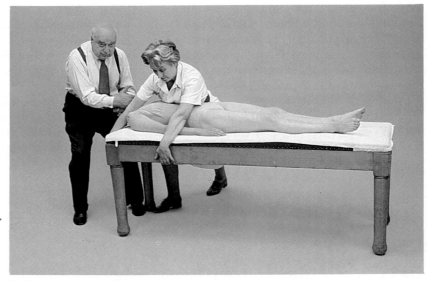

11.60

Fig 11.60 *Starting position. The operator will swing round to side-flex the patient's neck while the assistant prevents trunk movement.*

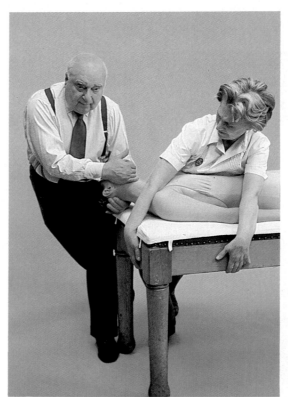

11.61

Fig 11.61 *Mid-action. The operator's entire weight is borne by his left leg which remains in the starting position. But his trunk has already swivelled round, following the backward sweep of his right leg (scarcely visible behind the leg of the couch).*

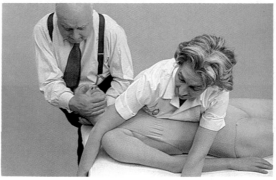

11.62

Fig 11.62 *Finishing position. The final impulse is delivered by the operator's forearm, as he pulls his elbow sharply into his side.*

Antero-posterior glide during traction

This method is adopted if limitation of extension holds out as the only painful movement. An assistant grasps the feet and the patient's head is maintained in the neutral position throughout, that is, neither in flexion nor extension (*Figure 11.63*). The operator fixes his lower leg against the couch and leans heavily backwards. He applies traction via the hand at the occiput which also furnishes the support for the patient's head (*Figure 11.64*). As the chin bears the brunt of the manipulation it can be protected by sponge rubber padding.

Strong downwards pressure is exerted momentarily on the chin not by movement of the hands so much as by the operator flexing his knees (*Figure 11.65*). This contrives a backward gliding of each cervical vertebra on the next. The patient is re-examined.

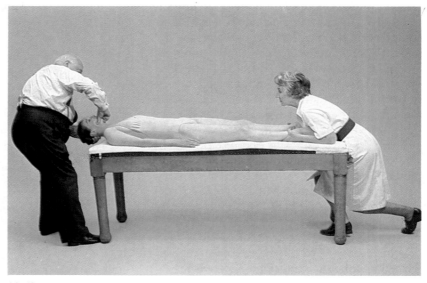

11.63

Fig 11.63 *Starting position. As with other cervical manipulations, the traction engenders centripetal force. This ensures that if the loose fragment moves at all, it moves centrally.*

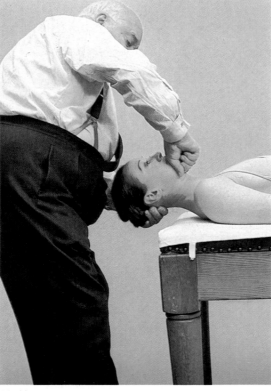

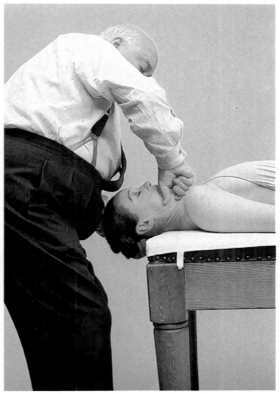

Figs 11.64, 11.65 *Starting and finishing positions. The manipulator's hands are above each other in the vertical plane; the patient's head remains horizontally aligned throughout. The manipulation consists of a single downwards thrust.*

11.64   **11.65**

Lateral gliding

Lateral gliding (*Figure 11.66*) serves principally to remove any residual ache after otherwise complete reduction. An assistant clasps the patient's trunk immobile against her abdomen.

The head is held in the neutral position. The operator's thumbs (with the thumb nail horizontal) are aligned on the patient's mandibles to keep the head in line with the body and prevent side flexion (*Figure 11.67*).

There is no traction. The operator presses sideways with one thumb and maintains the patient's head in line with her body by pressing in the opposite direction with the thenar eminence of his other hand. By simultaneously swinging his body at the hips he generates a pure gliding movement from side to side (*Figures 11.68; 11.69*) repeated several times each manipulation. Re-examination ensues.

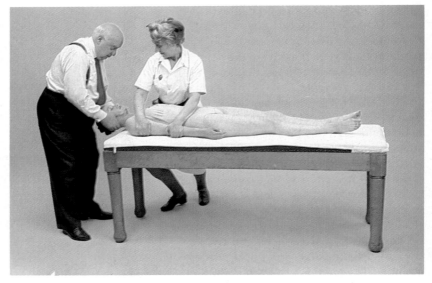

11.66

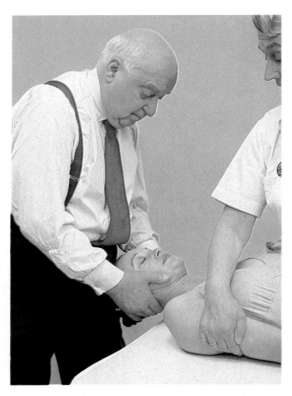

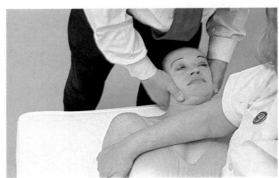

11.68

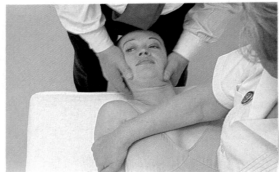

11.69

Fig 11.66 *Starting position, group. Traction is not required; the physiotherapist prevents the patient's trunk from side-flexing.*

Fig 11.67 *Starting position, detail.*

Figs 11.68, 11.69 *The movement is repeated a number of times. Note the operator swings his hips. Despite appearances, it is a relatively gentle manoeuvre.*

Traction with leverage

Traction with leverage (*Figure 11.70*) is a useful technique for central cervical disc protrusions that have set up central pain which is referred bilaterally, sometimes accompanied by pins and needles in hands and/or feet. As well as abolishing the immediate pain, this manipulation forestalls osteophytic growth which may, in the long run, threaten the spinal cord. The method is strongly contraindicated by signs (but not symptoms—see page 153) of spinal cord interference.

An assistant holds on to the patient's feet, and a layer of sponge is placed under the patient's occiput. With both feet against the legs of the couch, the operator holds the patient's head marginally flexed; he then leans backwards, the traction sustained by the hand under the mandible (*Figure 11.71*).

He bends his knees, extending the patient's neck to the neutral position with a jerk, his lower hand acting as a fulcrum (*Figure 11.72*). In this way he doubles his distracting force.

The patient is re-examined.

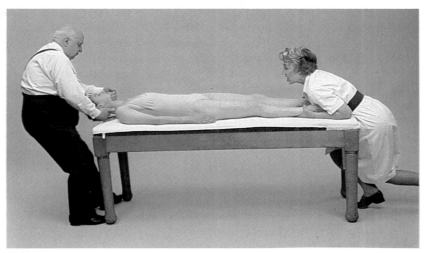

11.70

Fig 11.70 *Starting position. A safe manipulation if cord symptoms (but **not** signs) are present. Distraction is the strongest possible; there is no rotation.*

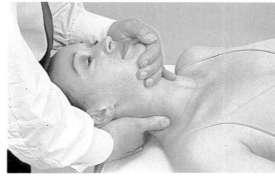

Fig 11.71 *Starting position, detail. The right hand acts only as a fulcrum; the left hand does all the work.*

11.71

Fig 11.72 *The manipulator all but sits down, achieving immense distraction.*

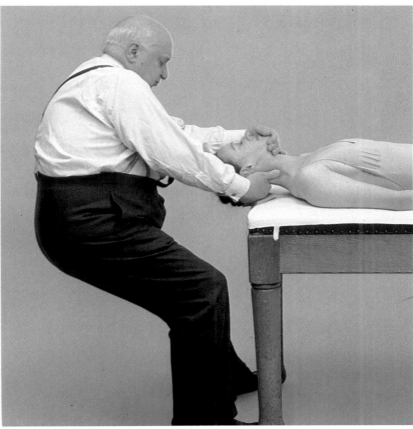

11.72

Acute torticollis

A special tactic must be deployed to where a young patient (generally under 30) suffers acute torticollis as the result of a nuclear protrusion. The patient cannot bring her head up to the vertical, far less rotate it in the direction that hurts. First, the standard manipulations, Rotations 1 and 2, are utilised to get her head back to the neutral position; thereafter the technique known as 'Bateman's'

follows to encourage full range.

The head is rotated in the painful direction until it hurts a little (*Figure 11.73*) and is supported in this position for some five minutes (*Figure 11.74*). It then transpires that further range is attainable (*Figure 11.75*) so the patient's head is supported in the new position (*Figure 11.76*) and full rotation is progressively achieved in this manner in about an hour. This method may be modified (*mutatis mutandis*) for any restriction of side flexion.

Relapse frequently sets in by the next day in which case the procedure is repeated, this time with lasting benefit. Alternatively, reduction is now practicable in the normal way.

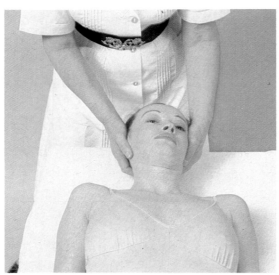

11.73

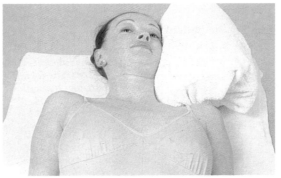

11.74

Figs 11.73, 11.74, 11.75, 11.76 *Full rotation can be restored step-by-step in the course of an hour. Normally acute torticollis in patients over 30 is treated in the ordinary way.*

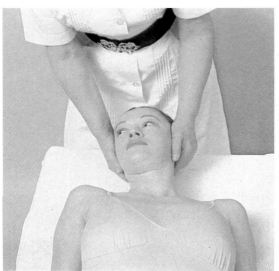

11.75

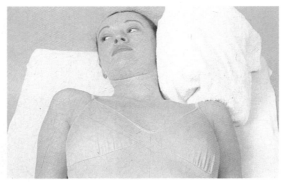

11.76

Differential diagnosis

Numerous conditions other than disc displacements may produce cervical, scapular or brachial symptoms. Each disorder is of itself rare and may be readily distinguished from a cervical disc lesion. Manipulation is at best useless and at worst dangerous for these cases. Capsular conditions have been briefly noted on page 154. Other possibilities include the following:

(1) Pancoast's tumour should be considered if the only painful movement is side flexion away from the painful side. Horner's syndrome and a first thoracic palsy are present and elevation of the scapula is limited. An X-ray is required.

(2) Neurofibroma. Any patient who seems to have a cervical disc lesion causing root pain in the limb for longer than six months should be suspected of a neurofibroma. The patient's age, a cough hurting down the arm, primary posterolateral onset, duration of brachial pain, extent of weakness, bilateral development, cord symptoms and cord signs may all prove diagnostic.

(3) Basilar ischaemia. Temporary ischaemia without thrombosis can be the consequence of pressure on the vertebral arteries. Vertigo on neck extension is a common complaint. Manipulation with rotation could cause traumatic spasm where the atlas compresses the vertebral artery and may end in death.

(4) Drop attacks result from congenital ligamentous laxity or a deformed odontoid process. They may permit such instability that both vertebral arteries can be momentarily occluded and the patient is apt to fall to the ground for no apparent reason. Drop attacks mean that manipulation is out of the question.

(5) An osteophyte may occasionally grow obliquely over the course of years to transfix a nerve root at the foramen. The resultant osteophytic root palsy is attended by little pain; in severe cases, the osteophyte should be drilled away with a dental burr.

(6) Neuralgic amyotrophy begins as a central pain succeeded by bilateral and then unilateral brachial pain—the muscles are affected regardless of root derivation. Spontaneous recovery occurs within six months of onset; full neck movements with violent pain provide a diagnostic contrast.

(7) In addition to nerve root impingement or an upper motor neuron lesion, pins and needles in the hand may result from:

(a) Acroparaesthesia—pins and needles occupy all ten digits in elderly patients. The symptoms come and go in erratic fashion day and night, and do not actually last for more than an hour at a time. A bilateral displacement may be responsible. In default of cord signs, manipulation sometimes gets rid of the symptoms (see page 161).

(b) Thoracic outlet syndrome—bilateral pins and needles recur at 2 am followed by matutinal numbness lasting a few minutes. The syndrome is an affection of the lower trunk of the brachial plexus, not the nerve roots, and is associated with a cervical or first rib squeezing the T1 and C8 roots during the day (*Figure 11.77*) as they pass under the clavicle.

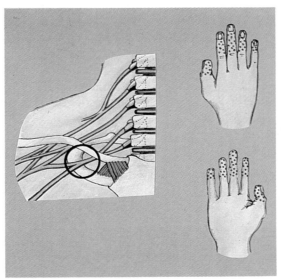

11.77, 11.78

Figs 11.77, 11.78 *The thoracic outlet syndrome. Daytime pressure on the nerve roots produces nocturnal pins and needles in both aspects of all five digits. By day the clavicle drops; at night the brachial plexus is freed from compression, evoking the symptoms.*

No symptoms are evoked at the time; the pins and needles (*Figure 11.78*) are a release phenomenon, occurring after the pressure is removed. The treatment is to teach the patient to keep the shoulder elevated at all times.

(c) Carpal tunnel syndrome—unilateral pins and needles in the anterior aspect of three-and-a-half digits. There is no paraesthesia above the wrist. The treatment is dealt with on page 65.

Appendix II gives a summary of other conditions capable of producing pins and needles in the hand.

Root signs

During the examination, root signs are looked for in a logical order, working down the arm for the sake of completeness. Here they are marshalled together root by root and in each case it is the *maximum* signs that are given, that is, all the signs that could be caused by a fully developed root palsy. In practice it is unlikely all will be encountered simultaneously; even one of the listed symptoms is indicative.

It will be remembered that in addition to pain in the dermatome, the symptoms may be preceded or accompanied by scapular pain referred from the dura mater.

C1 root pressure
Rare. No disc at this level. Cancer is the probable cause, producing pain in the dermatome (*Figure 11.79*) and weak, painful and limited neck rotation.

C2 root pressure
Rare. No disc at this level. Cancer is the probable cause, producing pain in the dermatome (*Figure 11.80*) and numbness at mid-neck.

C3 root pressure
Rare. Pain in the dermatome (*Figure 11.81*). Numbness in the cheek.

C4 root pressure
Rare. Pain in the dermatome (*Figure 11.82*). Numbness at point of shoulder.

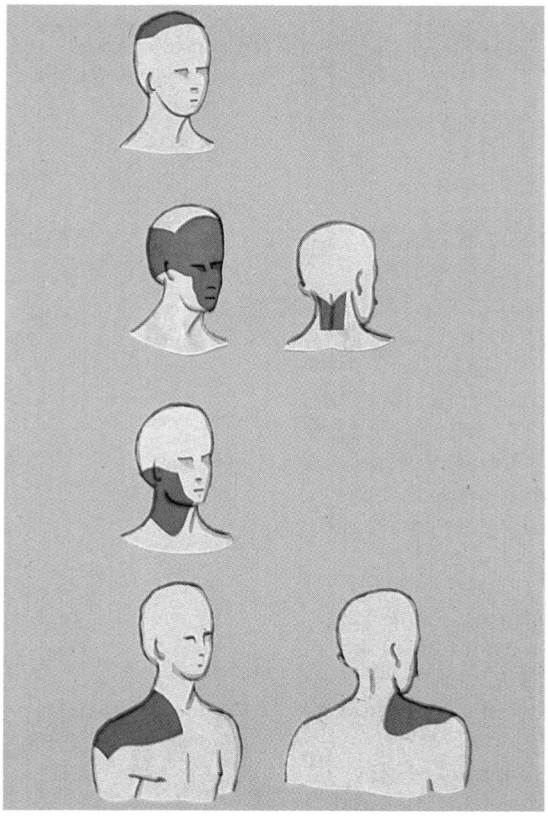

A C2, C3 and C4 root palsy weakens scapular elevation.

C5, C6, C7 and C8 root pressure
Displacements at these levels are commonplace and the maximum root signs are dealt with in detail opposite.

T1 root pressure
Rare. Most patients with symptoms apparently attributable to interference with this root are, in fact, the victims of some other disorder such as a cervical rib, a pulmonary sulcus tumour, secondary vertebral neoplasm or pressure on the median or ulnar nerve trunk.

T2 root pressure
In practice never occurs.

Figs 11.79, 11.80, 11.81, 11.82 *The cervical dermatomes. C1 (top), C2 (upper centre), C3 (lower centre), C4 (bottom). There are no discs to cause C1 or C2 root pressure; disc lesions compressing the C3 or C4 roots are rare. But dural extrasegmental reference can and frequently does produce pain in these areas.*

11.79, 11.80, 11.81, 11.82

C5 root pressure

Disc lesions fairly common. Pain in the dermatome (*Figure 11.83*). Pins and needles are normally absent.

Weak deltoid, supraspinatus—resisted abduction.

Weak biceps—resisted elbow flexion.

Weak infraspinatus—resisted lateral rotation.

Biceps jerk—absent or sluggish.

Brachioradialis jerk—absent, sluggish or inverted.

Differential diagnosis

In addition to a C4 disc lesion, consider:

(1) Lesion at the shoulder (eg supraspinatus tendinitis etc, see page 39).
(2) Rupture of the infraspinatus or supraspinatus tendon. The latter is the more common; weakness and no pain result.
(3) Palsy of the axillary nerve after dislocation

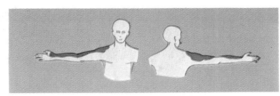

11.83

Fig 11.83 The C5 dermatome, front and back.

at the shoulder (weakness but no pain).
(4) Traction palsy of the fifth cervical root.
(5) Neuritis of the spinal accessory, long thoracic or suprascapular nerve (pain and weakness—see page 45).
(6) Myopathy deleteriously affecting the serratus anterior and both spinatus muscles complicated by capsular pain from the shoulder.
(7) Secondary malignant deposits in the humerus.
(8) Diaphragmatic pleurisy.

C6 root pressure

Disc lesions fairly common. Pain in the dermatome (*Figure 11.84*). Pins and needles in the thumb and index finger.

Weak extensores carpi radialis—resisted wrist extension.

Weak brachialis and biceps—resisted elbow flexion.

Weak subscapularis (occasionally)—resisted medial rotation.

Biceps jerk—sluggish or absent.

Differential diagnosis

In addition to a C5 disc lesion consider:

(1) The carpal tunnel syndrome (see page 65).

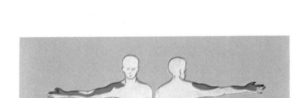

11.84

Fig 11.84 The C6 dermatome, front and back.

(2) The thoracic outlet syndrome (see page 163).
(3) Tendinitis or partial rupture of the biceps muscle (see page 44).
(4) Radial nerve pressure palsy at mid-humerus.
(5) Tennis elbow (see page 54).

C7 root pressure

Disc lesions extremely common. Probably 90% of cervical disc lesions causing a root palsy are at the sixth level compressing the seventh root. Pain in the dermatome (*Figure 11.85*). Pins and needles are usually felt in the index, long and ring fingers.

Weak latissimus dorsi—resisted arm adduction.

Weak triceps—resisted elbow extension.

Weak common flexor muscles—resisted wrist flexion.

Triceps jerk—rarely affected.

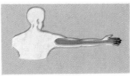

11.85

Fig 11.85 The C7 dermatome.

Differential diagnosis

In addition to a C6 disc lesion consider:
(1) Lead poisoning (always bilateral).
(2) Carcinoma of the lung.
(3) Golfer's elbow (see page 57).
(4) Tricipital tendinitis.
(5) Fracture of the olecranon.

C8 root pressure

Disc lesions fairly common. Pain in the dermatome (*Figure 11.86*) and also in the lower scapular area and the back or inner side of the arm and the inner forearm. Pins and needles in the long, ring and little finger.

Weak thumb adduction.
Weak thumb extension.
Weak ulnar deviation.
Weak adduction of the index finger.

Differential diagnosis

In addition to a C7 disc lesion consider:
(1) Cervical rib.
(2) The thoracic outlet syndrome (see page 163).
(3) Malignant deposits at the seventh cervical or first thoracic vertebra. Weakness is severe, pain is slight. The seventh cervical

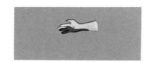

Fig 11.86 *The C8 dermatome.*

11.86

and first thoracic root are often also involved.
(4) Pancoast's tumour (see page 163).
(5) Angina, normally characterised by pain in the pectoral area spreading down the upper limb to the ulnar aspect of the hand.
(6) Traction palsy of the lower two roots of the brachial plexus.
(7) Frictional ulnar neuritis at the elbow (see page 58).
(8) Pressure on the ulnar nerve at the wrist.
(9) Thrombosis of the subclavian artery.

CHAPTER TWELVE

THE THORACIC SPINE

Disc lesions account for a higher proportion of thoracic pain than is often realised.

Clinically the thoracic spine is divisible into three sections, the first consisting of T1 and T2 which is examined with the cervical spine because the nerve roots serve the upper limbs. This leaves from T3 to T6, where displacements are extremely unusual, and from T6 to T12, where they are relatively frequent. Reduction is easy, relapse is commonplace.

Both posterior and anterior thoracic pain may stem from a disc lesion.

The dura mater

As at other spinal levels, the mechanism of pain is dural. A protrusion may compress the dura mater centrally, giving rise to unilateral extrasegmentally referred pain (*Figure 12.1*).

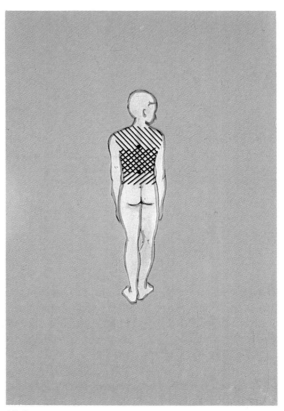

Fig 12.1 *The maximum extent of dural extrasegmental reference. A T6 protrusion (upper marker) can produce pain up to the base of the neck and down to the waist. T12 (lower marker) can refer pain up to T6 and down to the sacrum.*

12.1

The nerve roots

Alternatively, a posterolateral displacement produces root pain referred anteriorly. At T1 and T2 (both rare) the symptoms may be felt in the arm; root pain at lower levels causes symptoms experienced at the side or front of the trunk (*Figures 12.2; 12.3; 12.4*).

A cervical disc lesion is the routine cause of pain felt at upper thoracic levels; it is discomfort below the sixth thoracic dermatome that might arise from a thoracic disc lesion. At these levels diagnosis is often difficult and best approached from two aspects, the absence of visceral disease balancing and confirming signs of an articular disorder.

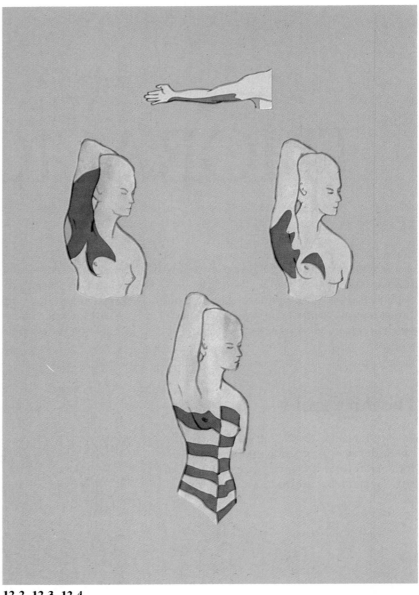

Figs 12.2, 12.3, 12.4 *The dermatomes. T1 (top), T2 and T3 (centre left and centre right). T4–T12 (bottom).*

12.2, 12.3, 12.4

History

Displacements

The mode of onset for a disc lesion is various, ranging from sudden ('thoracic lumbago') to posterior thoracic backache coming on slowly. In cases of primary posterolateral protrusion, the unilateral pain will be confined to the front of the chest or the abdomen—a highly misleading phenomenon; compression of the T11 or T12 roots provokes discomfort in the iliac fossae perhaps radiating to the testicles. Root pain may linger on indefinitely (*cf.* cervical and lumbar spines).

A deep breath usually hurts more than coughing. But symptoms of pleural, intercostal, muscular and costal provenance will also be increased so that respiratory exacerbation serves to rule out cardiac pain only.

Articular signs are seldom obvious and neurological signs conspicuous only by their absence. There are no tests for conduction (ie weakness) or mobility of the nerve roots and analgesia is not met with often. As at other levels, pain from a disc lesion will be dependent on posture and activities.

Examination

The upright spine is scrutinised in a good light for any bony irregularity and will, at the end of the physical examination, be palpated prone for deformity and the stiffness of ankylosing spondylitis.

Dural signs

The examiner looks for dural signs. Neck flexion (*Figure 12.5*) stretches the dura mater at both cervical and thoracic levels. Pain on neck flexion is therefore common to a defect at either level, but if the other neck movements are full and painless, attention is diverted to the thoracic joints. However, scapular approximation (*Figure 12.6*) pulls on the thoracic extent only of the dura mater via the first and second thoracic nerves; pain may be elicited from a central or lateral thoracic disc lesion.

Pain from stretching the first thoracic root (*Figure 12.7*) via the ulnar nerve incriminates only the T1 or T2 roots. In practice, disc lesions at either level are great rarities and are never accompanied by neurological signs; so if weakness is present too, the possibility of serious disease should be looked into.

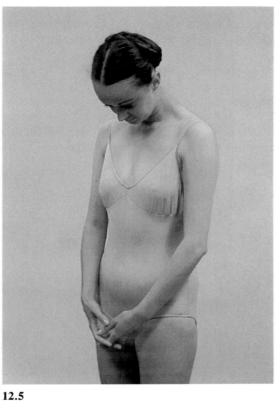

12.5

Fig 12.5 *Neck flexion: painful whether the lesion is at cervical or thoracic levels.*

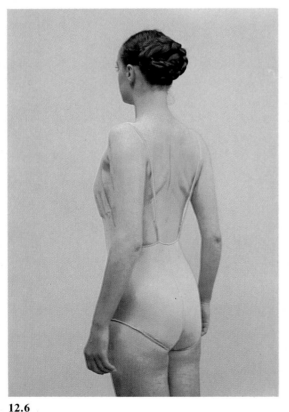

12.6

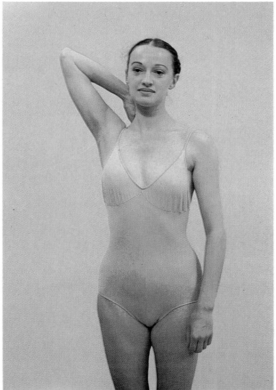

12.7

Fig 12.6 *Scapular approximation: painful if the lesion is thoracic.*

Fig 12.7 *T1 stretch; painful if the lesion is at T1 or T2.*

Joint signs

Articular signs are now sought by a series of active movements, largely passive in their diagnostic significance because of the effect of body weight. Extension is tested first (*Figure 12.8*).

The two side flexions follow (*Figures 12.9; 12.10*). Bilateral limitation in the young suggests serious disease but in the elderly may be attributable to no more than mobility dwindling with the passage of time.

The patient rotates first one way and then the other (*Figures 12.11; 12.12*) and finally flexes (*Figure 12.13*) her thoracic spine. A displacement generally causes asymmetrical pain and/or limitation on two, three or four movements.

The movement most likely to hurt with a disc lesion is the extreme of passive rotation (*Figures 12.14; 12.15*), achieved by holding the patient's knees between the examiner's to fix the pelvis; indeed, in a minor protrusion this may be the only painful movement.

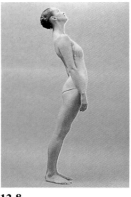
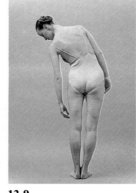
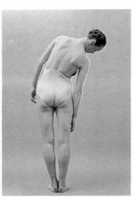

12.8 **12.9** **12.10**

Fig 12.8 *Extension.*

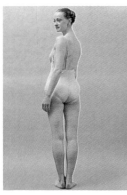
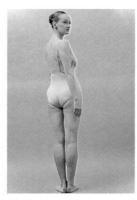
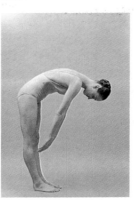

12.11 **12.12** **12.13**

Figs 12.9, 12.10 *The active side flexions.*

Figs 12.11, 12.12 *The active rotations.*

Fig 12.13 *Active flexion.*

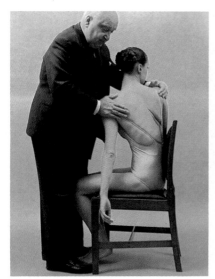
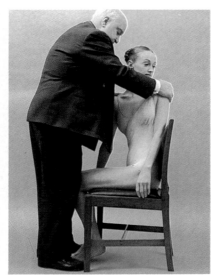

12.14 **12.15**

Figs 12.14, 12.15 *The passive rotations.*

Resisted movements

At the thoracic spine, resisted movements have particular significance as the muscles of the thorax and abdomen can and do suffer strain. For the resisted rotations (*Figures 12.16; 12.17*), the examiner grasps the patient's shoulders and inhibits movement of her pelvis by clamping her knees between his.

The side flexions are resisted (*Figures 12.18; 12.19*) by the patient bending outwards against the operator's arm while counterpressure is applied at her hip.

Movement is prevented at sternum and knee when resisted flexion is tested (*Figure 12.20*). The final resisted movement is extension (*Figure 12.21*).

Contractile structures that may be affected include the following:

Pectoral muscles—pain on resisted adduction felt at the front of the chest.

Intercostal muscles—pain on breathing.

Latissimus dorsi—pain on resisted adduction felt at the back of the chest.

Inferior posterior serratus—rare; pain on resisted rotation.

Rectus abdominis—pain on resisted flexion.

Oblique abdominal muscles—pain on resisted rotation.

All respond well to massage (see also page 18).

Muscular lesions do not radiate pain from the posterior thorax to the anterior (or vice versa); such distribution is sufficient on its own to acquit the muscles.

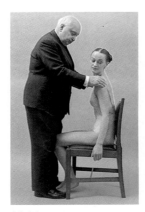
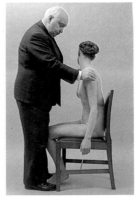

12.16   12.17

Figs 12.16, 12.17 *The resisted rotations.*

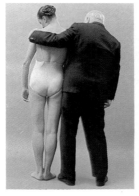
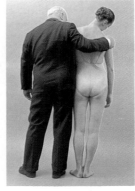

12.18   12.19

Figs 12.18, 12.19 *The resisted side flexions.*

Fig 12.20 *Resisted flexion.*

Fig 12.21 *Resisted extension.*

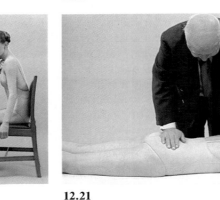

12.20   12.21

Cord signs

Finally, the patient's plantar response is tested (*Figure 12.18*). Sometimes the only signs of cord interference are pins and needles in both lower limbs on neck flexion but such cases do not always progress; they may remain unaltered for decades.

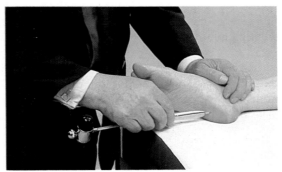

12.22

Fig 12.22 *Plantar response.*

Findings

Differential diagnosis

A disc lesion must be differentiated from the many other sources of thoracic pain. Some are noted briefly below.

(1) Visceral disorders are not influenced by thoracic movements.

(2) A neuroma clinging to the tissues on one side of the patient's spine will painfully limit side flexion away from that side; that is, side flexion away from the painful side hurts which is the opposite of the expected finding with a disc lesion. A spreading patch of cutaneous analgesia also arouses suspicion; the initial symptoms may be confined to the posterior thoracic area.

(3) Adolescent osteochondrosis is normally painless but produces mounting kyphosis at the affected joint. It may precipitate a disc lesion.

(4) Adult osteochondrosis is painless but limits extension.

(5) Senile osteoporosis is painless until pathological wedging takes over. This may cause symptoms lasting three months (see also page 218).

(6) Ankylosing spondylitis produces a pain that comes and goes, continuing for years irrespective of what the patient does; often the ache is at its worst on waking. Normally the lumbar spine becomes rigid before the thoracic joints stiffen; a flat lumbar spine associated with an upper thoracic kyphosis is suggestive. Treatment consists of phenylbutazolidine, indomethacin or prednisone.

(7) Osteitis deformans, aortic aneurysm, tuberculous caries and secondary malignant deposits set up pain arising from diseased bone.

(8) Fracture of a rib results in localised pain lasting six weeks at most. Symptoms from fracture of a vertebra cease at the end of three months.

(9) Neuritis of the spinal accessory, long thoracic or suprascapular nerve produces constant unilateral scapular pain for three weeks (see page 45).

(10) To start with, neuralgic amyotrophy causes bilateral upper thoracic pain. Subsequently the symptoms spread down one or both arms (see page 163).

(11) The diaphragm is derived from C3, C4 and C5 with the pain normally confined to the C4 dermatome. Pain arising from that part of the pleura not in contact with the diaphragm is felt in the chest. A Pancoast's tumour will invade the chest wall. In epidemic myalgia the pain is bilateral and accompanied by fever.

(12) The heart is mainly derived from the first, second and third thoracic segments.

(13) Pain from early thrombosis of the lower aorta is occasionally felt only in the lower thorax. Venous thrombosis recovers in a month or two.

Visceral embryology

For the convenience of those faced with thoracic or abdominal pain, a list of the approximate segmental derivations of the viscera is appended.

Heart	C8–T4
Lungs	T2–5
Oesophagus	T4–5
Stomach and duodenum	T6–8
Liver and gall bladder	T7–8 right
Pancreas	T8 left
Small intestine	T9–10
Appendix and ascending colon	T10–L1
Epididymis	T10
Ovary, testis and suprarenal	T11–12, L1
Bladder fundus, Kidney, Uterine fundus	T11–L1
Colonic flexure	L2–3
Sigmoid colon and rectum, Cervix, Neck of bladder, prostate and urethra	S2–5

Caution

A finding of painful and limited side flexion away from the painful side with both rotations free should always create suspicion of serious trouble. This is because rotations are the movement most likely to hurt with a disc lesion so if rotary range is full and painless, with another movement hurting, the physician is put on his guard by the discrepancy. Neoplasm or neuroma may be present.

Capsular lesions

The capsular pattern is designated by equal and severe limitation of movement in every direction. This indicates tuberculosis (rare), cancer, or ankylosing spondylitis.

Displacements

Thoracic disc lesions respond well to manipulation—success is almost invariable. It is the predisposition to recurrence that constitutes the problem (solved by the use of sclerosants—see page 181), although many patients can be kept continuously comfortable by attending for manipulative reduction on each relapse.

Treatment

All the findings that, at cervical and lumbar levels, show manipulation will fail have no bearing at the thoracic spine. All thoracic disc displacements are manipulated. Two assistants are required and a low couch is used. The only contraindications are:

(1) Signs of spinal cord pressure.
　　However, in cases marked merely by paraesthetic feet, sustained traction may be attempted. The procedure is as for lumbar traction (see page 206).
(2) If the patient is on anticoagulants.

　　The general remarks in Chapters 2 and 10 should be noted. Sessions last 20 minutes or so and varying techniques of increasing intensity may have to be tried; maximum benefit normally accumulates in one or two sessions.
　　The manipulations parallel those employed at the lumbar spine save that two assistants apply manual traction.

Manipulation

Before the session begins, passive extension is tested with the patient prone. Each joint is pressed towards extension with a slight jerk in the hope it will hurt more at one location than another or that greater resistance will be encountered. This identifies the exact level of the lesion. But often the same amount of stiffness is detected at several adjacent levels, in which case for the first manipulation pressure is brought to bear on the middle one. By contrast, the rotation strains involve the entire thoracic spine and not just one joint.

Extension during traction—1

The first manipulation consists of no more than a sharp downwards thrust during traction. One assistant grasps the hands and the other the feet (*Figure 12.23*). They pull strongly in opposite directions for a few seconds before and during the manipulation.

The ulnar border of the operator's palm is angled so that the centre of the fifth metacarpal bone presses on the spinous process at the affected joint (*Figure 12.24*). Reinforcement is now given with the other hand (*Figure 12.25*).

A sharp downwards jerk of a very small amplitude is imparted towards extension, keeping the arms straight (*Figure 12.26*). Then the patient is re-examined. At the upper thorax, considerably more force is required.

In elderly patients it is not difficult to fracture a rib, and rotary techniques (see pages 176–180) should be preferred.

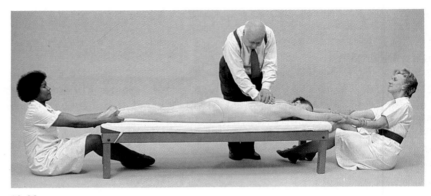

12.23

Fig 12.23 *The two assistants pull in opposite directions.*

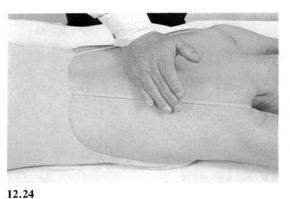

12.24

Fig 12.24 *The hand is slanted to confine pressure to the affected level.*

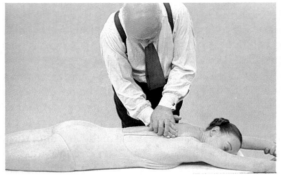

12.25

Fig 12.25 *The operator reinforces with his other hand and presses gently while the traction takes effect.*

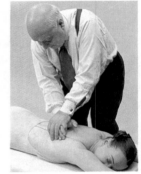

12.26

Fig 12.26 *The overthrust. A downwards jerk is transmitted via the arms.*

Re-examination: an example

The examiner checks that the movements previously found to have full painless range (e.g. side flexion, flexion and one rotation) are still normal.

It may be found that the original painful limitation of extension (*Figure 12.27*) has now improved (*Figure 12.28*).

Likewise, the original limitation of rotation (*Figure 12.29*) may have diminished (*Figure 12.30*). In such a case the manipulation has helped, and subject to the qualifications on page 142 it is therefore repeated until reappraisal registers no further improvement. But if it has not done good, the manoeuvre is tried again at an adjacent joint and the patient again re-examined.

The next ploy would be to repeat the same manipulation just to one side of the spinous process at the affected level thereby adding an element of rotation.

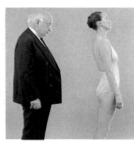

12.27   12.28

Figs 12.27, 12.28 *Re-examination. Extension before the manipulation (left) and after (right). The manipulator notes any changes in the signs.*

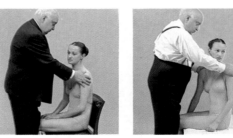

12.29   12.30

Figs 12.29, 12.30 *Re-examination. Rotation before (left) and after (right) the manipulation. The patient reports on any change in symptoms, including on taking a deep breath.*

Extension during traction—2

This manoeuvre exerts a different thrust; the two pertinent vertebrae are rotated, again during traction supplied by two assistants (*Figure 12.31*). Often reduction can be accomplished by use only of this and the previous methods.

The operator extends the wrist of one hand, bringing the pisiform bone into prominence and placing it to the near side of the spinous process just above the site of displacement. The thumb of his other hand is abducted, drawing it backwards to make the trapezio-first-metacarpal joint stand out; then this is laid on the far side of the spinous process just below the affected level (*Figure 12.32*).

The operator now presses down with a sharp jerk, pushing the hand which is further away from him distally and his near hand proximally (*Figure 12.33*). The patient is re-examined and if improvement has resulted the manipulation is repeated.

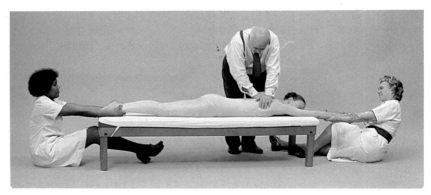

12.31

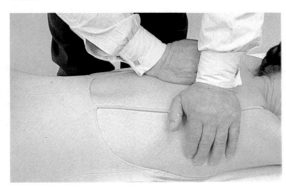

12.32

Fig 12.31 *The operator's hands are crossed to produce a rotation thrust. Note one assistant has braced her knee against the couch and the other wedged her foot against its leg.*

Fig 12.32 *Both hands are motive; they are pushed in opposite directions.*

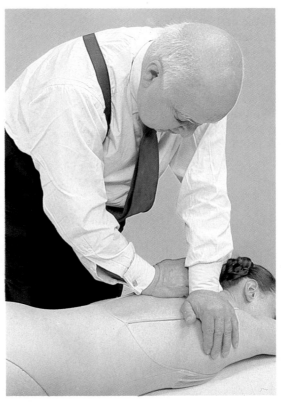

12.33

Fig 12.33 *The overthrust. The operator leans right over the patient.*

Rotation strains

For the rotations, the exact site of the displacement is no longer of interest as the entire extent of the thoracic spine is manipulated with the strain falling on the blocked joint. The manipulations are arranged in order of increasing force.

Rotation during traction—1

This is employed once the previous measures cease to afford benefit or in the unlikely event that they prove excessively painful. The patient's trunk is rotated, first in the direction that does not bring on the pain, irrespective of which side the pain is felt.

The assistant at the feet grasps only the uppermost leg and will, at the moment of overpressure, participate by swinging it in the same direction in which the manipulator forces the pelvis. The assistant at the upper end pulls on both arms, again in the direction of the manipulation (*Figure 12.34*).

The manipulator will use a downward thrust of his body weight to force one arm backwards and the other forwards. He places one hand on the patient's buttock and the other against the prominent border of her scapula (*Figure 12.35*). The operator twists the patient's thorax as far as possible before the traction starts, and pauses there for a couple of seconds until it takes effect (*Figure 12.36*).

He then rotates his thorax utilising his body weight to impell the patient's thorax towards, and her pelvis away from, himself with a strong jerk (*Figure 12.37*). The patient is re-examined and if improvement is apparent the manoeuvre is repeated.

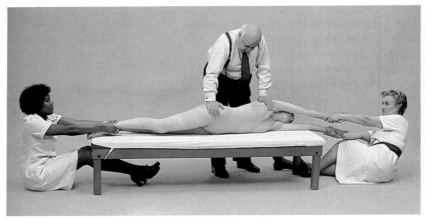

12.34

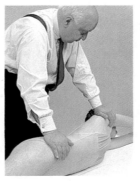

12.35

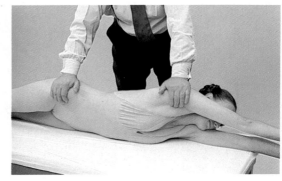

12.36

Figs 12.34, 12.35, 12.36 *Starting position. The thorax is twisted as far as possible before the traction begins.*

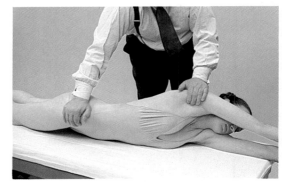

12.37

Fig 12.37 *Finishing position. Further rotation is forced. Note how the armpit has come up while the pelvis is now flat on the couch.*

Rotation during traction—2

This manipulation is the reverse of its predecessor; the pelvis is pulled towards the operator and the thorax thrust away. The assistant at the foot grasps the uppermost leg only and will pull it in the same direction as the manipulator forces the pelvis (*Figure 12.38*).

The physician hooks the fingers of one hand about the anterior superior spine of the patient's ilium. The heel of his other hand is lodged against the lateral aspect of her thorax; it is over this arm that body weight is poised (*Figure 12.39*).

The operator twists the patient's thorax as far as it will go (*Figure 12.40*) and then waits a few seconds for traction to open the joints.

The hand on the pelvis is then drawn sharply upwards and towards the operator, while the thoracic hand is pushed downwards and away (*Figure 12.41*). The movement is assisted by

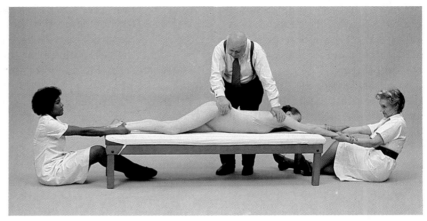

12.38

rotation of the manipulator's thorax, thus taking full advantage of his body weight. The patient is re-examined.

Fig 12.38 *The pelvis is to be lifted and the shoulder held down.*

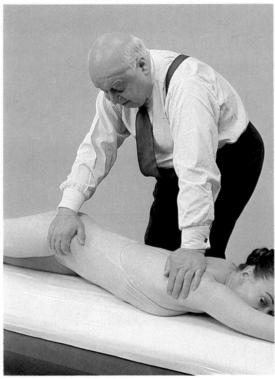

12.39

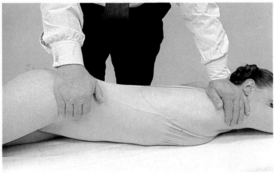

12.40

Figs 12.39, 12.40 *Starting position. The operator's body weight keeps the upper thorax flat on the couch.*

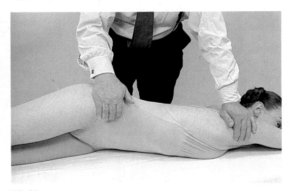

12.41

Fig 12.41 *The overpressure. Rotation is clearly seen; note the expanse of abdomen, with both thighs now visible.*

Rotation during traction—3

Stronger purchase can be obtained by using the patient's thigh. This manipulation is seldom called for but is useful if one rotation remains obstinately painful. The assistants apply traction (*Figure 12.42*).

One hand keeps the patient's upper trunk flat on the couch while the other holds her knee off the couch, rotating the thorax (*Figure 12.43*). The assistants pull.

After a couple of seconds the manipulator draws the patient's knee sharply upwards towards himself without letting her thorax move (*Figures 12.44; 12.45*).

During this phase the operator's body weight is used to maintain pressure on the thorax while the upward pull on the thigh is accomplished only by the strength of his arm. The patient is re-examined. This method pays particular dividends when a small physiotherapist has to deal with a large patient.

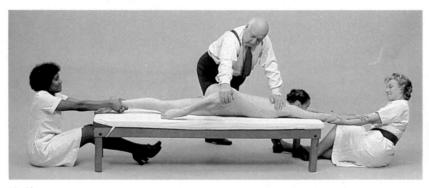

12.42

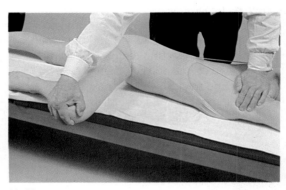

12.43

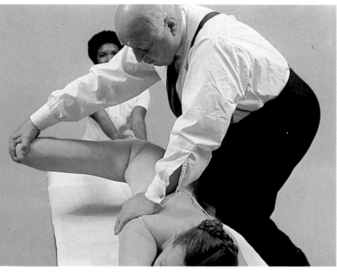

12.44

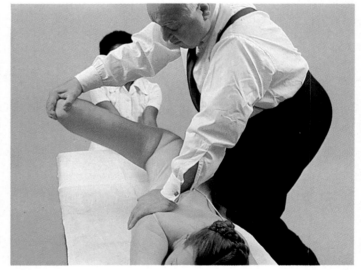

12.45

Figs 12.42, 12.43, 12.44 *Starting position. Again the body weight is over the scapula, pinning the upper thorax in the saggital plane.*

Fig 12.45 *The overpressure.*

Rotation during traction—4

Maximum mechanical advantage is obtained by this manipulation which lengthens the thoracic lever. The patient lies face upwards while two assistants generate strong traction for the few seconds preceding and during the manipulation (*Figure 12.46*).

The projecting lateral edge of the patient's scapula is pinned to the couch while her knee is flexed to a right angle. Her trunk is rotated until the resistance that heralds the end of the range (*Figure 12.47*).

The patient's knee is smartly pressed towards the floor (*Figure 12.48*). During the manipulation, the operator's body weight is balanced over the patient's shoulder to keep her immobile on the couch. The patient is re-examined.

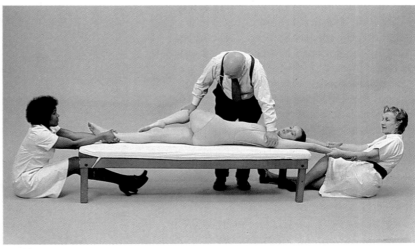

12.46

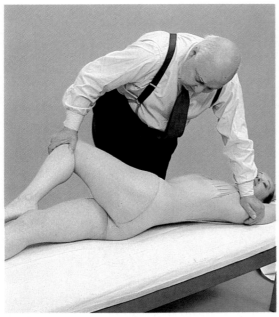

12.47

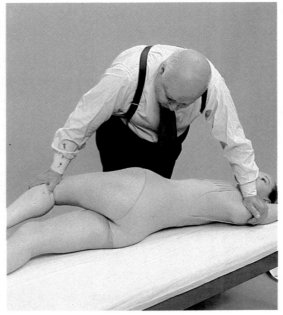

12.48

Figs 12.46, 12.47 *Starting position. This is the strongest rotation strain. The force is greatly enhanced both because the hands are applied to opposite sides of the patient's body and because the thrust is downwards.*

Fig 12.48 *The overpressure is strong but controlled.*

Upper thoracic rotation during traction

This is suited only to the rare upper thoracic protrusion. Traction is applied by the assistants, the physiotherapist at the head grasping the patient's head (*Figure 12.49*). The patient's forearm is placed behind her back.

The manipulator's hands are clasped through the circle of the patient's arm. The heel of his near hand presses down on the sixth to eighth thoracic levels; the other forearm is exerted against her shoulder, raising it off the couch (*Figure 12.50*).

The operator then side-flexes his thorax, lifting the patient's shoulder girdle up while delivering a rotation thrust with his lower hand (*Figures 12.51; 12.52*). This simultaneously rotates and extends the patient's upper thoracic joints during traction.

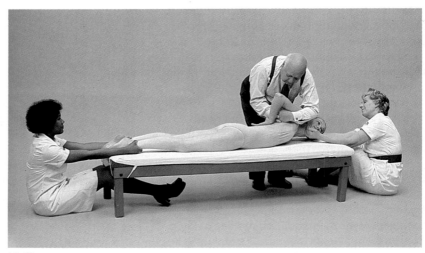

12.49

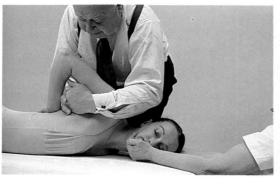

12.50

Figs 12.49, 12.50, 12.51 *Starting position. The operator links his hands through the circle of the patient's internally rotated arm.*

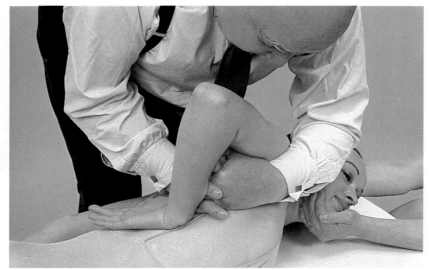

12.51

Fig 12.52 *The overpressure. The operator presses down on the rib cage with his right hand, while adducting his elbow to raise the front of the thorax. The movement is best noted by diminution of background area between the operator's arm and chest.*

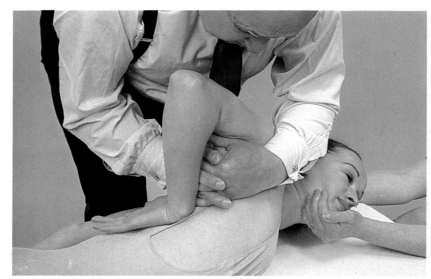

12.52

Recurrence

Recurrence at regular intervals must be expected and normally requires no more than renewed manipulative reduction. A corset at the thoracic spine is seldom effective.

Repeated relapse can be countered by sclerosant therapy.

Sclerosants

A chemical irritant is injected into the posterior ligaments about the joint containing the displacement. Tissue contracture results and the ligaments shorten in a period of about two months, producing increased stability at the joint. This diminishes the liability to intervertebral displacement. It is, naturally, of the essence that the displacement is reduced prior to the injection.

The solution (1ml) is injected into each ligamento-periosteal junction at both ends of the supraspinous ligaments; in addition, the facet joints to either side are infiltrated.

The solution, known as P2G, consists of:

phenol 2–2.5%
dextrose 20–25%
glycerine 20–25%
pyrogen-free water to 100%

In the syringe 4ml of this fluid is mixed with 1ml of 1:50 procaine solution in saline.

A 5ml syringe is used. Considerable pressure is required to force the fluid into the tough ligamentous attachments. Localisation prior to manipulation will generally have indicated the level but normally two ligaments are injected for good measure; in cases of doubt three may be infiltrated.

After the injection the patient is sore for the rest of the day. A total of three injections are given to each ligamento-periosteal site at weekly intervals and the patient is warned not to flex her thoracic spine until the sclerosis is fully established at the end of two months.

The patient lies prone and a grid is drawn on her back. One line runs down the mid-line intersected by three others at the mid-points between the spinous processes. The lateral boundaries of the grid overlie the facet joints about 1.5cm from the mid-line (*Figure 12.53*).

First the ligamento-periosteal junctions of the supraspinous ligaments are infiltrated. The needle is thrust vertically downwards where the cross-bar intersects the mid-line. After 1cm the needle is turned and angled proximally until it touches bone, and P2G 1ml is deposited along the underside of one spinous process (*Figure 12.54*). The needle is then partially withdrawn and the tip tilted distally to complete the injection along the superior ridge of the other spinous process (*Figures 12.55; 12.56*).

The adjacent levels are now infiltrated using the same technique.

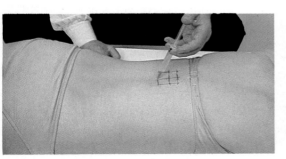

12.53

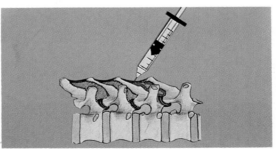

12.54

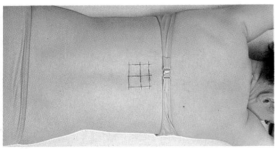

12.55

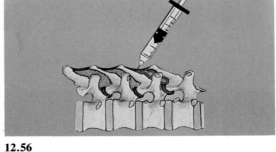

12.56

Fig 12.53 *The grid. The cross-bars are at the mid-point between tips of the spinous processes.*

Figs 12.54, 12.55, 12.56 *To infiltrate the supraspinous ligaments, the angle of insertion must be altered. Beads of fluid are injected all along the ligamento-periosteal junction.*

Next the facet joints are treated. The insertion is made vertically at the intersection of the cross-bar and the lateral line (*Figures 12.57; 12.58*). The needle hits bone at a depth of about 3cm and the edges of the joint are sought. A series of droplets is injected along its length, and the procedure repeated at the other side (*Figures 12.59, 12.60*) and then at the adjacent joints.

Patient and physician reconvene next week and the week after that for re-injection. If examination shows a displacement is present it is reduced by manipulation before infiltration.

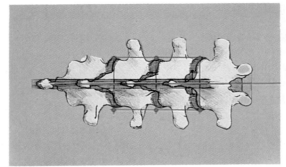

12.57

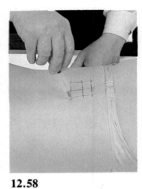

12.58

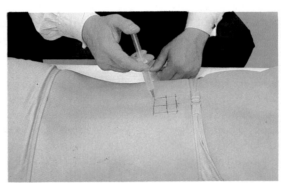

12.59

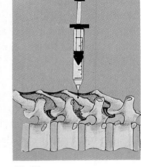

12.60

Fig 12.57 *The outer intersections on the grid overlie the facet joints.*

Figs 12.58, 12.59, 12.60 *Injection to the facet joints on both sides. A series of droplets are delivered at each requisite level.*

CHAPTER THIRTEEN

THE LUMBAR SPINE

Clinical examination shows that the great preponderance of lumbar disorders are attributable to disc lesions. Often this diagnosis is considered to be applicable only to severe cases with pain down the leg and with neurological deficit; in fact intervertebral displacements can be responsible for the mildest backache as well as for intermediate and severe symptoms. Here, as elsewhere at the spine, a displacement of disc material may move either posteriorly to compress the dura mater (*Figure 13.1*) giving rise to extrasegmental pain or laterally to compress the dural sleeve of a nerve root, which precipitates pain in the appropriate dermatome and weakness in the relevant muscle group.

At the cervical and thoracic levels treatment is simple: by and large, most and all displacements respectively are manipulated. At the lumbar spine the patient may require manipulation, traction, epidural local anaesthesia, sclerosants or a corset. In addition, a great deal can be done by way of prophylaxis. The correct response to each case depends not only on the examination but also on the patient's history which is of paramount importance. Only a tiny proportion of cases go to operation.

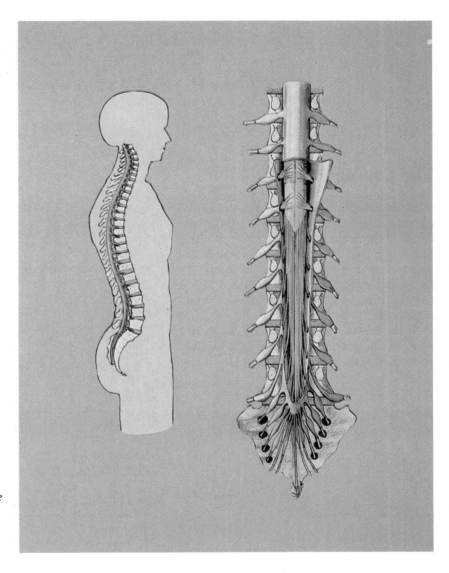

Fig 13.1 *The dura mater is a sensitive structure. The dural sheath to the nerve roots continues to the distal end of the intervertebral foramen; hence the phenomenon of root pain from disc pressure.*

The dura mater

A displacement of disc material compressing the dura mater will cause pain felt anywhere from the back of the trunk to the scapulae, anteriorly at the abdomen or groins, at the side of the sacrum or upper buttock, at the coccyx or down both legs to the calves (*Figure 13.2*). Dural pain will not be felt in the ankle or foot. If extrasegmental, the radiation of pain has no necessary bearing on the level of the articular lesion, although often the pain is perceived locally.

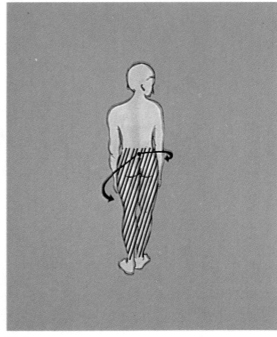

Fig 13.2 *Dural pain can be referred anywhere within this zone, but is less common down the legs. Note the feet are excluded.*

13.2

The nerve roots

A lateral disc displacement may interfere only with the dural sleeve of the nerve root or with the parenchyma as well. The former produces pain in any part of the dermatome; the latter weakness and/or paraesthesia. The roots commonly affected are L4, L5, S1 and S2; the corresponding dermatomes are illustrated in *Figures 13.3; 13.4; 13.5; 13.6.*

As the nerves emerge obliquely, any root signs may be polyradicular. The joint itself is insensitive to internal derangement.

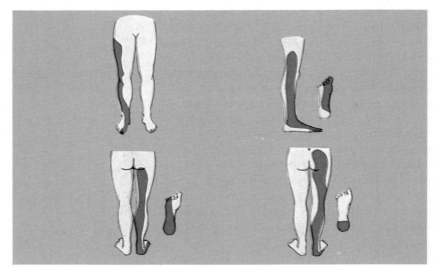

13.3, 13.4, 13.5, 13.6

Figs 13.3, 13.4, 13.5, 13.6 *The dermatomes of the commonly affected nerve roots. L4 (top left). L5 (top right). S1 (lower left). S2 (lower right).*

The disc

A displacement may be composed of cartilage or part of the *nucleus pulposus*. Nuclear material engenders backache or root pain of slow onset over some hours as the nucleus seeps through the cracked disc; since the displacement is semi-liquid and cannot be clicked back into place by manipulation, the treatment of choice is traction.

By the age of 60 the disc has become uniform throughout in substance and the nucleus has disappeared; thus in the elderly the question of whether a displacement is nuclear or cartilaginous is not at issue. At that age and after, all appropriate displacements are manipulated. Annular protrusions outnumber nuclear lesions by a factor of about two.

History

Displacements

The physician takes an exhaustive history, ascertaining—in chronological order—when the pain started, what brought it on, what the symptoms were then, what they are now, whether they spread, if so where to, whether the pain is constant or intermittent, whether a cough hurts, and whether the pain and the degree of disability are slight, moderate or severe. Based on this information he will decide:

(1) Whether it is a disc lesion or one of the uncommon causes of backache.
(2) On the type of any disc lesion present (hard/soft, large/small, central/unilateral, stable/unstable, primary posterolateral onset, etc.).
(3) On the type of patient and whether the described degree of pain and disablement tallies with his appearance and known daily activities.

History affords the clearest indications on how to treat a disc lesion. It also sorts out backache from other sources as only a few disorders (e.g. internal derangement) give rise to episodic pain and only intermittent internal derangement repeatedly fixes a joint within its range of movement. A lengthy history running back over the years of itself excludes serious progressive disease.

Pain from a disc lesion arises only from pressure exerted on the dura mater or the nerve root. So there is a threshold to the different events which can take place in the closed cavity lying in the mid-line of the lumbar area. 'All discs are alike and all other disorders are different' is a sound working maxim.

It will be found that pain from a disc lesion is connected with posture, activity and exertion. It can be brought on by, for example, digging. In due course a central protrusion tends to shift posterolaterally to the nerve root, producing symptoms in the limb. The initial minor protrusion interferes with the movement of the joint and not the nerve root so local pain and articular signs are thus at their most obvious when neurological signs are lacking. But when the protrusion has passed posterolaterally it interferes little with joint movement. Thus root pain and clear neurological signs supervene as the articular symptoms fade.

The mode of onset varies from a gradual ache to the abrupt fixation of lumbago. A cough is often painful. Sciatica unaccompanied by backache recovers of itself in 12 months, but there is no such time limit to backache.

Examination is conducted for:

(1) Bone signs.
(2) Joint signs.
(3) Dural signs.
(4) Nerve root mobility.
(5) Nerve root conduction.

Examination

After a careful history the patient undresses and the back is inspected in a good light. If an angular kyphosis is present, a vertebral body may have become wedge-shaped due to tuberculous caries, neoplasm or fracture. Localised osteitis deformans, senile osteoporosis and spondylolisthesis are often symptomless. The latter is frequently visible and palpable when the patient stands even though the radiograph taken with the patient lying shows no abnormality.

A displacement of disc material can produce characteristic deviation (*Figure 13.7*); if gross, it is more likely to result from a fourth rather than a fifth lumbar disc lesion because of the stabilising effect of the iliolumbar ligaments.

The posture of lumbago (*Figure 13.8*) indicates the sacrospinalis muscles cannot be in spasm as the patient is fixed in flexion not extension. However the muscles do contract normally to prevent the patient toppling further forwards.

The physician checks to see if the pelvis is horizontal (*Figure 13.9*) or oblique. Seven per cent of the population have a difference of 1.2cm or more in the length of their legs; usually this is nothing to worry about. All the same, if one leg is found to be shorter than the other the examiner slides a series of thin platforms under the sole of the short leg until the pelvis is level. In the event that this eases or abolishes the pain on standing, a raised heel should be worn indefinitely.

The patient points to the area of her pain. When a disc lesion results in local discomfort this is felt on a level with or just below the joint affected (generally L4 or L5). First and second lumbar disc lesions are extremely rare so care must be exercised against ascribing pain felt at upper and mid-lumbar levels to a disc.

If the pain spread down the leg, the physician establishes whether the pain in the back increased at the same time. If so, it is a danger signal showing the lesion is spreading (e.g.metastases) rather than shifting (e.g. a disc displacement). If the pain came on first in the leg (i.e. primary posterolateral onset) this contraindicates manipulation and indicates traction.

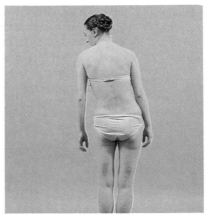

13.7

Fig 13.7 *A disc lesion at L4 may make the patient deviate. In genuine cases, the patient compensates by holding shoulders level and head upright.*

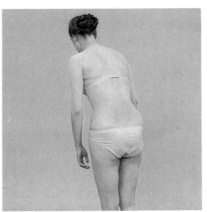

13.8

Fig 13.8 *Attribution of lumbago to errector muscle spasm is remarkable in view of the patient's flexed posture.*

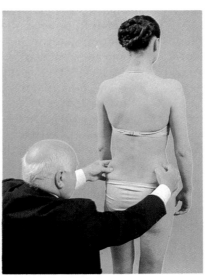

13.9

Fig 13.9 *Checking for lateral tilt of the pelvis. Inequality of leg length is not necessarily painful.*

Joint signs

The joint is now examined. There is no appreciable rotation at the lumbar spine and hence only four movements are undertaken; they are active but, because of the body weight, are passive in their diagnostic import. Passive extension (*Figure 13.10*) is the first.

Both side flexions are performed (*Figures 13.11; 13.12*). All serious diseases of the lumbar spine result in equal limitation of both side flexions.

Flexion (*Figure 13.13*) is the movement most likely to be limited by a lumbar disc lesion. A painful arc may be noted as the displacement is shifted by alteration in the angulation of the joint surfaces. This is pathognomonic of a disc lesion and excludes neurosis, since a patient suffering psychogenic symptoms is unlikely to allege his pain disappears as flexion increases.

Alternatively, the patient may deviate during flexion. The deviation, which materialises as the patient seeks to minimise traction on the dura or nerve root, is also pathognomic.

A displacement will block part of the joint causing pain and/or limitation (unequal in different directions) on some but not all movements. However, in lumbago all four movements are apt to hurt, but the degree of pain and limitation still differ for each movement (*cf.* the capsular pattern).

The patient now moves to the couch and her manner of so doing should correspond with her disablement. So in suspected malingering the patient is enjoined to swing herself round with legs extended (*Figure 13.14*). If this does not hurt, it amounts to a finding both of 90° of painless trunk flexion and of full painless straight-leg raise. A genuine patient will manoeuvre with caution (*Figure 13.15*).

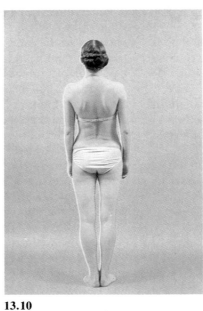

13.10

Fig 13.10 *Extension. The lumbar movements may evoke or alter the symptoms. Range may be full or limited.*

Figs 13.11, 13.12 *The side flexions. Consider if any limitation is capsular or non-capsular.*

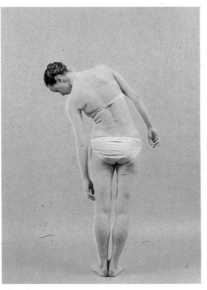

13.11

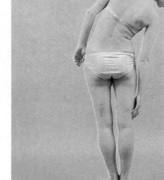

13.12

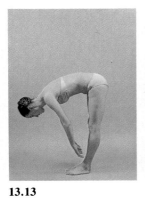

13.13

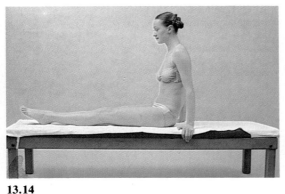

13.14

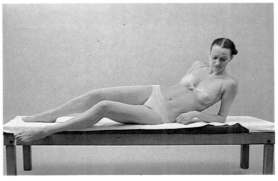

13.15

Fig 13.13 *Flexion is left till last, as an ache persisting afterwards might obscure the response to other movements.*

Fig 13.14 *Getting onto the couch. Postures achieved by the unsupervised patient can be revealing. The position above is inconsistent with limited flexion.*

Fig 13.15 *A genuine patient may have to move very carefully.*

Dural signs: straight-leg raising

The patient lies supine and her straight-leg raise is tested (*Figure 13.16*).

Raising the leg with the knee extended pulls on the dura mater via the sciatic nerve running down the back of the leg. Straight-leg raise thus stretches the dura (*Figures 13.17; 13.18; 13.19*). If the normal mobility of the membrane is impeded by a central disc protrusion then straight-leg raise will cause pain and may be limited bilaterally.

Likewise, straight-leg raising pulls on the L4, L5, S1 and S2 nerve roots, one or two of which may be fixed by a lateral disc protrusion. In such a case there will be pain and unilateral limitation.

Straight-leg raising is thus a test for dural mobility (bilateral limitation) and nerve root mobility at L4, L5, S1 and S2 (unilateral limitation). In practice, L4 root pressure sometimes gives rise to bilateral limitation.

Pain on full straight-leg raising suggests a small protrusion and is also common in elderly patients' sciatica and after laminectomy. Much backache (unlike lumbago) produces no limitation of straight-leg raising. A painful arc can be explained by a protrusion so small that the dura mater or nerve root merely catches against it and slips over.

Limited straight-leg raising may be accompanied by neurological signs established later. This double finding indicates a greater degree of pressure involving the parenchyma as well as the sheath of the nerve root, and has important bearings on treatment.

If neck flexion (*Figure 13.20*) increases the pain, involvement of the dura is confirmed because the tissue whose mobility is impaired must run from the neck to the calf. Attention is thereby confined to the dura mater and its continuation as the sciatic nerve.

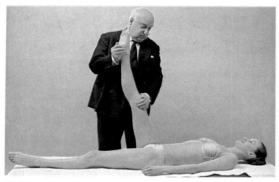

13.16

Fig **13.16** *Straight-leg raising. The larger the protrusion, the greater the limitation. Full range shown.*

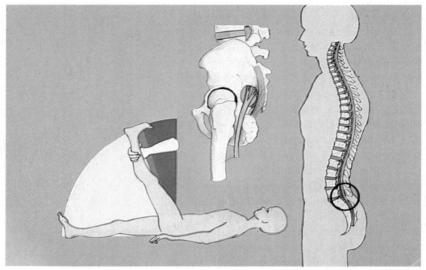

13.17, 13.18, 13.19

Figs **13.17, 13.18, 13.19** *Flexing the hip with the knee extended (left) pulls on the dura mater (right) via the sciatic nerve (centre).*

Fig **13.20** *Neck flexion pulls the dural tube upwards by an average of 3cm. It may exacerbate pain.*

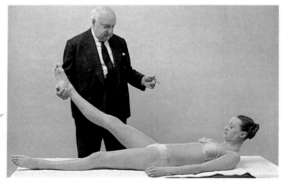

13.20

Root signs

Next the sacroiliac joint, the hip joint and the external aspect of the lumbar nerve roots are examined. A disc lesion interfering not just with mobility of the nerve root (i.e. painful limitation of straight-leg raising) but also with motor conduction of the parenchyma will produce muscle weakness. So the resisted movements of the leg will prove weak rather than painful; the signs may be referable to more than one root. Except in acute lumbago none of the following movements will increase pain from a displacement.

The anterior sacroiliac ligaments are stretched (*Figure 13.21*) by downward and outward pressure applied to the anterior superior spines of the ilia. Should this bring on the pain—as opposed to merely proving uncomfortable centrally—the sacroiliac joint is examined in detail.

Resisted hip flexion (*Figure 13.22*) may be weak—the L2 or L3 root—or possibly painful, implicating the psoas. The patient presses her thigh upwards with the operator's counterpressure restraining her shoulder.

For resisted dorsiflexion the patient pushes her foot upwards against the doctor's resistance (*Figure 13.23*); if this is weak the L4 root is incriminated.

Impairment of conduction of the L4 or L5 root is indicated by painless weakness on resisted extension of the hallux (*Figure 13.24*).

Painless weakness on resisted eversion (*Figure 13.25*) suggests a lesion of the L5 or S1 roots.

The knee jerk (*Figure 13.26*) may be absent or sluggish in L3 lesions.

The patient turns over and her ankle jerk is tested (*Figure 13.27*); if absent or sluggish, this denotes involvement of the S1, S2 or occasionally the L5 root.

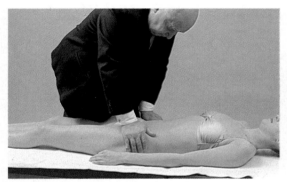

13.21

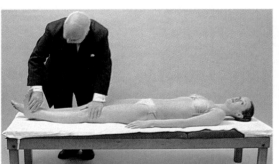

13.23

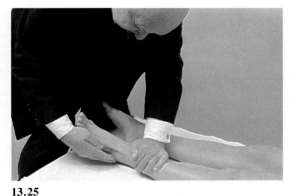

13.25

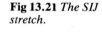

13.22

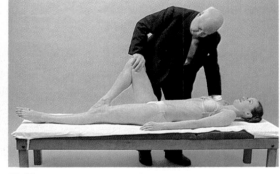

13.24

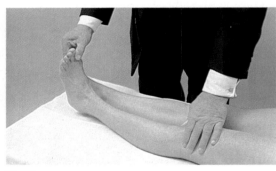

13.26

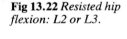

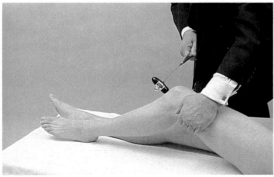

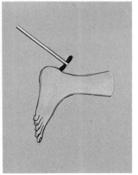

13.27

Fig 13.21 *The SIJ stretch.*

Fig 13.22 *Resisted hip flexion: L2 or L3.*

Fig 13.23 *Resisted dorsiflexion: L4.*

Fig 13.24 *Resisted toe extension: L4 or L5.*

Fig 13.25 *Resisted eversion: L5 or S1.*

Fig 13.26 *The knee jerk: L3.*

Fig 13.27 *The ankle jerk: S1 or S2.*

The mobility of the third lumbar root is checked by passive knee flexion in prone-lying (*Figure 13.28*), a procedure analogous to straight-leg raising. The root is stretched via the femoral nerve which passes to the front of the knee (and is thus relaxed by straight-leg raising itself). In L3 lesions, passive knee flexion tends to be painful at full range rather than limited.

Weakness of the quadriceps muscles is assessed by resisted knee extension as the patient tries to force her leg downwards (*Figure 13.29*). This tests the integrity of the L3 nerve root; the normal patient is stronger than the examiner.

Weakness of the hamstrings showing impairment of conduction down the S1 or S2 nerve roots is detected on resisted knee flexion; the patient presses her leg upwards (*Figure 13.30*). This time the examiner is stronger than the normal patient.

The patient is asked to squeeze her buttocks together and the examiner tests the bulk of the muscles by pinching the gluteal mass (*Figure 13.31*). Wasting is attributable to involvement of the S1 or S2 roots.

The strength of the calf muscles is assessed by asking the patient to stand on tip-toe on one leg at a time (*Figure 13.32*). The nerve roots are S1 and S2. In practice this test is normally earmarked for the beginning of the examination when the patient is still standing.

Finally, analgesia is sought on the dorsum of the foot and the toes.

An L4 distribution occupies the big toe only, L5 the big toe and the two adjacent toes and S1 the outer two toes. The underside of the heel is S2.

Although the spinal cord itself terminates at L1, the plantar reflex (*Figure 13.33*) should be tested as a matter of course; if intermittent claudication is suspected, pulsation at the ankle is checked.

During the examination the physician runs through the root signs working down the limb in an order suited to the patient's convenience. On pages 219–222 the signs are displayed root by root in summary form.

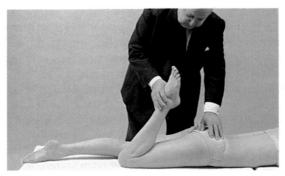

13.28

Fig **13.28** *Passive knee flexion: L3.*

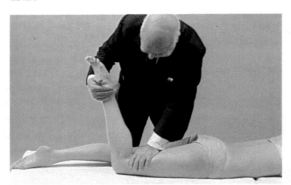

13.29

Fig **13.29** *Resisted knee extension: L3.*

Fig **13.30** *Resisted knee flexion: S1 or S2.*

Fig **13.31** *Gluteal wasting: S1 or S2.*

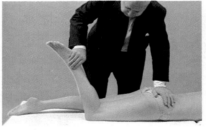
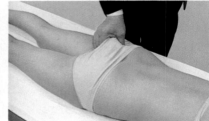
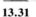

13.30   **13.31**

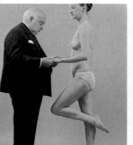
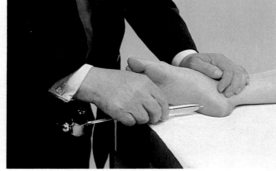

13.32   **13.33**

Fig **13.32** *Calf muscles: S1 or S2.*   Fig **13.33** *Plantar reflex.*

Findings

Capsular lesions

All serious disorders of the lumbar spine result in limitation of movement in all directions (*Figures 13.34; 13.35; 13.36*). But because the amount of flexion and extension attainable by a normal individual are so markedly different, the capsular pattern is most easily recognised by equal limitation of both side flexions. Even with no flexion of the lumbar spine itself the patient may still be able to touch her knees by bending at the hip (*Figure 13.37*).

Tuberculosis, neoplasm, chronic osteomyelitis, recent fractures, ankylosing spondylitis and osteitis deformans all produce the capsular pattern; all are visible radiographically.

A practiced eye is required to detect the capsular pattern since the range of side flexion ordinarily diminishes with age. Maximum side flexion attainable in youth can be favourably contrasted with that achieved by those of advancing years, even in the absence of any affection (*Figure 13.38*). Clinical judgement will assess what is normal for any age group.

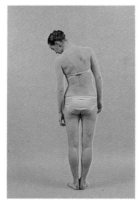
13.34

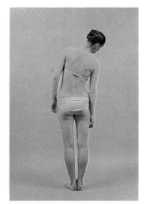
13.35

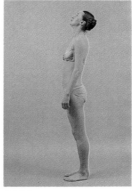
13.36

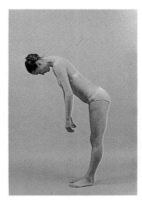
13.37

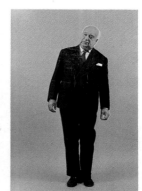
13.38

Figs 13.34, 13.35, 13.36, 13.37 *The capsular pattern in a young adult. The most distinctive feature is the equal limitation of side flexions. Flexion itself is largely achieved by movement at the hips (Fig 13.37).*

Fig 13.38 *Limitation of side flexion is a normal finding in the elderly.*

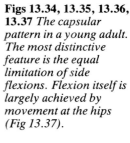

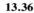

The radiograph

A number of conditions occur which, although visible radiographically, either never cause pain or only sometimes cause it. In the former category come Schmorl's nodes, osteoarthrosis, osteophytosis (unless posterior) and adolescent osteochondrosis. Spondylolisthesis and osteoporosis may sometimes produce symptoms of themselves.

But their detection on the X-ray should not lead to abandonment of the search for an alternative cause of pain until the physician is certain the history and findings on clinical examination so warrant.

A large number of non-disc lesions give rise to pain. These conditions, including the above, are outlined at pages 218–219.

Displacements

A lumbar disc lesion may be characterised by:
(1) A history consistent with a displacement.
(2) Pain and limitation of the lumbar movements in the non-capsular pattern characteristic of a displacement.
(3) Dural symptoms and signs.
(4) Nerve root symptoms and signs (impaired mobility).

(5) Nerve root symptoms and signs (impaired conduction).

Often items (3), (4) and (5) will be absent, leaving the diagnosis to be founded on history and the movements alone, reinforced by attendant congruous negative findings.

The propensity of the various spinal levels

for disc lesions is in the approximate proportions of:

    L1:   1:10,000
    L2:   1:1000
    L3:   1:20
    L4 and L5: Account for the remainder (i.e. nearly all disc lesions) about equally.

At L3 and above, a disc lesion (rare) protruding laterally may impinge on one root only of corresponding number. A disc lesion at L4 may affect either the L4 or the L5 root or both.

A disc lesion at L5 may compress one or two of the L5, S1 and S2 roots.

Both the S3 and S4 roots (caution) may be threatened by either the L4 or the L5 disc. The various combinations are tabulated on page 219.

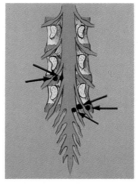

13.39

Fig 13.39 *The root(s) compressed at each level vary with the precise site of displacement.*

Disc lesions: anomalies

The behaviour of disc lesions at L1 and L2 (both very rare) is unconventional. The protrusions are nearly all nuclear. The pain arises gradually when a certain posture is maintained and disappears when the posture is altered. Lesions at these levels do better with traction than with manipulation.

The so-called 'mushroom phenomenon' responds neither to traction nor to manipulation. The patient is elderly and the intervertebral disc largely eroded so that the gap between the vertebrae, originally standing at about 1cm, is now in the region of 1mm. This means the posterior longitudinal ligament is extremely lax and any posterior protrusion of residual disc material bulges it out with ease to compress the dura mater.

The history is distinctive. The pain starts after the patient has stood for a while and the body weight has compressed the joints. Disc material then protrudes posteriorly. The symptoms may consist of either backache with dural pain spreading to both limbs, or unilateral root pain without backache. The pain stops almost at once when the patient relieves the joint from weightbearing by lying down.

Confirmation of the diagnosis may be obtained if the pain ceases immediately on bending forwards; this tightens the posterior longitudinal ligament thus reducing the protrusion instantly. The patient is over 60. The condition (pain on standing) must be differentiated from spinal claudication (pain on walking).

The central backache can be relieved by arthrodesis and the root pain by an injection of steroid suspension at the nerve root itself.

Treatment

Summary

There are three main conservative treatments for a lumbar disc lesion:

(1) Manipulation (see pages 194–205).
(2) Traction (see pages 206–209).
(3) Epidural local anaesthesia (see pages 210–214).

Relapse may be dealt with either by sclerosants (see page 215) and/or a corset (see page 217), both administered after reduction of the displacement. Only a tiny proportion of cases require—or are appropriate for—the drastic remedy of surgery.

Manipulation

Manipulation of the lumbar joints follows exactly the same principles as elsewhere and the general remarks in Chapters 10 and 12 should be noted. But the joints are so large and strong that manual traction makes no impact and accordingly is discarded; hence there is no need for assistants. Sessions last 20 minutes or so and after each manipulation the patient is re-examined to assess progress.

Various techniques of increasing strength may be tried. Most benefit materialises during the first two sessions; it is rare that a fourth encounter brings further improvement.

A low couch about 15 inches high is required. It must be firm.

Absolute bars to manipulation

(1) Spinal cord signs (but these will be absent as the cord ends at L1).
(2) Signs of impingement on the fourth sacral root. Sacro-perineal numbness or weakness of the bladder or anus are danger signals. Pain is felt in the perineum, rectum and scrotum. All these symptoms, which emerge during the history, suggest that the posterior ligament is bulging considerably and is possibly partly ruptured. Manipulation might rupture it completely and allow massive extrusion of the entire disc.
(3) Bilateral sciatica unaccompanied by backache. The posterior ligament is attacked from both sides by a disc lesion and may be ruptured by manipulation.
(4) Spinal claudication implies considerable distortion of the posterior ligament; manipulation should be avoided. Walking causes pins and needles in both feet which cease as soon as the walking stops.
(5) Anticoagulant treatment contraindicates manipulation as intraspinal haematoma formation has been reported.

Note also:

(1) Hyperacute lumbago renders manipulation intolerable. The patient is rigid with pain:
    (a) When asked to lie prone it takes some minutes to roll over.
    (b) Gentle pressure to the patient's back sets up unbearable pain.
    Induction of epidural local anaesthesia should be carried out *stat.* (see page 210). Reasonably severe lumbago responds well to manipulation, often with immediate relief.
(2) Pregnancy should be disregarded for the first four months. For the next four, supine and side-lying rotations may be used, but during the last month manipulation is best avoided.

(3) In a case of genuine organic symptoms coupled with psychogenic exaggeration, manipulation may be cautiously attempted having first warned the patient that a 'post-manipulative crisis' may strike briefly some hours following recovery. Cases of pure neurosis should be left well alone.

Manipulation may not succeed

The sole indication for spinal manipulation is a cartilaginous disc displacement. About one-third of lumbar displacements are nuclear, except in patients over 60 where all are cartilaginous. Primary posterolateral protrusions (i.e. sciatica without immediately preceding backache) all appear to be nuclear.

Manipulation will not avail in the following cases:

(1) Pain down the leg with root signs (i.e. weakness, sluggish or absent reflex or analgesia). The protrusion is too large.
(2) Root pain (unaccompanied by significant backache) which has been down the leg for six months or more in a patient under 60.
(3) Sciatica with lumbar deformity. If there is root pain with little or no backache (*cf.* backache with slight sciatica) together with considerable lateral deviation at the lumbar spine when the patient stands normally, manipulation usually fails. The protrusion is too large. Side flexion barely reaches the vertical and shoots a pain down the lower limb.
(4) Sciatica without backache, with the patient fixed in slight flexion, normally proves intractable except by laminectomy. Any attempt to stand erect sends twinges down the lower leg. The protrusion is too large.
(5) The patient is under 60 and:
    (a) Any trunk movement other than flexion increases or brings on the pain in the lower limb.
    (b) Side flexion in a patient with backache hurts on the side towards which the patient leans.
    In both cases the displacement is probably nuclear and will benefit from traction.
(6) Post-laminectomy. Manipulation seldom succeeds although there is no harm in trying, particularly if there is a fresh protrusion at another joint. But traction stands a good chance.
(7) If there is sciatic pain without backache and the reasonably intense root symptoms are subsiding, it is best to steer clear of both manipulation and traction. The patient is over the worst and epidural local anaesthesia is the route to follow.

Rotation strains

Despite engagement of the articular processes at each facet joint to limit rotation, a rotation strain is a highly effective way of securing reduction at low lumbar levels. The manipulator always embarks on a session with Rotation Strain—1 and then progresses as necessary to the more severe rotations. However with the elderly or those suffering minor protrusions, following incomplete reduction by Rotation Strain—1 it may be thought best to move on to the milder extension strains.

For all rotation strains the patient lies on her painless side. This means the distracting force opens the joint on the bad side thus allowing the displacement room to move. When maximum benefit has been afforded by any particular manoeuvre, the patient is rotated in the opposite direction although still lying on her painless side. If the pain seems to be central, straight-leg raise usually elucidates the situation by proving painful unilaterally. In the absence of any indicator, the manipulator proceeds by trial and error.

Rotation strain—1

The patient lies on her painless side, with her upper thigh flexed to bring the femoral trochanter into prominence (*Figure 13.40*). The manipulation consists of twisting the patient's trunk during distraction.

The manipulator uses one hand to push the trochanter forwards and the other to force the front of the shoulder downwards: this preliminary measure rotates the patient's trunk in opposite directions.

As the manipulator leans forward the body weight is used to secure additional rotation and also to distract the lumbar joints. Distraction is achieved as one hand is impelled sideways towards the patient's head and the other hand sideways towards her feet (*Figure 13.41*).

A physiotherapist of slighter build may have to lean forwards very considerably to achieve the same effect (*Figure 13.42*).

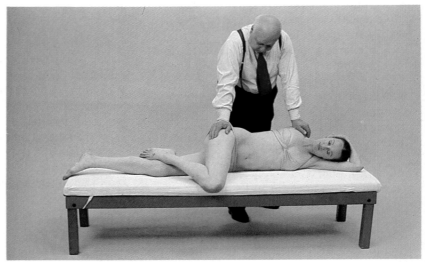

13.40

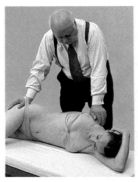 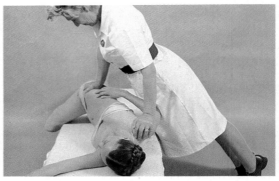

13.41 **13.42**

Fig 13.40 *Starting position. The patient's trunk will be rotated in opposite directions. Note the low couch and the absence of any assistants.*

Figs 13.41, 13.42 *Starting position. The hands are in contact with the skin to avoid slippage. Note how a physiotherapist of lighter build uses all her body weight.*

After a few seconds of sustained pressure, the overstrain is applied by the manipulator jerking his body forwards to increase momentarily both rotation and distraction (*Figures 13.43, 13.44*).

The patient is re-examined and if benefit has resulted the manoeuvre is repeated. If not, succeeding variants are tried. It is worth remembering that when a patient returns for a second treatment after improvement at the first it may be best to omit Rotation Strain—1 and go straight to which ever variant was previously found the best.

Caution
If the manipulation sets up pain felt in the lower limb, the rotary methods are dispensed with and the manipulations towards extension tried instead. If they too shoot pain down the lower limb, manipulation ceases altogether.

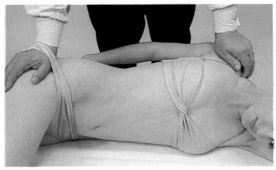

13.43

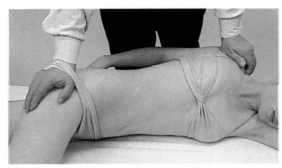

13.44

Figs 13.43, 13.44
Starting and finishing positions.

Re-examination: an example
If straight-leg raise was previously limited this is now reassessed; a decrease in limitation (*Figures 13.45a, 13.45b*) indicates a corresponding diminution of the displacement and would encourage the operator to try the same manoeuvre again, before progressing to stronger measures if necessary. Straight-leg raise is a highly sensitive indicator and full painless range may well be attained before reduction is complete. If this happens—or if straight-leg raise was full and painless to start with—the patient is tested by her lumbar movements, checking both that the bad ones are better and the good ones no worse. If a cough was originally painful the patient is asked to cough again.

Subject to the general remarks on page 142, if the patient is improved the procedure is repeated and the patient re-examined. In due course, after maximum benefit has been attained, the manipulator progresses to Rotation Strain—2.

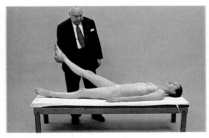

Figs 13.45a

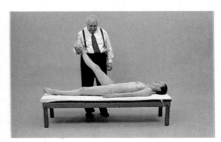

13.45b

Figs 13.45a, 13.45b
Re-examination. Straight-leg raising before (left) and after the manipulation (right) is a sensitive indicator of progress. Once it is full, the lumbar movements are tested instead.

Rotation strain—2

This is the reverse of its predecessor: during distraction the pelvis is forced towards the operator and the shoulder away (*Figure 13.46*). The patient lies on her pain-free side.

The operator curves one hand round the anterior iliac spine and places the palm of his other hand on her upper thorax against the spine of the scapula (*Figure 13.47*).

The manipulator leans forwards over the patient, stretching her thorax and pelvis apart by pushing outwards. Rotation is gradually increased (*Figure 13.48*).

To apply his overpressure the manipulator jerks his body downwards and simultaneously forces his arms further apart and into rotation, drawing the iliac spine in towards him and thrusting the scapula down and away (*Figure 13.49*).

The patient is re-examined and if improvement is evident the manoeuvre is repeated. If not, a stronger rotation strain may be obtained by Rotation Strain—3.

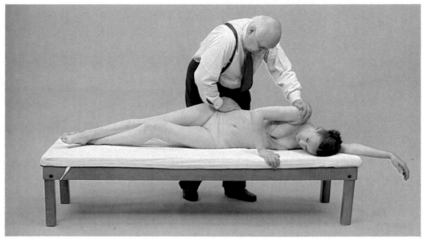

13.46

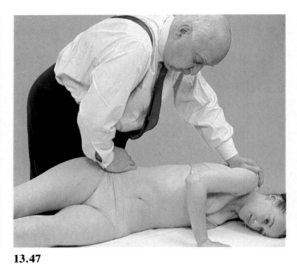

13.47

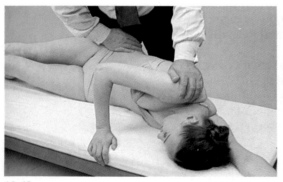

13.48

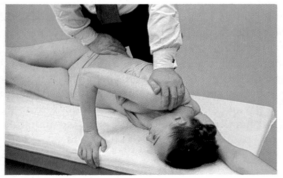

13.49

Figs 13.46, 13.47
Starting position. The operator takes the patient to the extreme of comfortable range.

Figs 13.48, 13.49
Starting and finishing position. The forceful overthrust momentarily pushes the patient's shoulder towards her ear and her pelvis towards supination.

Rotation strain—3

Both this manipulation and its successor, Rotation Strain—4, are contraindicated in patients with arthritis of the hip and in the elderly with whom the strength of the femur is unreliable. This caveat applies because the thigh is enlisted as a lever; it is held horizontally and pulled into extension towards the manipulator while the shoulder is pinned to the couch. The patient is lying on her painless side (*Figure 13.50*).

The operator's knee abuts against the patient's lower buttock to steady her on the couch. One hand bears down on the shoulder; the body weight is applied here while the other hand fully extends and adducts the hip joint (*Figure 13.51*).

The overpressure is applied by the manipulator maintaining pressure on the patient's shoulder while he rotates his thorax and jerks the thigh sharply upwards (*Figure 13.52*). The patient is re-examined.

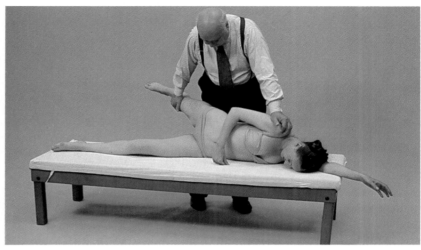

13.50

Figs 13.50, 13.51 *Starting position. Extension of the hip is most clearly shown in Fig 13.50.*

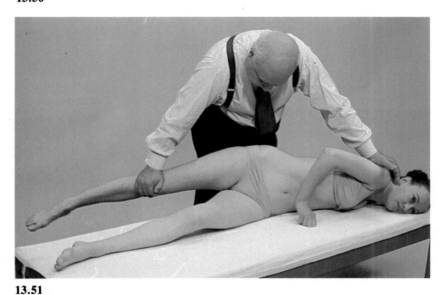

13.51

Fig 13.52 *Finishing position. Note how the movement is assisted by the operator leaning towards the patient's head; he swivels his thorax to achieve added extension of the patient's hip.*

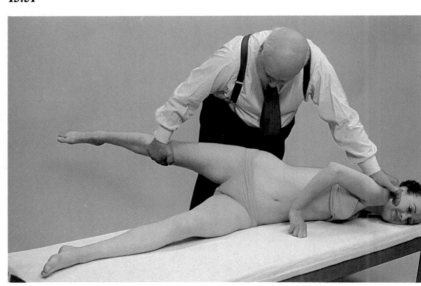

13.52

Rotation strain—4

This manipulation, like Rotation Strain—3, affords maximum rotation but little distraction and similarly should be avoided with the elderly or those with arthritis of the hip. Again the thigh is used as a lever, but this time it is forced downwards (*Figure 13.53*).

The patient lies face upwards, well towards the side on which the manipulator stands and he employs his knee to steady her trunk and keep her on the couch. Then he flexes her hip to a right angle and applies his other hand to her shoulder. It is over this arm that his body weight is concentrated in order to ensure the patient's thorax is maintained flat on the couch (*Figure 13.54*).

Muscular force is used to press the knee sharply towards the floor and rotate the lumbar spine (*Figure 13.55*).

The patient is re-examined and the manoeuvre repeated if benefit has accrued. In patients who hold the spine vertical without lumbar deviation it is often best to start with the hip flexed to rather less than a right-angle.

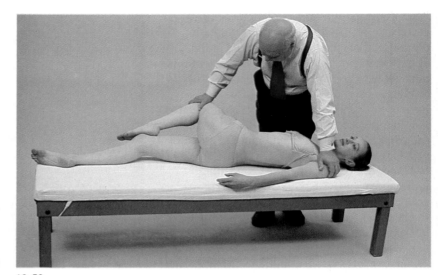

13.53

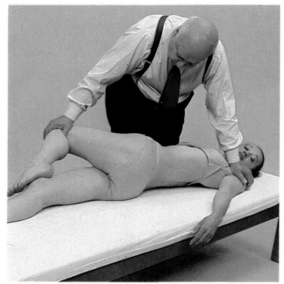

13.54

Figs 13.53, 13.54 *Starting position. The body weight is balanced over the patient's shoulder, clamping it to the couch.*

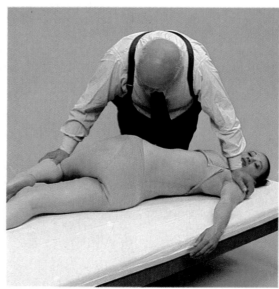

13.55

Fig 13.55 *Finishing position. The operator half-turns as his hands are thrust downwards and apart.*

Rotation strain—5

This is a variation on Rotation Strain—4. Downward pressure is again delivered to the thigh at the knee, but this leg is also used to achieve side flexion transmitted via the other leg hooked over (*Figure 13.56*).

For the starting position the patient flexes her knees and crosses her legs, the leg on the painless side uppermost. The operator stands opposite the painful side and places his hand on the lower knee. The other hand is on the patient's shoulder, fixing the upper part of the trunk flat on the couch; it is over this arm that the body weight is poised (*Figure 13.57*).

The downward pressure on the knee is stepped up until tissue resistance is felt heralding the end of range. During this stage the patient's free knee is kept in position by pressure against the operator. Sharp overstrain then forces the knee further downwards, rotating the lumbar spine while simultaneously achieving side flexion towards the painless side (*Figure 13.58*).

The patient is re-examined. The manipulation is often successful for those with considerable lateral deviation. For the other methods of correction of lateral deviation the reader is referred to page 205.

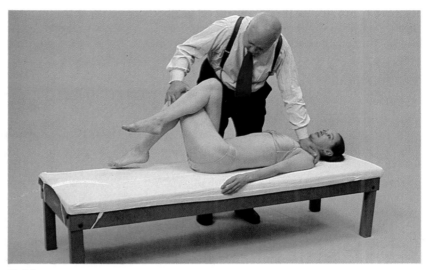

13.56

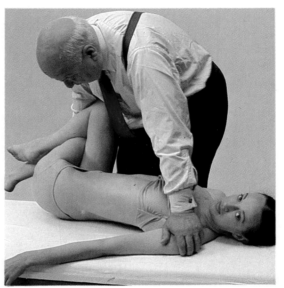

13.57

Figs 13.56, 13.57 *Starting position. This time it is the hip on the good side which is flexed over the other leg and used as a lever.*

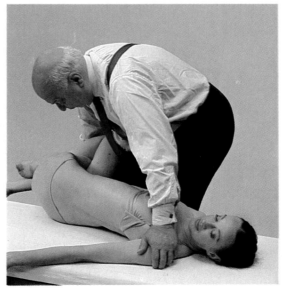

13.58

Fig 13.58 *Finishing position. The operator's body pressure against the good thigh fixes the lumbar spine in side flexion, while the rotation is imparted by a sharp thrust on the bad knee.*

Extension strains

The extension strains are best reserved for the elderly or those with a minor protrusion. It is unlikely they will engineer much improvement on a patient who has already been through the rotary methods, but they may be useful for the new or more nervous patient.

Forced extension—1

This manipulation consists of pressing down sharply at the site of the displacement (*Figure 13.59*).

One hand is placed so that the mid-shaft of the fifth metacarpal bone engages against the prominence formed by the spinous process of the relevant vertebra (*Figure 13.60*). This will almost certainly be L4 or L5.

The other hand is used for reinforcement (*Figure 13.61*). Only the ulnar border of the lower hand is in contact with the patient, thus localising the pressure.

The manipulator leans on the patient's back for a few seconds to secure some extension and then bends his head and thorax abruptly forwards using body weight to give the final jerk. As he does so each upper limb is kept rigid, to act as a stiff rod communicating the thrust of the manipulator's trunk (*Figure 13.62*). The patient is re-examined.

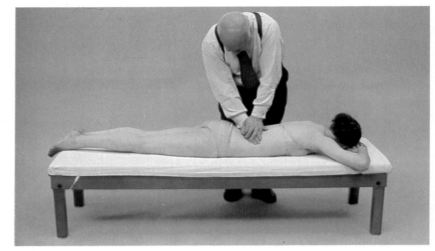

13.59

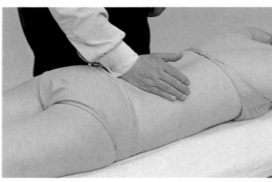

13.60

Figs 13.59, 13.60, 13.61 *Starting position. One hand is tilted; the other is cupped over it.*

Fig 13.62 *The overthrust. The manipulator leans sharply forwards.*

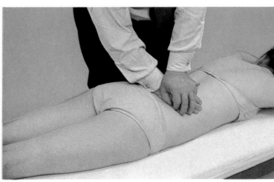

13.61

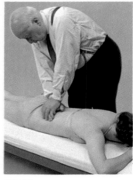

13.62

Forced extension—2

This manipulation is all but identical to Forced Extension—1 except that the operator's hands are placed further over, away from the patient's mid-line (*Figure 13.63*). This means that the weight of the thrust is medial as well as downwards and thus produces a significant amount of rotation.

The operator stands on the patient's bad side; it is this side of the joint which will be opened.

Both hands are applied to the patient's good side with the forearm just short of pronation.

The other hand is again used for reinforcement (*Figure 13.64*) and the operator leans right over the patient and presses until all the play has been taken out of the joint.

He then jerks his head and thorax downwards, keeping his arms rigid to apply the overpressure which is directed towards himself (*Figure 13.65*).

The patient is re-examined. If some benefit has been secured the procedure is repeated, and subsequently the pressure is administered to the other side of the mid-line.

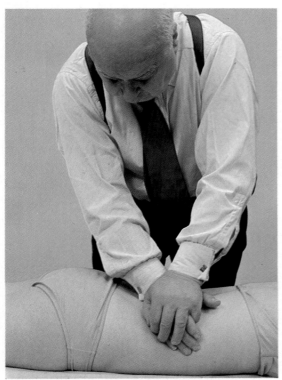

13.63

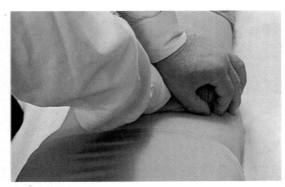

13.64

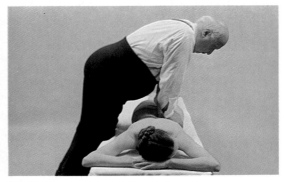

13.65

Fig 13.63 *Starting position. The hands are well to the side of the mid-line.*

Fig 13.64 *Configuration of the hands.*

Fig 13.65 *The overpressure. The operator uses all his body weight.*

Forced extension—3

A stronger extension strain can be obtained by using the thigh as a lever (*Figure 13.66*). This is particularly productive where partial reduction has already been achieved, but the technique should not be adopted if previous extension strains have resulted in no improvement.

The operator stands on the side away from the patient's pain. The ulnar border of one hand bears down just above the posterior spine of the ilium, while the hip is extended and strongly adducted to open the lumbar joints (*Figure 13.67*).

The lumbar hand is pressed down and the knee hand pulled sharply up. The movement is assisted by the manipulator leaning heavily towards the patient's head (*Figure 13.68*).

The patient is re-examined. If some benefit has accrued the movement is repeated.

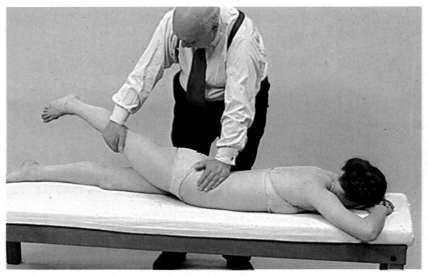

13.66

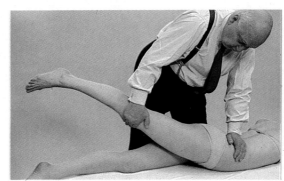

13.67

Figs 13.66, 13.67 *Starting position. The operator's right hand pulls up, his left hand pushes down well lateral to the spine.*

Fig 13.68 *Finishing position. The operator pulls the thigh up and towards himself.*

13.68

Forced extension—4

This is a stronger version of the previous manipulation, suitable for dealing with a heavily-built patient. The added force is obtained by using the knee to apply downward lumbar pressure (*Figure 13.69*). Like its predecessor, this manipulation is omitted if previous extension strains have resulted in no benefit.

The manipulator stands on the patient's painful side, and the hip is again strongly adducted and extended to its utmost, lifting the patient's pelvis off the couch (*Figure 13.70*).

The overthrust is applied by pressing down with the knee while raising the patient's thigh towards further extension and adduction (*Figure 13.71*).

The patient is re-examined and, if necessary, the final extension manipulation is employed.

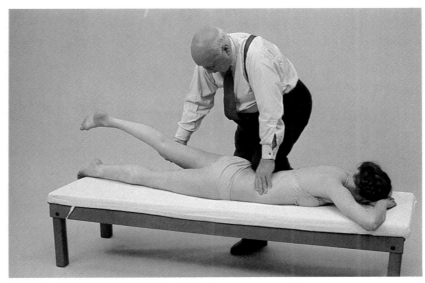

13.69

Figs 13.69, 13.70 *Starting position. Note that the operator's knee clamps the patient's trunk to the couch; his right hand is in supination so the thigh can be adducted during extension of the hip.*

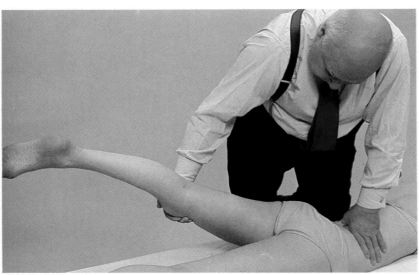

13.70

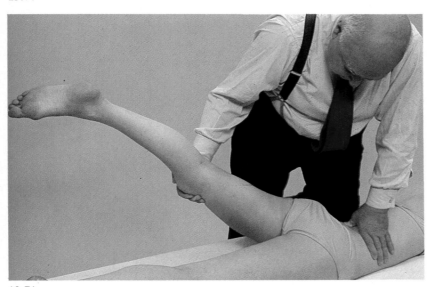

13.71

Fig 13.71 *Finishing position.*

Forced extension—5

The patient lies prone with her trunk
side-flexed as far as possible towards the
painless side: this opens the joint space on the
affected side. Manipulation forces extension
with further distraction (*Figure 13.72*).

The operator stands on the patient's good
side, with his forearms crossed. The heel of the
lower hand is on the iliac crest and the heel of
the upper pushes upwards under the lowest
ribs (*Figure 13.73*).

The manipulator forces his hands in opposite
directions by leaning his trunk forwards.
Keeping his elbows rigid he then jerks his
thorax downwards, imparting a sudden
extension thrust at the fourth lumbar level
together with momentary further distraction
(*Figure 13.74*). The patient is re-examined.

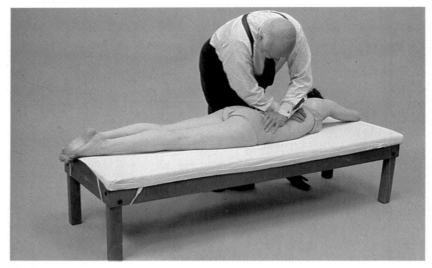

13.72

Figs 13.72, 13.73
*Starting position. The
patient is side-flexed
towards the operator.
The hands are crossed
and firmly applied to the
patient's trunk.*

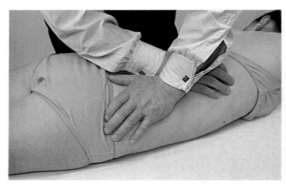

13.73

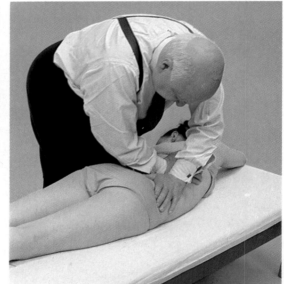

Fig 13.74 *Finishing
position. The operator's
hands are forced in
opposite directions as he
leans sharply forwards.*

13.74

If, altogether, the extension strains have
been fruitful then the rotation strains—if not
previously employed—are tried.

If the patient is no better it is probably

worthwhile trying the rotation strains
nonetheless, although the physician may have
to reconsider his original diagnosis of a
cartilaginous displacement.

Correction of lateral deviation—1

Correction of lateral deviation may be called for where manipulation has eased the pain but side flexion in one direction remains limited. This often comes out when the patient stands for a few moments and the tilt to one side quickly reappears. Extension may also be limited.

The patient lies on her back and flexes both hips. Her legs are crossed. If the deviation is towards the right, the right thigh is uppermost (*Figure 13.75*).

By simultaneously pulling on the near knee and pushing on the far, full lumbar side flexion is achieved in the previously blocked direction (*Figures 13.76; 13.77*). The rotary movement is repeated several times to develop range; then on the fourth or fifth twist, the extreme of range is held for a good minute or so. This goes on a number of times for, say, 10 minutes until the spine stays vertical after the patient has stood for a while.

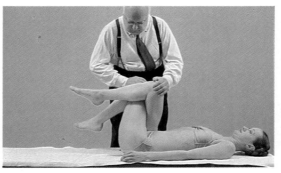

13.75

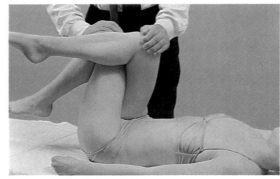

13.76

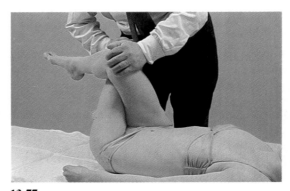

13.77

Fig 13.75 *Sometimes side flexion remains obstinately limited; the patient may stand crooked. The starting position for this corrective manipulation entails crossing the patient's legs with the thigh on the limited side uppermost.*

Figs 13.76, 13.77 *The legs are repeatedly swung from side to side; side flexion will gradually increase and the corrected position should be held to consolidate range.*

Correction of lateral deviation—2

The patient stands and the manipulator puts his hands round the patient's pelvis, placing his chest against the patient's arm (*Figure 13.76*). He pulls the pelvis towards himself in the direction it will not go and repeats this movement several times (*Figure 13.77*). He then keeps the patient in the laterally corrected position for a couple of minutes, during which time lordosis is restored by the patient repeatedly and increasingly extending her lumbar spine.

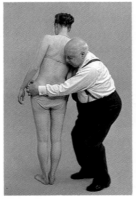

13.78

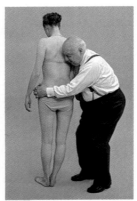

13.79

Figs 13.78, 13.79 *As the patient's pelvis is hugged towards the operator, his shoulder forces her spine upright. While in the corrected position, the patient actively achieves extension.*

Traction

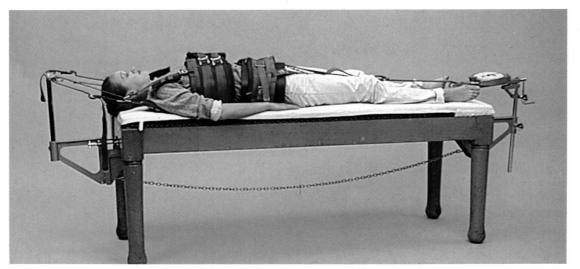

13.80

Fig 13.80 *Lumbar traction for nuclear displacements. Sessions must be daily, the traction must be sustained (not intermittent) and in the range of 35 to 80 kg. It is a comfortable treatment.*

Traction is the treatment of choice for small nuclear protrusions (*Figure 13.80*). Whereas a fragment of cartilage can be clicked back into position by manipulation, the nucleus is soft and will be influenced only by suction.

To be effective the traction must conform to particular specifications.

(1) The distracting force must be the greatest the patient can stand without discomfort—35kg/80lb would be the minimum for a small woman and 80kg/180lb the greatest for a really large man. Cautious resort to lesser poundage will, at best, fail to secure maximum distraction and, at worst, produce nothing at all.
(2) The traction must be sustained for periods of half-an-hour. Intermittent traction will not achieve reduction, as is seen below.
(3) The traction must be given daily—that is, five times per week minimum. Its object is to suck the intervertebral protrusion back further during one session than it comes out before the next.
(4) Two weeks' treatment are usual before the full benefits are manifest. Only very seldom are more than four weeks necessary.

Traction has three effects all conspiring towards the same end:

(1) The lumbar vertebrae are distracted; X-rays have shown an increase in width of each lumbar joint of 2.5mm. This increase in distance between the articular edges allows more room for a displacement to return to its original site and may actually disengage a protrusion just too large to shift during mere avoidance of compression by recumbency.

(2) A sub-atmospheric pressure is induced in the joint when the bones move apart. This tends to suck back any protrusion to the centre of the joint.
(3) The posterior longitudinal ligament is tautened. This pushes the protrusion anteriorly towards the centre of the joint.

Before each session, the patient is re-examined to see if any improvement has resulted from the previous day's treatment. In a suitable case some amelioration may be evident after the first few sessions and should continue steadily thereafter. If no improvement is apparent after a week or ten days, it is worthwhile debating whether things might be improved by altering the patient's posture on the couch (e.g. lying face down), or by changing the position of the straps.

Traction and bed-rest
The intention of traction is to obtain rapid reduction of the protrusion by distracting the joint surfaces mechanically. This is a positive purpose. Bed-rest merely avoids the compression stress on the spine entailed by upright posture. This is a negative purpose.

In patients under 60, bed-rest is usually successful in the end but achieves the same result as traction much more slowly. Traction brings the joint surfaces much further apart than is achieved by just lying in bed. In consequence a much greater centripetal force acts on the protruded part of the nucleus and recovery is greatly accelerated.

Bed-rest for patients with nuclear protrusions is an unnecessary waste of time and money. If the displacement is cartilaginous it should of course be manipulated.

Traction has the added advantage of enabling the patient to be up and about attending his business pending recovery.

Intermittent traction

Continuous traction fatigues the muscles. After a while they relax. Only then does the pull fall on the joint and distraction commence; it is not until three minutes after traction begins that electromyographic silence is attained. Hence pulls of shorter duration merely elicit the strength reflex and exercise the sacrospinalis muscles without separating the joint surfaces.

Indications for traction

The sole indication is a small nuclear protrusion at lumbar levels. The patient is thus under 60 as after that age the nucleus no longer exists.

Nuclear protrusions are characterised by gradual onset of pain often brought on by sitting or stooping. The aggravation may mount overnight after, for example, a day's gardening.

The following symptoms also imply a nuclear protrusion:

(1) Side flexion towards the painful side increases the pain. This applies only to patients under 60 with backache as opposed to lumbago.
(2) Trunk movements other than flexion bring on or increase pain down the lower limb.
(3) Primary posterolateral onset, that is, the pain struck first in the leg without previous backache. There is, however, a marked tendency in these patients to relapse following traction. In such cases it may be best to await spontaneous recovery assisted by epidural local anaesthesia.

Additionally, traction is more effective than manipulation in cases of:

(1) First and second lumbar disc lesions (very rare).
(2) Recurrence after laminectomy.
(3) Bilateral longstanding limitation of straight-leg raising in young adults (but up to three months daily traction may be required).

In cases of doubt, that is, where the protrusion is of indeterminate nature, manipulation should be tried first as it is much quicker. If manipulation fails, traction should not begin until the following day otherwise it may make the pain worse.

Contraindications

(1) Acute lumbago strongly contraindicates traction. Severe backache is no bar, but lumbago with fixation in flexion or twinges in the back on trunk movement means traction must not be attempted.
   The traction itself will not hurt. However the moment the pressure is eased even slightly, agonising pain is engendered and it may take the patient some hours to get off the couch.
(2) Sciatica with gross lumbar deformity, whether fixation of flexion or side flexion, will be similarly painful on traction. Laminectomy is required.
(3) Patients with gross emphysema, heart disease, a thoracoplasty or any severe respiratory disorder may not be able to tolerate the band about the thorax.

Traction is also to be avoided in the presence of S4 root signs (see page 222) and will fail in the following instances:

(1) With neurological deficit (as opposed to mere root pain). The protrusion is too large; manipulation will not work either and epidural local anaesthesia is the likely countermeasure.
(2) Where sciatica (as distinct from backache with some leg pain) has lasted more than six months. Nor will manipulation prove effective unless the patient is over 60 in which case any displacement must be cartilaginous. The physician can either await spontaneous recovery or consider an injection of epidural local anaesthetic (which is also the treatment of choice where an attack of sciatica is already subsiding and the patient is over the worst).

Equipment

A purpose-built traction table is not a necessity—a standard couch can be adapted by means of a special attachment. In addition, a proper harness is required with supplementary padding for added comfort (*Figure 13.81*).

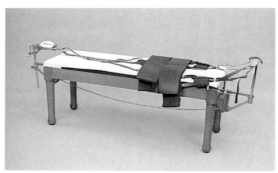

13.81

Fig 13.81 *The apparatus. Accessories that can be hand-bolted on to a standard couch are more than adequate.*

Technique

The patient is examined at each attendance before the treatment, since the physical signs immediately after traction are an unreliable guide. Lumbar movement and straight-leg raise are assessed (*Figure 13.82*).

The straps are done up very tightly with great attention paid to the positioning of the padding. Then the patient is covered with a blanket and the pressure is slowly raised over the course of some five minutes (*Figures 13.83; 13.84*).

The distracting force is the maximum the patient can bear painlessly. Traction is a comfortable process and the patient should never feel pain. If it hurts, something is wrong: the case is either unsuitable or the treatment has been marred by bad technique.

The patient stays on traction for half-an-hour but the physiotherapist remains within call. After the first few minutes some of the distracting force will be lost and the poundage should be topped up.

When the treatment ends, the force is wound down very slowly, taking up to five minutes. Traction appliances with a ratchet which releases all the distraction at once are diligently avoided; anything other than slow diminution of pressure can produce severe twinges.

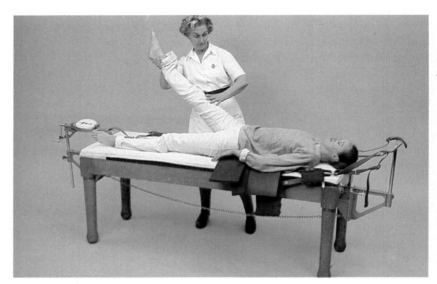

Fig 13.82 *Re-examination before treatment. After the traction the lumbar movements should be avoided while the spine settles down.*

13.82

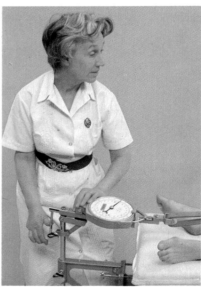

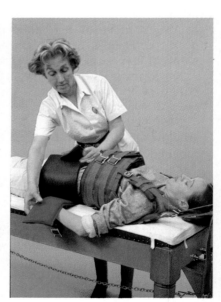

Figs 13.83, 13.84 *The high poundage demands plenty of soft padding under both the thoracic and the pelvic harness. The pressure is wound up slowly.*

13.83

13.84

The patient is left for some minutes to regain her normal length before compressing the joint by standing. She is shown how to get off the couch by rolling on to her side (*Figure 13.85*) and then putting her feet over the edge of the couch and rising sideways to a sitting position.

The patient must always bend at the knees when picking up her footwear. Use of a chair minimises stooping when the shoes are put on (*Figure 13.86*).

The first treatment should be given with caution, particularly in patients with lumbago that has only just lost its twinges. For comfort's sake, the patient should not consume a large meal before the session and should be encouraged to keep as relaxed and as still as possible during the stretch; coughing must be avoided.

Treatment is given daily until reduction has been secured; this normally takes one to three weeks, although sometimes a fourth week is justified if improvement is continuing. If ten adequate sessions have done no good, traction should be discontinued (except in cases of longstanding bilaterally limited straight-leg raise in young adults). When the patient is nearly well, a painful arc on straight-leg raising becomes apparent. Many patients begin to get better only during the second week.

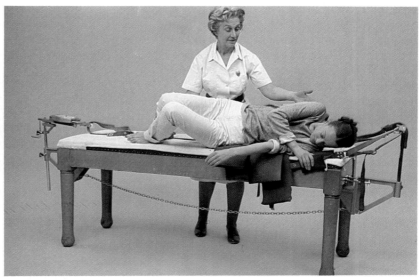

13.85

Fig 13.85 *After the treatment. The patient rolls into the sitting position to avoid lumbar flexion.*

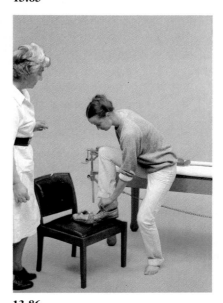

13.86

Fig 13.86 *Prophylactic education. No lumbar treatment is complete without cautioning the patient against unnecessary flexion strains.*

The patient's position

It is standard practice to start the treatments with the patient on her back. Unless re-examination shows this posture not to work, it is maintained for subsequent attendances. But if the traction has not begun to prove effective after a few days, this poses the question of a different approach.

Probably the easiest way to alter the pull on the spinal joints is to raise or lower the attachments at one or both ends of the couch. Where the apparatus does not permit such flexibility, the same effect may be achieved by altering the strapping or the patient's posture.

There is a theoretical maximum of eight different positions. The patient may lie face down or face up, and whether prone or supine the straps may be applied in four different ways. They can be fastened to either the top or the underside of the thoracic and lumbar harnesses. Thus both straps may be pulling from the underside, both may be pulling from the upper side, the lumbar strap may be up and the thoracic strap down and vice versa. The variation in direction of pull may be minimal but in difficult cases it can mean all the difference between success and failure.

Epidural local anaesthesia

Epidural local anaesthesia is the treatment of choice for an irreducible lumbar displacement. This means its application is restricted to large displacements that cannot be shifted by manipulation or traction. Most patients thought to require laminectomy merely need this injection to get well and stay well.

A solution of 1:200 procaine 50ml is injected via the sacral hiatus into the neural canal (*Figure 13.87*). This bathes the external aspect of the dura mater and nerve roots in anaesthetic, so although the displacement remains in position the patient can no longer feel the pain. In suitable cases—with a couple of further injections if necessary—full and lasting relief is to be expected.

It is a simple outpatient procedure.

Results

Immediately following a successful injection the patient regains painless (though not necessarily full) lumbar mobility and full and painless straight-leg raise.

After the first hour or so the symptoms may or may not return. A week should elapse before assessing the long-term results of the injection unless severe pain makes it imperative to see the patient sooner.

The upshot of the injection is very variable during the days immediately following infiltration. Some patients lose their symptoms for a couple of days and then relapse whereas others get well and stay well. A few undergo increased pain for a day or two and then improve rapidly.

The injection should be repeated at the end of a week if either:

(1) The patient's pain is diminished.
(2) His lumbar mobility or straight-leg raise has improved (even though the pain remains unaltered).

A total of three further injections may be required at, for example, weekly or two-weekly intervals.

If there is no improvement at the end of the first week, treatment by injection is abandoned. Alternatively, if at that date the patient has full painless range then no further treatment is called for except in the event of subsequent deterioration.

In 1963 Coomes (see page 141) estimated the relative value of recumbency and epidural local anaesthesia in a series of 50 patients. All had sciatica with severe pain and signs of impaired conduction along the nerve root. Half were hospitalised and the others received one or two

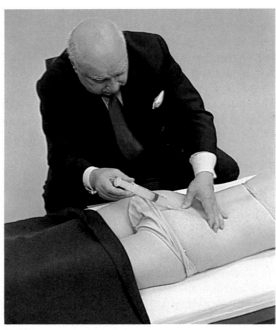

13.87

Fig 13.87 *Injection of procaine via the sacral hiatus anaesthetises the lower extent of the dura mater. Often the relief from pain is permanent.*

injections and rested at home. The conclusion was that the injected patients had largely recovered in ten days, whereas the recumbent took 30 days to reach the same degree of comfort. In Canada, Fraser (1976) contrasted the duration and cost of acute lumbago treated by epidural local anaesthesia and by traditional measures (e.g. recumbency, traction in bed, heat, analgesics) and came up with figures of 3.8 days for the injection and 15.6 for the other methods.

Anaesthetic

The solution is 1:200 procaine 50ml in normal saline without adrenaline—pure water must not be used otherwise really severe pain results for about 24 hours. Only surface anaesthesia is needed, as a stronger solution would go on to penetrate the dural sleeve causing temporary paralysis.

Procaine achieves better results than the more modern anaesthetics.

Indications

The injection is the main weapon for disposing of root pain with absent or sluggish reflex, one or more weak muscles or analgesic skin (not mere pins and needles).

Indications are:

(1) *Hyperacute lumbago*. Both manipulation and traction are strongly contraindicated; the patient experiences severe twinges on the slightest movement and is generally immobilised in bed. The injection affords

immediate, complete relief for about 90 minutes during which free mobility of the joint is restored and spontaneous reduction begins. The patient must get home and into bed before the end of this interlude; he should lie prone. Not much pain returns and by the following morning the patient is normally well enough for reduction to be secured by manipulation.

(2) *Root pain with neurological signs*. Neither manipulation nor traction will work.

It will be borne in mind that the injection does not work so well on:

(a) Patients over 60, but good results can be obtained.

(b) Third lumbar disc lesions (relatively rare) with root pain.

(3) *Root pain without neurological signs*. There are six cases where the injection is useful:

(a) Root pain that has continued for too long. Root pain should clear up spontaneously in a year at most. Epidural local anaesthesia is indicated if the pain—usually accompanied by limited straight-leg raise—obstinately refuses to go.

(b) Primary posterolateral disc protrusions. The displacement is nuclear so manipulation will fail, and although traction succeeds there is a high rate of recurrence. The injection is only successful when the protrusion has steadied in the position of maximum displacement, designated by the limitation of straight-leg raise becoming stable (usually with a range of 30°–45°).

(c) Recurrent sciatica after a root palsy. Relapse at the same level from sciatica with neurological signs is uncommon following recovery, whether achieved spontaneously or brought about by an epidural injection. However, if the pain revives within a year then epidural local anaesthesia is given; it is more often successful than treating the attack as a new displacement by starting off again with manipulation or traction.

(d) Root pain without physical signs. A patient may complain of root pain and yet have full painless range of both straight-leg raise and lumbar movements. If the history suggests a disc lesion, epidural local anaesthesia is induced diagnostically and in many cases secures full lasting relief. The cause of pain may be bruising of the dural sleeve persisting from a past disc lesion.

(e) Recovering sciatica. If sciatic pain without backache and the reasonably intense root symptoms are subsiding, it is best to steer clear of manipulation and traction. The patient is over the worst and suffers from little more than an ache in the limb and limited straight-leg raise.

(f) Nocturnal cramp. Severe cramp in the calf of the affected leg coming on each night may wake a patient long after sciatica has ceased. Epidural local anaesthesia serves to desensitise the nerve root; it may need to be repeated some six months later.

(4) *Pregnancy*. In the last month of pregnancy, the injection is to be preferred to manipulation or traction.

(5) *Intractable backache*. A low lumbar disc lesion which, in the absence of contraindications, proves refractory to both manipulation and traction should be treated by epidural local anaesthesia. The constant ache may be lastingly abolished or diminished.

(6) *Chronic backache*. A chronic constant backache may present with no articular signs. Manipulation of such a disc lesion will fail whereas the injection may relieve the dural bruising.

(7) *Matutinal or nocturnal backache*. The patient can do everything, even heavy work by day, but is regularly woken in the small hours or early morning by backache severe enough to force him out of bed. The symptoms last for about an hour and examination during the day reveals nothing. The only diagnostic indication may be that *during his attack* a cough causes pain.

(8) *Diagnostic*. It is chiefly in early cases with slight symptoms and physical signs difficult to interpret that local epidural anaesthesia helps diagnostically. It is also useful in patients with uncharacteristic backache and in medico-legal disputes. If, following the injection, the symptoms abate and full straight-leg raise is found to be practicable, the lesion must be connected with the exterior surface of the dura mater or the lower lumbar nerve roots. They are the only tissues rendered anaesthetic.

Laminectomy and epidural local anaesthesia
Operation can leave the patient with a permanently weakened back. As the worst that can result from an unsuccessful injection is for the patient to be no better, it makes sense to try epidural local anaesthesia before surgery—the more so since conservative treatments are less likely to prove effective after the operation. This argument is further bolstered on grounds of time and expense—minimal in the case of the injection—and also because the results compare well.

Statistical corroboration
Ombregt's findings (International Symposium on Low Back Pain, Antwerp, 12/6/82) amply

substantiate the indications for the injection arrived at on clinical grounds. Over a period of two years he injected 94 patients; of these, 69 were restored to full painless range. A total of 208 injections were given without side-effects.

Ombregt's findings were classified as follows:

1. Hyperacute lumbago. Five cases. All painfree within five days. The injection was supplemented by one to four sessions of manipulation.
2. Backache. Twenty one cases, producing 12 recoveries and nine failures. Chronic low back pain thus remains a difficult problem. The category was subdivided as follows:

    (a) Intractable backache (i.e. manipulation and traction failed to secure adequate or any relief). Nine cases. Three failures, three painfree after injection and subsequent manipulation, three painfree after injection alone.

    (b) Chronic backache with no clear articular signs. Nine cases. Three well (previous mean duration of pain two and a half years) and six no better (previous mean duration of pain four years).

    (c) Matutinal backache. Three patients, all rendered painfree.
3. Root pain without neurological deficit. Twenty three cases. Nineteen recoveries and four failures, subdivided as follows:

    (a) Root pain for six months or longer (previous mean duration of pain 20 months). Thirteen cases. Ten painfree within average of 5.1 weeks after an average of 2.7 injections each. Three no better.

    (b) Primary posterolateral onset. Four cases. All recovered after one to two injections.

    (c) No results from traction or backache. Six cases. Five recoveries, one failure.
4. Root pain with neurological deficit. Thirty nine cases. Thirty one recoveries, eight no better. Of the failures, four required laminectomy. Of the 33 patients with L5, S1 or S2 palsies, a total of 29 were rendered painfree; but one of the two L3 palsies was unimproved as were three out of the four L4 palsies.
5. Root pain, post-laminectomy. Six cases.

Two well (12 months elapsed since operation), four no better (4–12 years elapsed since surgery).

Contraindications

These are remarkably few:

(1) *Sensitivity to local anaesthetic.* Inquiry should be made of any history of adverse reaction to procaine. If a patient does state he is sensitive to procaine, it is more probable that adrenaline is the trouble and a test injection should be made into, for example, the buttock.

(2) *Strict asepsis must be observed.* Introduction of bacteria into the neural canal would be disastrous and the injection must be postponed if the neighbouring skin is not clear from sepsis. Should a needle have to be inserted twice, a fresh one must be used.

(3) *The proper procedure should be followed:*

    (a) The injection is never given under general anaesthesia. The patient cannot then report on any untoward symptoms.

    (b) Only 50ml is run in slowly over the course of some minutes.

    (c) The physician checks that the needle has not penetrated the theca. An injection into the cerebrospinal fluid would prove fatal.

It is probably best to wait a few days after a myelogram before epidural local anaesthesia is induced. A pre-1950 laminectomy militates against success as diffuse fibrosis—which the anaesthetic cannot penetrate—resulted from the talcum powder in which the surgeons' gloves were then packed. A post-1950 laminectomy or arthrodesis of any period have no such deleterious consequences.

Dangers of epidural injection have been greatly exaggerated. In the 50,000 injections given by the author a total of four patients were encountered with a semi-permeable dura mater and developed a paraplegia lasting two hours. Two of these cases were recorded 25 years ago before central sterilisation and may have been attributable to some pollution in the water in which the instruments lay. No case of sepsis has yet occurred.

Technique

The object of the injection is to insert the needle through the sacral hiatus and inject 50ml of 1:200 procaine into the sacrum. As the injection proceeds the fluid ascends to the third lumbar level, thus anaesthetising the dura mater and nerve roots (*Figure 13.88*).

The patient lies prone with buttocks exposed. The physiotherapist sterilises the skin at the lower sacrum and intergluteal cleft and then assists by holding the buttocks stretched well apart (*Figure 13.89*).

The doctor is seated on the left and uses his left hand to palpate for the two cornua, two bony prominences just to either side of the mid-line at the fourth sacral level (*Figure 13.90*). The gap between the cornua indicates the position of the sacral hiatus through which the needle will be inserted. A small amount of the procaine solution is injected into the overlying skin.

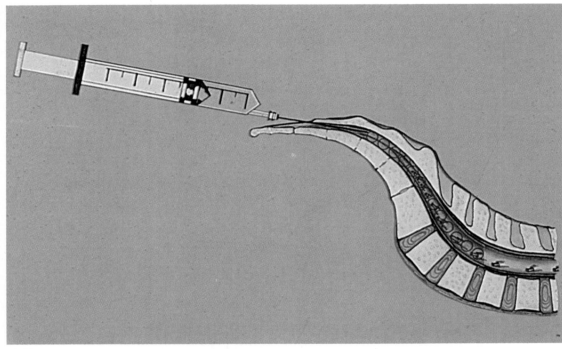

Fig 13.88 *Injection into the neural canal. The needle stops well short of the theca; the anaesthetic rises to L3.*

13.88

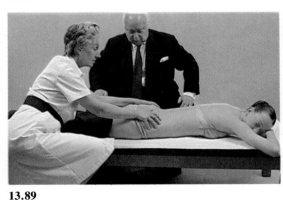

13.89

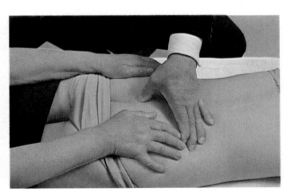

13.90

Fig 13.89 *The physiotherapist's arms are horizontal, out of the physician's way, as she holds the gluteal masses apart.*

Fig 13.90 *Palpating for the cornua.*

An ordinary lumbar puncture needle with stylet is passed through the anaesthetic area of skin and on into the intercornual space (*Figure 13.91*).

The difficult part of the insertion is to assess correctly the angle at which to thrust the needle further. If it is blocked by hitting bone, a different angle must be tried. While palpating for the cornua the physician will have gauged the slope on the flat surface presented by the fifth sacral segment. This gives some guidance on the angle at which to insert the needle; it varies widely from patient to patient.

In the ordinary case the needle passes in without hindrance to some 4–5cm. In most patients the theca ends at the lower level of the first sacral vertebra and the needle must stop short of this line.

The stylet is now withdrawn (*Figure 13.92*). If cerebrospinal fluid escapes, the dura mater extends to an abnormally low level and the needle lies intrathecally. The physician notes the level at which the flow ceases as he withdraws the needle, and the injection is deferred until the following day by which time the puncture will have sealed.

If nothing flows back, the injection commences. If blood issues, the needle lies in a vein or haematoma and must be edged into a harmless position.

The injection proceeds very slowly: infiltration of the entire amount takes from 5–10 minutes. At first the patient feels an ache at each side of the mid-sacrum; later the symptoms are reproduced in the leg. Finally the pain ceases.

The injection raises the pressure in the cerebrospinal fluid, which is transmitted upwards to the brain. The first indication of a labile cerebral circulation is often faltering speech, so throughout the infiltration the physiotherapist chats to the patient to make her talk. If the patient complains of giddiness—or of intolerable pain—the injection is stopped for a few minutes before resuming slowly.

Aspiration is repeated every 10ml to make sure the tip of the needle has not moved.

If the needle has missed the space between the cornua, it will lie extrasacrally, and as the injection continues a swelling would be felt rising at one side of the sacral spinous processes. Throughout the first half of the injection the operator's left hand rests on the sacrum in order to detect any mound appearing there (*Figure 13.93*).

After the injection, the patient lies prone for 20 minutes, the physiotherapist remaining with her. This is an essential precaution as it is only by the end of this time that any adverse effects would have appeared. The patient can now go home, returning next week for re-examination. For results and the appropriate follow-up procedure see page 210.

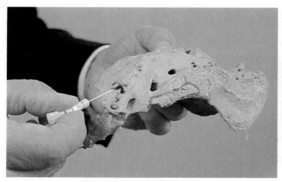

13.91

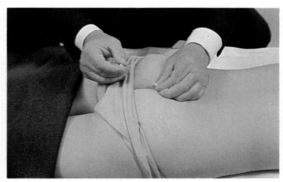

13.92

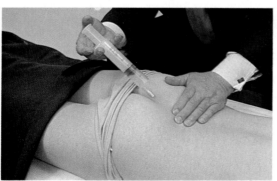

13.93

Fig 13.91 *The angle of insertion is a matter of fine judgement and experience.*

Fig 13.92 *Withdrawing the stylet. Were the theca penetrated, cerebrospinal fluid would escape.*

Fig 13.93 *A faulty insertion can lead to the needle lying superficial to the sacrum; the physician feels for any extrasacral swelling.*

Prophylaxis

At the lumbar spine there are three main methods of prophylaxis:

(1) Ligamentous sclerosants.
(2) Corset.
(3) Posture.

All three approaches depend on enhanced lumbar stability in the correct position.

Sclerosants

For general information on intention, method and sclerosant solution the reader is recommended to the corresponding section on the thoracic spine at page 181. It will be remembered any displacement must first be reduced.

The ligaments are infiltrated at both ends at their point of insertion to periosteum; no fluid is introduced unless the tip of the needle is felt to impinge against bone. At each point, 1ml solution is injected.

Injections are given at weekly intervals and the following ligaments are infiltrated.

(1) The first week: the supraspinous and interspinous ligaments at the fourth and fifth lumbar levels.
(2) The second week: the ligaments around the facet joints.
(3) The third week: the deep lumbar fascia.

The injections smart as the solution goes in. Then the local anaesthetic takes effect, and the ache ceases for at least an hour. After that the pain returns, but by the next day the symptoms have ceased.

The patient returns a week later for re-examination and the succeeding injection. If any displacement is found, manipulative reduction is carried out immediately. Only when this is complete is the patient ready for the next infiltration.

Until the tissue contracture is established, the patient must avoid flexing her back. Contracture takes about six weeks; thereafter the tendency to relapse is greatly diminished, although after some years the injections may have to be repeated.

The first injection: supraspinous and interspinous ligaments

A skin drawing is not required; the physician palpates for the declivity between the spinous processes and the needle is inserted half-way between the fifth spinous process and the first sacral spinous process. First the tip points superiorly until it meets bone and a series of droplets are deposited along the inferior surface of the fifth lumbar spinous process (*Figures 13.94; 13.95*).

Then the needle is half withdrawn and the procedure repeated along the upper surface of the first sacral spinous process (*Figure 13.96*).

The entire procedure is repeated at the fourth lumbar level.

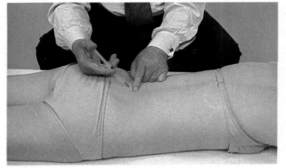

13.94

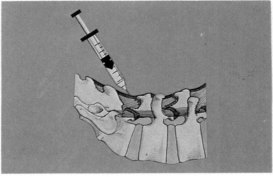

13.95

13.96

Figs 13.94, 13.95, 13.96 *One ml P2G is injected along the ligamento-periosteal junctions at L4 and L5. Injections are never made unless the physician is clinically certain the displacement is reduced.*

The second injection: facet ligaments

This time a skin drawing is made (*Figure 13.97*). The long side-to-side line is a marker running between the iliac crests; the L4/5 joint lies directly underneath. The mid-line is intersected by three cross-bars, each half-way between the spinous processes. The lateral boundaries of the grid are some 2.5cm to either side of the mid-line and overlie the facet joints (*Figure 13.98*).

The needle is inserted directly downwards at the corner of the grid (*Figure 13.99*) and should encounter tough ligamentous resistance before reaching bone. Then 1ml is injected partly into the ligament and partly into the joint.

The process is repeated on the other side (*Figure 13.100*) and then at the other level (*Figure 13.101*).

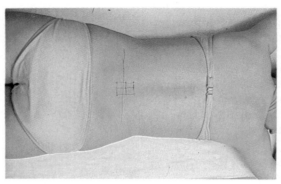

13.97

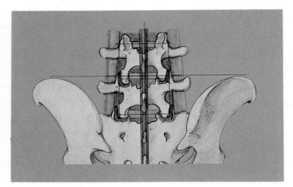

13.98

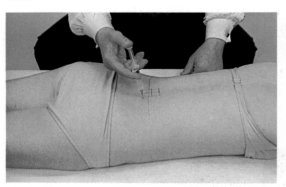

13.99

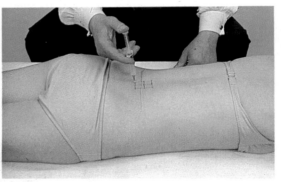

13.100

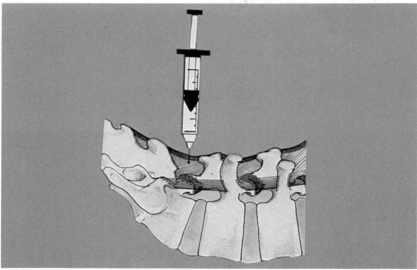

13.101

Figs 13.97, 13.98 *The grid is identical both for injection of the facet ligaments and the deep lumbar fascia (see next page). Sites of infiltration for both are shown on Fig 13.98.*

Figs 13.99, 13.100, 13.101 *The needle enters vertically at the outer corners of the grid to inject 1ml P2G into capsule and ligaments of the facet joints.*

The third injection: deep lumbar fascia

The final injection is given a week later into the medial edge of the deep lumbar fascia. A spot is chosen level with the relevant spinous process on the boundary of the grid (*Figure 13.102*) and the needle is thrust in until it runs into the lamina (see *Figure 13.98*). It is half-withdrawn and inserted obliquely until the bony lamina is no longer tangible; the medial edge of the deep lumbar fascia lies just laterally. Then 1ml is injected in a single load.

The procedure is duplicated on the other side and at the adjacent level (*Figures 13.103; 13.104*).

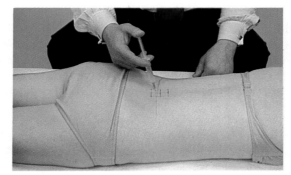

13.102

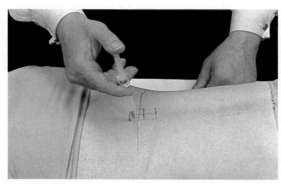

13.103

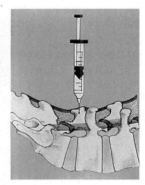

13.104

Figs 13.102, 13.103, 13.104 *One ml P2G is injected into one spot at each of the four medial edges.*

A corset

Recurrent attacks from an unstable fragment of disc may be prevented by use of a properly made corset. This is much to be preferred to the plaster cast which, apart from many other drawbacks, cannot be sufficiently tight to take effect. It must be emphasised that a corset is not a means of reducing a displacement; it is a method for maintaining reduction once it has been achieved.

The corset is made of cloth with two posterior steels accurately moulded to the patient's lumbar curve. An exact fit of the steels is essential.

The corset extends as far above as below the level requiring support and must span at least 12 inches. It can be worn indefinitely, but to be really effective the corset must be tight enough to prevent lumbar movement.

Posture

Nachemson's findings (see page 140) have demonstrated that the intervertebral pressure is at its greatest when the patient flexes her spine. Moreover, when the spine is in flexion the disc is pushed posteriorly (i.e. towards the dura mater) by the tilt on the surfaces of the vertebrae. As these two effects frequently combine to produce a displacement, the moral is clear. The patient must:

(1) Flex her trunk as little as possible, particularly when lifting.
(2) Maintain her lumbar lordosis.

These precepts should govern her deportment throughout life, whether at work or in the home, standing, sitting, lying or lifting. The regimen, together with its rationale and implications, must be driven home.

Differential diagnosis

A large number of non-disc lesions give rise to pain in the back, groin or lower limb; even in the aggregate, they are much less common than a disc lesion. Some are considered briefly below.

Afebrile osteomyelitis
In acute cases, the history resembles lumbago but straight-leg raise is full. If the condition is chronic, the pain encroaches for some weeks with no diagnostic signs until the onset of bilateral limitation of side flexion. In both cases the capsular pattern is found.

Ankylosing spondylitis
The symptoms are irregular irrespective of activity; an X-ray of the sacroiliac joints is diagnostic. The capsular pattern is present. See also page 76.

Aortic occlusion
The pain occurs only on walking; usually claudication in one or both limbs overshadows the minor backache.

Brucellosis
The symptoms are a chronic backache with minor fever. In the later stages an X-ray is diagnostic.

Fractured transverse process
The unilateral pain follows direct injury to the back and abates after two weeks. Resisted side flexion usually hurts and an X-ray is diagnostic.

Fractured vertebral body
The central pain is constant for the first few weeks but ceases after a month or so. At first the capsular pattern is marked and a kyphos is palpable at the level of the fracture. An X-ray is diagnostic.

Gastric ulcer adherent to the lumbar spine
The symptoms are connected both with posture and eating. An X-ray of the stomach is diagnostic.

Ligamentous overstretching
The symptoms seem to occur only in spondylolisthesis.

Neoplasm, lumbar
The history is of steady aggravation (unlike disc lesions) and of major root signs and minor root pain (disc lesions present the reverse) in a distribution not corresponding to any one root. The capsular pattern and an X-ray are both informative.

Neoplasm, sacral
Full painless lumbar range is accompanied by gross weakness of the muscles of one or both feet, but in the average case there is no root pain. An X-ray is diagnostic.

Neuroma, lumbar
The condition is rare and should be considered, for example, if the history is unusual or if L1 or L2 root signs are discovered. The capsular pattern is sometimes present and a myelogram reveals the growth.

Neurosis
The alleged history, signs and symptoms are inconsistent and contradictory.

Nutritional osteomalacia
The gait—a characteristic waddle—puts the physician on the right track.

Osteitis deformans
Movement of the lumbothoracic spine is restricted and the pain pervades the entire back. An X-ray is diagnostic.

Osteoporosis, senile
Pain results only if the condition is accompanied by a disc lesion or if the wedging comes on suddenly, in which case the ache is severe for a week or two and goes after a couple of months. An X-ray is diagnostic. Sometimes repeated micro-fractures cause pain.

Osteochondrosis, adolescent
The condition appears to be harmless of itself. In 1962 Ross (see page 143) X-rayed the spine of 5000 police candidates aged 20. He found evidence of osteochondrosis in two-thirds but only 4.2% of this group had experienced backache.

Osteophytosis, posterior
In contrast to anterior osteophytosis, pain may result from compression of the dura mater by a posterior osteophyte. An X-ray is diagnostic.

Spinal claudication
Walking (*cf.* standing) causes backache, typically with pins and needles in both feet.

Spondylolisthesis
Spondylolisthesis may be painless or may be responsible for a disc lesion at the unstable joint. In the latter case there is an enhanced liability to relapse for slight reasons. Alternatively, pain can result from the

sustained stretching of the intervertebral ligaments. The ache is then central and largely unconnected with lumbar movements, but if the nerve roots are caught against the bony ridge of the vertebra below then root pain is engendered (generally bilateral with pins and needles).

Tuberculous caries
Kyphos is detectable where bone is eaten away; there is fixation and pain here and at adjacent levels. The X-ray is diagnostic and the capsular pattern is present.

Vertebral hyperostosis
Elderly patients with an ache in the entire trunk and marked limitation at every spinal joint may be the victims of vertebral hyperostosis. An X-ray is diagnostic.

Referred pain
Pain referred to the back from, for example, an intra-abdominal or pelvic viscus will allow full painless range of lumbar movement.

The lumbar nerve roots

Monoradicular and polyradicular symptoms

The table below sets out the roots which may be affected by a disc lesion at any given level:

L1 disc	L1 root only
L2 disc	L2 root only
L3 disc	L3 root only
L4 disc	L4 root by itself
	L4 and L5 roots together
	L5 root by itself
	S3 root by itself (extremely rare)
	S4 root by itself

L5 disc	L5 root by itself
	L5 and S1 roots together
	S1 root by itself
	S1 and S2 roots together
	S2 root by itself
	S3 root by itself (extremely rare)
	S4 root by itself

Lumbar root signs

The maximum root signs at each level are detailed below. A disc lesion may affect two roots simultaneously (see above); involvement of three would arouse grave disquiet.

L1 root pressure
Disc lesions at both L1 and L2 are very rare and root pressure even rarer, as the nerve roots emerge high up and pass well lateral to the disc.

Pain in the dermatome (*Figure 13.105*) and numbness in the groin.

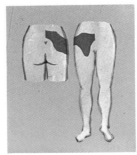

Fig 13.105 *The L1 dermatome.*

13.105

L2 root pressure

A displacement at L2 is commoner than L1, although still highly unusual.

Pain in the dermatome (*Figure 13.106*).
Weak psoas—resisted hip flexion.
Analgesia from groin to knee.
In addition to a disc lesion consider:

(1) Secondary malignant deposits (psoas grossly weak *and* spinal movements grossly limited).
(2) Meralgia paraesthetica (analgesia at outer aspect of thigh; the lumbar movements have no bearing on the pain).

Pain at the front of the thigh may also be caused by lesions of the hip joint, psoas, abductor and quadriceps muscles, psoas bursa, femur or a loose body in the hip joint.

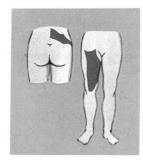

13.106

Fig 13.106 *The L2 dermatome.*

L3 root pressure

Disc lesions are fairly common at the L3 joint. As the nerve root is stretched by lumbar extension and relaxed on flexion, extension is the movement predisposed to hurt in the thigh. Pain in the dermatome (*Figure 13.107*).

Weak quadriceps—resisted knee extension.
Weak psoas—resisted hip flexion.
Painful prone-lying knee flexion.
Pain at front of knee on full straight-leg raise (occasionally).
Sluggish or absent knee jerk.
Analgesia from patella to ankle.
For alternative causes of pain at the front of the thigh see L2.

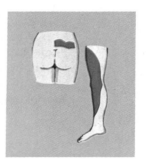

13.107

Fig 13.107 *The L3 dermatome.*

L4 root pressure

Disc lesions abound at both the L4 and L5 joints; in either case the pattern may be polyradicular. Thus a lateral displacement pinches the L4 root, one protruding just at the edge of the posterior longitudinal ligament (i.e. more medially) pinches L5 and a large displacement will compress both roots. Pain in the dermatome (*Figure 13.108*).

Weak tibialis anterior—resisted dorsiflexion.
Weak extensor hallucis—resisted extension of the hallux.
Analgesia at outer part of lower leg running to the big toe.
Limitation of straight-leg raise (occasionally bilateral).
Jerks unaffected.

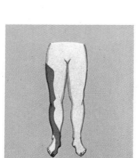

13.108

Fig 13.108 *The L4 dermatome. Both L4 and L5 include the big toe.*

L5 root pressure

The L5 root can be compressed by either the L4 or the L5 disc. The pattern may be polyradicular. Pain in the dermatome (*Figure 13.109*).

Weak extensor hallucis—resisted extension of the hallux.

Weak peronei—resisted eversion of the foot.

Weak gluteus medius—resisted abduction of the thigh.

Analgesia at outer leg running to the inner three toes.

Unilateral limitation of straight-leg raise.

Sluggish or absent ankle jerk.

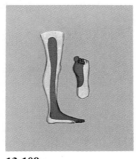

13.109

Fig 13.109 *The L5 dermatome.*

S1 root pressure

The S1 root can be affected by the L5 disc. The pattern may be polyradicular. Pain in the dermatome (*Figure 13.110*).

Weak peronei—resisted eversion of the foot.

Weak calf muscles—rising on tip-toe.

Weak hamstrings—resisted knee flexion.

Wasting of, and inability to contract, the gluteal mass.

Unilateral limitation of straight-leg raise.

Sluggish or absent ankle jerk.

Analgesia of the outer two toes, the outer foot and the outer leg as far as the lateral aspect of the knee.

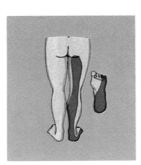

13.110

Fig 13.110 *The S1 dermatome.*

S2 root pressure

This is as for S1 except:

(1) The peronei are not involved.
(2) The analgesia ends under the heel, not extending to the foot.

The dermatome is shown in *Figure 13.111*.

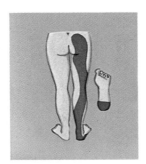

13.111

Fig 13.111 *The S2 dermatome.*

S3 root pressure

It is highly unusual for other roots to be affected at the same time as the S3 root and pain in the dermatome (*Figure 13.112*) is the only symptom. There is no muscle weakness, no limitation of straight-leg raise, no analgesia, and the bladder and rectal functions are normal—as are the jerks.

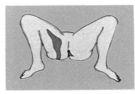

13.112

Fig 13.112 *The S3 dermatome.*

S4 root pressure

The S4 root may be compressed by either the L4 or the L5 disc protruding centrally, unlike other roots which are only threatened by lateral protrusions. S4 root pressure is an absolute bar to manipulation (see also page 193) and even traction is not wholly safe. Pain is felt in the saddle area, scrotum or vagina (*Figure 13.113*) with analgesia of the anus, loss of rectal expulsive power and difficulty in passing or retaining urine. By contrast the articular signs may be unobtrusive and it is thus the history rather than the examination which alerts. Permanent bladder paralysis may ensue if the condition is left untreated and immediate

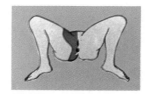

Fig 13.113 *The S4 dermatome.*

13.113

laminectomy is the rule. Bilateral sciatica threatens the posterior longitudinal ligament, rupture of which might endanger the S4 root.

Rectal, penile, scrotal, testicular, vaginal and bladder disorders are by far the commonest causes of fourth sacral pain.

PART FOUR

APPENDICES

I THE DERMATOMES

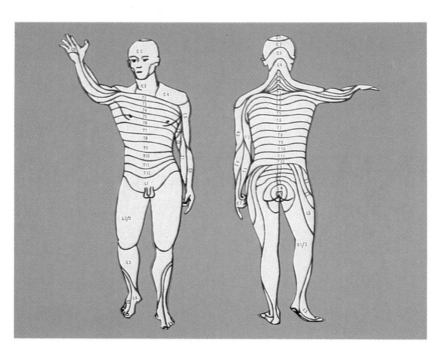

I.1, I.2

Figs I.1, I.2 *The dermatomes*

After the first month, the fetus starts to divide into about 40 segments. With the passage of time each segment becomes differentiated into dermatome (skin), myotome (muscles and other soft tissues) and scleratome (bone and fibrous septa). The dermatomes govern the distance that pain arising from any point in the myotome may travel distally.

The shape of each dermatome varies considerably from one individual to another. Those illustrated on this and the ensuing pages are substantially based on the work of Foerster who, in 1933, mapped out the dermatomes anew. But minor refinements are incorporated where clinical experience has consistently shown discrepancies with the original.

The opening diagrams are included by way of a general overview, as they depict only the central part of many of the skin segments and cannot represent the considerable areas of overlap.

The dura mater refers pain not on a segmental but on an extrasegmental basis. The areas to which pain may be referred from a cervical, thoracic and lumbar disc lesions are illustrated in Figures I.24, I.25 and I.26.

Figs I.3, I.4, I.5, I.6 *The upper cervical dermatomes. C1 (top), C2 (upper centre), C3 (lower centre), C4 (bottom).*

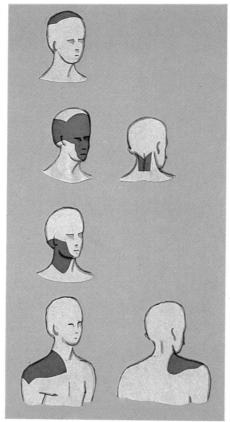

Figs I.7, I.8, I.9, I.10 *The lower cervical dermatomes. C5 (top), C6 (upper centre), C7 (lower centre), C8 (bottom).*

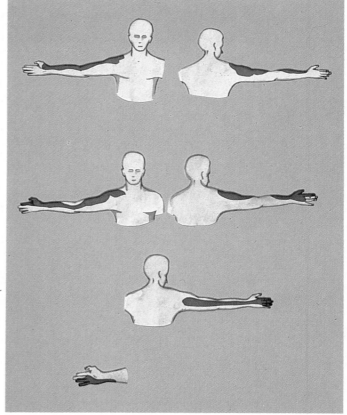

I.3, I.4, I.5, I.6

I.7, I.8, I.9, I.10

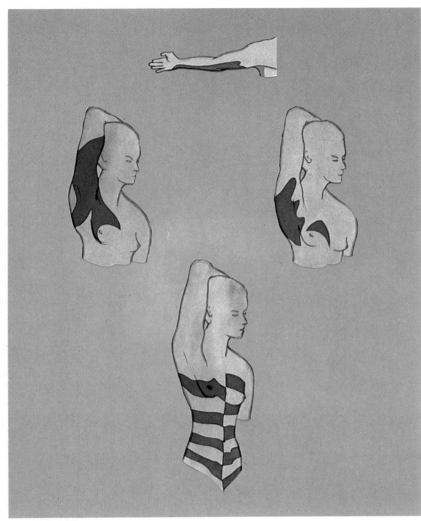

Figs I.11, I.12, I.13, I.14
*The thoracic
dermatomes. T1 (top),
T2 (centre left), T3
(centre right), T4–12
(bottom).*

**Figs I.15, I.16, I.17,
I.18, I.19** *The lumbar
dermatomes. L1 (top
left), L2 (top centre), L3
(top right), L4 (lower
left), L5 (lower right).*

I.11, I.12, I.13, I.14

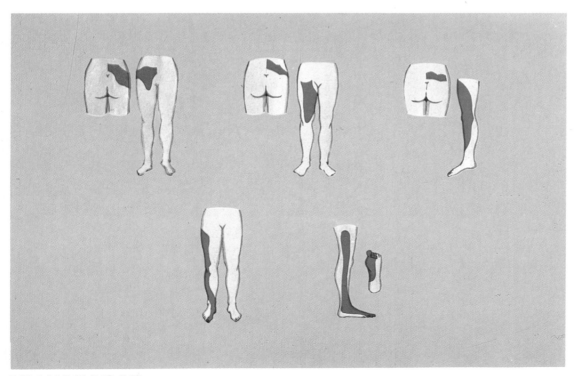

I.15, I.16, I.17, I.18, I.19

Figs I.20, I.21, I.22, I.23
The sacral dermatomes. S1 (top left), S2 (top right), S3 (lower left), S4 (lower right).

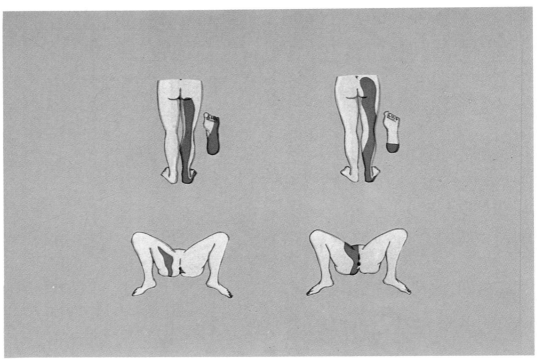

I.20, I.21, I.22, I.23

Figs I.24, I.25, I.26
Extrasegmental reference. The areas in which pain may be felt as a result of interference with the dura mater at cervical (left), thoracic (centre) and lumbar levels (right).

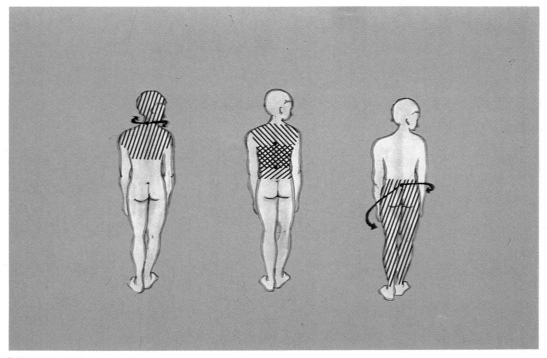

I.24, I.25, I.26

II PINS AND NEEDLES

Pins and needles in all four limbs characterise disorders such as peripheral neuritis, diabetes, pernicious anaemia and central cervical disc lesions.

Pressure on the spinal cord: no pain; pins and needles referred extrasegmentally.

Pressure on the dural sleeve to a nerve root: pain; numbness; pins and needles (neither edge nor aspect).

Pressure on a nerve trunk: no pain; pins and needles (a release phenomenon; aspect but no edge).

Pressure on a small nerve: no pain; numbness; slight pins and needles (aspect and edge).

Where symptoms are present, the whole nerve must be examined from the spine distally. The lists below set out the various areas (often with alternatives) that can be affected by pins and needles caused by different types of lesion; the indications given are probabilities not certainties.

The hand

When an area that does not correspond to any one nerve is described, the lesion must lie above the differentiation of the brachial plexus.

C5 disc lesion (C6 root): Thumb, index and long finger. Thumb and index finger (the more common).

C6 disc lesion (C7 root): Index, long, ring and little finger. Index, long and ring finger (the most common). Index and long finger. Long finger alone. Long and ring finger.

C7 disc lesion (C8 root): Long, ring and little finger. Ring and little finger.

Carpal tunnel syndrome: Thumb, index, long and radial side of the ring finger; palmar surface.

Cervical rib (compressing the lower trunk of the brachial plexus prior to division into median and ulnar nerve): All five digits of one hand. Thumb, index, long and radial side of the ring finger.

Median nerve, compression: Thumb, index, long and radial side of the ring finger; palmar surface.

Radial nerve, compression: As above, dorsal surface.

Cervical central disc lesion: All five digits of both hands.

Thoracic outlet syndrome: All five digits of one hand. All five digits of both hands.

Ulnar nerve, compression: Little finger and ulnar side of ring finger.

Numbness of the thumb alone is likely to be caused by occupational pressure on the digital nerve at the outer side of the thumb, whereas pins and needles normally stem from contusion of the thenar branch of the median nerve.

The thigh

L2 root pressure: front of thigh.
L3 root pressure: front of thigh.
L4 root pressure: outer side.
L5 root pressure: outer side.
S1 root pressure: back of thigh.

S2 root pressure: back of thigh.
Meralgia paraesthetica: outer side only.
Pregnancy or large uterine fibromyoma: outer side.

Lower leg

S1 root pressure: back of calf.
S2 root pressure: back of calf.
Entrapment of the saphenous nerve just below the knee: along front of leg to big toe.

Entrapment of the tibial nerve as it emerges half-way down the tibia: down front of leg and first and second toes.

The feet

The cause of pins and needles in the feet usually lies in the spine.
Cervical disc lesion: Cord signs (bilateral).
Thoracic disc lesion: Cord signs (bilateral).
Lumbar disc lesion: Root pressure (unilateral, see list below).
Spinal claudication: Lack of arterial blood supply on walking (bilateral).
Spondylolisthesis: Root pressure (bilateral).

Root pressure

L4 root: The hallux.
L5 root: First, second and third toes, inner half of the sole, dorsum of whole of foot.
S1 root: Outer two toes and outer half of the sole.
S2 root: Plantar aspect of the heel (and the whole of the back of the leg up to the buttock.

Pressure on the popliteal nerve at the neck of the fibula produces pins and needles in the foot.

III THE CAPSULAR PATTERNS

Shoulder
So much limitation of abduction, more than that of lateral rotation, less than that of medial rotation.

Elbow
Flexion usually more limited than extension, rotations full and painless except in advanced cases.

Wrist
Equal limitation of flexion and extension, little limitation of deviations.

Trapezio-first metacarpal joint
Only abduction limited

Sign of the buttock
Passive hip flexion more limited and more painful than straight-leg raise.

Hip
Marked limitation of flexion and medial rotation, some limitation of abduction, little or no limitation of adduction and lateral rotation.

Knee
Gross limitation of flexion, slight limitation of extension.

Ankle
More limitation of plantiflexion than of dorsiflexion.

Talocalcanean joint
Increasing limitation of varus until fixation in valgus.

Mid-tarsal joint
Limitation of adduction and internal rotation, other movements full.

Big toe
Gross limitation of extension, slight limitation of flexion.

Cervical spine
Equal limitation in all directions except for flexion which is usually full.

Thoracic spine
Limitation of extension, side flexion and rotations, less limitation of flexion.

Lumbar spine
Marked and equal limitation of side flexions, limitation of flexion and of extension.

IV FACTSHEETS

The shoulder

Summary

A straightforward joint producing clear findings. History of little importance diagnostically. Exclude neck as source of pain before proceeding to examination of shoulder. Nearly all shoulder structures are of C5 derivation.

For convenience, the acromio– and sternoclavicular joints are included in the following table.

Examination

Active elevation I: willingness.
Passive elevation: joint capsule, psychogenic limitation.
Active elevation II: painful arc (lesion lies in a pinchable position).
Passive abduction: glenohumeral range (cf active elevation I).
Passive lateral rotation: joint capsule.
Passive medial rotation: joint capsule.
Resisted abduction: supraspinatus.
Resisted adduction: pectoralis major, latissimus dorsi (both rare).
Resisted lateral rotation: infraspinatus.
Resisted medial rotation: subscapularis.
Resisted elbow flexion: biceps.
Resisted elbow extension: triceps (rare).

Capsular pattern

Some limitation of medial rotation (except in a very mild case), greater limitation of passive abduction, greatest limitation of passive lateral rotation.

End-feel

Hard on elevation suggests arthritis.

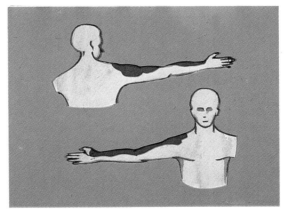

IV.1

Fig IV.1 *The C5 dermatome.*

DIAGNOSIS	SIGNS AND SYMPTOMS	TREATMENT
A. Pain on passive movement		
I. Capsular conditions Traumatic arthritis	Trauma plus capsular pattern. Patient aged 45 or over	Stage 1: stretch Stage 2: injection 2 ml steroid suspension *or* distract Stage 3: stretch
Steroid sensitive arthritis	Capsular pattern, no trauma	Injection 2 ml steroid suspension
Osteoarthrosis	Normally symptomless of itself	No treatment warranted
2. Non-capsular conditions Acute subdeltoid bursitis	Incapacity to abduct arm, rapid onset	Stage 1: morphine plus injection 2 × 5 ml steroid suspension (NB possible subacromial extent) Stage 2: figure of eight bandage
Chronic subdeltoid bursitis	Painful arc only	Injection 0.5% procaine 5–10 ml, possibly subacromial

B. Pain on resisted movement		
Supraspinatus – 4 sites	Painful resisted abduction with/without painful elevation and/or painful arc (localising signs)	Injection 1 ml steroid suspension *or* massage (except at musculotendinous junction, where only massage is effective)
Infraspinatus – 3 sites	Painful resisted lateral rotation (NB localising signs)	Injection 1 ml steroid suspension *or* massage
Subscapularis – 2 sites	Painful resisted medial rotation (NB localising signs)	Injection 1 ml steroid suspension *or* massage
Biceps – 5 sites (2 at elbow)	Painful resisted elbow flexion and usually painful resisted supination	Glenoid origin: injection 2 ml steroid suspension Bicipital groove: massage Belly: massage
Acromioclavicular joint	Passive movements, especially adduction, painful at extreme of range	Injection 1 ml steroid suspension *or* massage
Sternoclavicular joint	Painful neck and scapular movements	Injection 1 ml steroid suspension

The elbow

Summary
The patient can normally distinguish between referred pain and pain of local origin. Commence with examination of neck and shoulder if necessary.

Capsular pattern
Flexion is more limited than extension; rotations are free except in advanced arthritis.

End-feel
A softer end-feel on extension suggests a displacement, as does a hard end-feel on flexion. A hard end-feel on pronation or supination suggests severe arthritis. A hard end-feel on extension is found both in the normal joint (full range) and in arthritis (limited range).

Figs IV.2, IV.3, IV.4
The C5, C6 and C7 dermatomes (top, centre and bottom). Nerve root pain or symptoms originating from the shoulder may be felt in the arm.

Examination

Passive flexion: joint capsule.
Passive extension: joint capsule.
Passive pronation: upper radio-ulnar joint or accessory sign for the biceps.
Passive supination: upper radio-ulnar joint or accessory sign for biceps.
Resisted flexion: biceps.
Resisted extension: triceps (rare).
Resisted pronation: accessory sign for common flexor tendon (golfer's elbow) or pronator teres (rare).
Resisted supination: biceps if resisted flexion also painful or supinator brevis (rare).
Resisted wrist flexion: golfer's elbow.
Resisted wrist extension: extensores carpi radialis (tennis elbow).

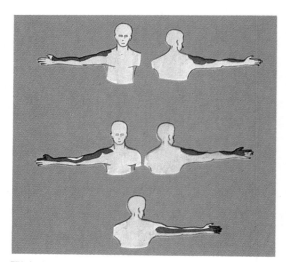

IV.2, IV.3, IV.4

DIAGNOSIS	SIGNS AND SYMPTOMS	TREATMENT
A. Pain on passive movement		
1. Capsular conditions Traumatic arthritis	Trauma plus capsular pattern	Injection 2ml steroid suspension *or* rest in flexion. No forced movement
Rheumatoid arthritis	Capsular pattern, no trauma	Injection 2ml steroid suspension. No forced movement
Osteoarthrosis	Normally symptomless of itself	No treatment warranted
2. Non-capsular conditions Displacement in adolescence	Intermittent attacks, limitation of extension or flexion	Operate
Displacement in adults	Intermittent attacks, limitation of extension or flexion	Manipulative reduction if extension limited
B. Pain on resisted movement		
Biceps – 5 sites (3 at shoulder)	Painful resisted flexion and painful resisted supination; if passive pronation also painful the site is at the tenoperiosteal junction	Lower musculotendinous junction: massage Lower tenoperiosteal junction: injection 2ml steroid suspension *or* massage
Tennis elbow – 4 sites	Painful resisted wrist extension	Tenoperiosteal junction (common): injection 1ml steroid suspension *or* massage and Mills's manipulation *or* tenotomy Belly (rare): injection 0.5% procaine 10ml Tendinous (very rare): massage Supracondylar (very rare): massage
Golfer's elbow – 2 sites	Painful resisted wrist flexion and sometimes painful resisted pronation	Tenoperiosteal site: injection 1ml steroid *or* massage Musculotendinous junction: massage

The wrist and hand

Summary
With the exception of pins and needles, symptoms are not referred appreciably.

Capsular patterns
Lower radioulnar joint: pain but no limitation on both passive rotations

Wrist: equal limitation of flexion and extension
Thumb: limitation of passive abduction, pain on passive backward movement during extension.
Interphalangeal joints: about equal limitation of flexion and extension with rotations painful at extreme of range.

Examination

Wrist

Passive pronation: capsule, radioulnar joint.
Passive supination: capsule, radioulnar joint.
Passive wrist flexion: capsule, wrist joint; dorsal ligaments.
Passive wrist extension: capsule, wrist joint; carpal subluxation.
Passive radial deviation: ulnar collateral ligament.
Passive ulnar deviation: radial collateral ligament.
Resisted wrist flexion: flexor tendons.
Resisted wrist extension: extensor tendons.
Resisted ulnar deviation: ulnar deviators.
Resisted radial deviation: radial deviators.

Thumb

Passive backward movement during extension: capsule, trapezio-first-metacarpal joint.
Resisted thumb extension: abductor longus and extensor brevis pollicis.
Resisted thumb flexion: flexor pollicis longus (rare).
Resisted thumb abduction: abductor longus and brevis (rare).
Resisted thumb adduction: thumb adductor (rare).

Fingers

Resisted finger abduction: interosseus muscles.
Resisted finger adduction: interosseus muscles.
Resisted finger extension: extensors.
Resisted finger flexion: flexors.
Passive finger extension: interphalangeal joints.
Passive finger flexion: interphalangeal joints.

The last four movements are normally performed for all fingers simultaneously.

DIAGNOSIS	SIGNS AND SYMPTOMS	TREATMENT
WRIST **A. Pain on passive movement**		
1. Capsular conditions Rheumatoid or traumatic arthritis, radioulnar joint	Capsular pattern	Injection 1ml steroid suspension
Arthritis, wrist 1. Traumatic	Capsular pattern plus fracture	Immobilisation
2. Rheumatoid	Capsular pattern	Immobilisation *or* injection 2ml steroid suspension
3. Osteoarthrosis		No treatment warranted
2. Non-capsular conditions Carpal capitate subluxation	Passive extension slightly limited, flexion full and painful	Manipulative reduction
Lunate capitate ligament	Passive wrist flexion painful at extreme of range	Massage
Radial collateral ligament	Painful passive ulnar deviation at extreme of range	Injection 1ml steroid suspension *or* massage
Ulnar collateral ligament	Painful passive radial deviation	Injection 1ml steroid suspension
Carpal tunnel syndrome	Pins and needles, 3½ digits	Injection 2ml steroid suspension (diagnostic and sometimes curative)

B. Pain on resisted movement		
Extensores carpi radialis	Painful resisted wrist extension and radial deviation	Injection 1ml steroid suspension *or* massage
Extensores carpi ulnaris	Painful resisted wrist extension and ulnar deviation	Injection 1ml steroid suspension *or* massage
Flexor carpi ulnaris	Painful resisted wrist flexion and ulnar deviation	Injection 1ml steroid suspension *or* massage
Flexor carpi radialis	Painful resisted wrist flexion and radial deviation	Injection 1ml steroid suspension *or* massage
Flexor digitorum – upper site	Painful resisted finger flexion	Injection 2ml steroid suspension *or* massage (except if rheumatoid)

THUMB
A. Pain on passive movement

Arthritis, trapezio-first metacarpal joint	Capsular pattern	Injection 1ml steroid suspension *or* massage

B. Pain on resisted movement

Abductor longus and extensores pollicis, tenosynovitis – 2 sites	Painful resisted extension and painful resisted abduction	Upper site: massage Lower site: injection 1ml steroid suspension
Flexor pollicis longus 1. Tenosynovitis – 2 sites	Painful resisted flexion	Upper site: injection 1ml steroid suspension *or* massage Lower site: injection 1ml steroid suspension
2. Trigger thumb	Thumb locks	Injection 1ml steroid suspension *or* operation

HAND
A. Pain on passive movement

Arthritis, finger joints	Capsular pattern	If rheumatoid, injection 0.5–1ml steroid suspension

B. Pain on resisted movement

Dorsal interossei	Painful resisted abduction	Massage
Palmar interossei	Painful resisted adduction	Massage
Flexor digitorum – lower site 1. Trigger finger	Finger locks	Injection 1ml steroid suspension *or* operation
2. Rheumatoid inflammation	Painful resisted finger flexion	Injection 1ml steroid suspension

The sacroiliac, buttock and hip

Summary
As symptoms in the buttock, thigh or hip are frequently referred from the spine, preliminary examination and history must exclude this possibility. The sacroiliac joint itself is rarely at fault.

The sign of the buttock
This indicates a major lesion. It is some limitation and pain on SLR and more limitation and pain on passive hip flexion.

Capsular pattern
Hip: marked limitation of medial rotation, some limitation of flexion and abduction.

End-feel
If the hip joint is normal, the end-feel on all four passive movements is elastic; in arthritis, the end-feel is hard. A prematurely empty end-feel on passive hip flexion accompanies the sign of the buttock.

Examination

Fig IV.5 *The area to which pain may be referred by a lumbar disc lesion compressing the dura mater.*

Fig IV.6 *The L3 dermatome. The hip is of L3 derivation.*

SIJ strain (supine): anterior sacroiliac ligaments.
SIJ strain (side lying): posterior sacroiliac ligaments.
SIJ strain (prone): anterior sacroiliac ligaments.
Passive hip flexion: joint capsule; the sign of the buttock; loose body; bursitis.
Passive medial rotation: joint capsule.
Passive lateral rotation: joint capsule; loose body; bursitis.
Passive hip extension: joint capsule.
Straight-leg raise: The sign of the buttock if passive hip flexion more limited and more painful.
Resisted hip flexion: psoas and quadriceps, malignant disease.
Resisted lateral rotation: gluteal bursitis (accessory sign); quadratus femoris.
Resisted medial rotation: gluteal bursitis (accessory sign).
Resisted abduction: gluteal bursitis (accessory sign).
Resisted extension: gluteal bursitis (accessory sign).

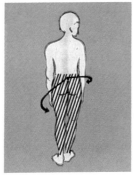

IV.5

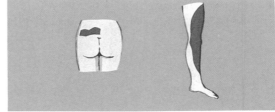

IV.6

Resisted adduction: adductors ('rider's sprain').
Resisted knee extension: quadriceps.
Resisted knee flexion: hamstrings.

DIAGNOSIS	SIGNS AND SYMPTOMS	TREATMENT
SACROILIAC		
Ankylosing spondylitis	Painful SIJ strain(s)	Phenylbutazone or indomethacin during attack
BUTTOCK		
Serious disorders e.g. osteomyelitis, ischiorectal abscess, etc.	The sign of the buttock	As appropriate
Psoas bursitis	Painful passive adduction in flexion, sometimes painful passive lateral rotation	Injection 0.5% procaine 50ml or possibly 5ml steroid suspension
Gluteal bursitis	Painful passive movements in a non-capsular way	Injection 0.5% procaine 50ml or possibly 5ml steroid suspension
Claudication	Pain on sustained active hip extension	Operation

HIP
A. Pain on passive movement

1. Capsular conditions Rheumatoid, traumatic or spondylitic arthritis	Capsular pattern	Injection 5ml steroid suspension
Osteoarthrosis	Capsular pattern	Early stage: stretch
Serious disorders in children, e.g. congenital dislocation, pseudocoxalgia, etc.	Mostly visible radiographically	As appropriate
2. Non-capsular conditions Loose body with or without osteoarthrosis	Severe momentary twinges	Manipulative reduction – 2 methods

B. Pain on resisted movement

Psoas	Painful resisted hip flexion when hip at right angles	Massage
Adductor longus	Painful resisted hip adduction	Tenoperiosteal junction: injection 2ml steroid suspension *or* massage Musculotendinous junction: massage
Rectus femoris	Painful resisted knee extension	Massage
Hamstrings	Painful resisted knee flexion	Ischial origin: injection 5ml steroid suspension Belly: injection 50ml local anaesthetic during first few days, thereafter massage plus Faradism

The knee

Summary
History is particularly important and in cases of traumatic origin must establish the precise strain imposed on the joint. Capsular limitation is often a secondary response to ligamentous sprain. The capacity for localization is good.

Capsular pattern
More limitations of flexion than of extension with rotations free.

End-feel
In arthritis the end-feel on passive flexion is usually hard.

Examination

Passive flexion: joint capsule.
Passive extension: joint capsule.
Valgus strain: medial collateral ligament.
Varus strain: lateral collateral ligament.
Passive lateral rotation: medial coronary ligament.
Passive medial rotation: lateral coronary ligament.
Forwards shearing: anterior cruciate ligament.
Backwards shearing: posterior cruciate ligament.
Lateral shearing: posterior cruciate ligament (secondary sign), meniscus.
Resisted flexion: hamstrings.
Resisted medial rotation and flexion: semitendinosus or popliteal muscles (rare).
Resisted lateral rotation and flexion: biceps.
Resisted extension: quadriceps.
   Test for fluid, heat, synovial thickening; consider cause of painless weakness, particularly on resisted extension.

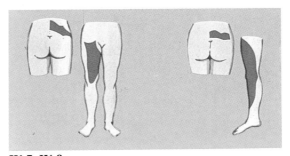

IV.7, IV.8

Figs IV.7, IV.8 *The L2 (left) and L3 dermatomes (right).*

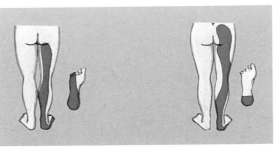

IV.9, IV.10

Figs IV.9, IV.10 *The S1 (left) and S2 dermatomes (right).*

235

DIAGNOSIS	SIGNS AND SYMPTOMS	TREATMENT
A. Pain on passive movement		
1. Capsular conditions Secondary traumatic arthritis	Trauma plus capsular pattern	Diagnose and treat causative lesion
Rheumatoid arthritis	Capsular pattern, no trauma	Injection 5ml steroid suspension
Osteoarthrosis	Visible radiographically	No treatment warranted
Baker's cyst	Cyst in upper calf following rheumatoid arthritis	Aspirate
Haemarthrosis	Capsular pattern, joint distended	Aspirate
2. Non-capsular conditions Medial collateral ligament	Painful passive valgus strain plus marked capsular pattern	Acute and subacute stage: massage in maximum flexion and maximum extension followed by gentle mobilisation Chronic stage: manipulative rupture
Stieda-Pellegrini's disease	Visible radiographically following valgus strain	No treatment
Medial coronary ligament	Painful passive lateral rotation plus capsular pattern	Massage
Cruciate ligaments – 4 sites (anterior cruciate, anterior or posterior end; posterior cruciate, anterior or posterior end)	Some/all passive movements painful at extreme of range	Injection 2ml steroid suspension
Meniscus	Immediate disabling pain, knee locks	Manipulative reduction probably followed by operation
Loose body with or without osteoarthrosis	Intermittent attacks, often full passive extension hurts and flexion is limited	Manipulative reduction – 4 methods
B. Pain on resisted movement		
Suprapatellar tendon	Painful resisted extension	Injection 2ml steroid suspension *or* massage
Infrapatellar tendon	Painful resisted extension	Injection 2ml steroid suspension *or* massage
Quadriceps expansion	Painful resisted extension	Massage
Hamstrings	Painful resisted flexion	Bellies: massage followed by Faradism
	Lesion at bicipital tendon if resisted lateral rotation also painful	Bicipital tendon: massage
Popliteal tendon	Painful resisted flexion and painful resisted medial rotation	Belly: massage Tendinous origin: injection steroid suspension *or* massage

The leg

Summary
Soft-tissue lesions of the leg present few
problems either of diagnosis or treatment.

Examination

Standing on tip toe: gastrocnemius and soleus.
Resisted dorsiflexion: tibialis anterior.
Resisted plantiflexion: gastrocnemius and
soleus.
Resisted inversion: tibialis posterior.

Resisted eversion: peronei.
  Short plantiflexor muscles may produce any
one of a number of conditions in the ankle or
foot.

DIAGNOSIS	SIGNS AND SYMPTOMS	TREATMENT
Pain on resisted movement Gastrocnemius – 'tennis leg'	Painful resisted plantiflexion, except when knee flexed	Injection 0.5% procaine 50ml *and* active exercises *and* raised heel and massage
Tendo Achillis	Painful resisted plantiflexion	Massage *or* injection 2ml steroid suspension
Intermittent claudication	Pain in calf on walking, relieved by rest	Operation
Peroneal tendon – 4 sites	Painful resisted eversion	Massage
Tibialis posterior – 3 sites	Painful resisted inversion	Support and massage *or* massage
Tibialis anterior	Painful resisted dorsiflexion and painful resisted inversion	Massage

The ankle and foot

Summary
Despite the intricacy of the foot joints, the
lesions are easy to identify and respond well to
treatment.

Capsular patterns
Ankle: more limitation of plantiflexion than of
dorsiflexion.
Talo-calcanean joint: increasing limitation of
varus until it fixes in valgus.

Mid-tarsal joint: limitations of adduction and
internal rotation, other movements full.
Big toe: gross limitation of extension, slight
limitation of flexion.

Examination

Passive dorsiflexion: ankle joint.
Passive plantiflexion: ankle joint, anterior
tibiotalar ligament.
Passive inversion during plantiflexion:
talofibular, calcaneofibular and mid-tarsal
ligaments.
Passive eversion during plantiflexion: deltoid
ligament.
Varus strain: tibiofibular ligament,
talocalcanean joint, calcaneofibular ligament.
Valgus strain: talocalcanean joint.
Mid-tarsal passive dorsiflexion: mid-tarsal
joint.

Mid-tarsal passive plantiflexion: mid-tarsal
joint.
Mid-tarsal passive adduction: mid-tarsal joint
(capsular pattern).
Mid-tarsal passive abduction: mid-tarsal joint.
Mid-tarsal passive medial rotation: mid-tarsal
joint (capsular pattern), calcaneocuboid
ligament.
Mid-tarsal passive lateral rotation: mid-tarsal
joint.
  The examination proceeds to the toes if
necessary. The resisted movements of the leg
must also be tested.

DIAGNOSIS	SIGNS AND SYMPTOMS	TREATMENT
ANKLE		
Pain on passive movement *1. Capsular conditions* Osteoarthrosis	Capsular pattern	Arthrodesis if warranted
2. Non-capsular conditions Anterior talofibular ligament – 2 sites	Painful passive inversion during plantiflexion	First day or so: injection 1ml steroid suspension. Thereafter massage only
Calcaneofibular ligament	Painful varus strain	First day or so: injection 1ml steroid suspension. Thereafter massage only
Calcaneocuboid ligament	Painful passive inversion and mid-tarsal medial rotation	First day or so: injection 2ml steroid suspension. Thereafter massage only
Adhesions, talofibular or calcaneocuboid ligaments	Pain following exertion	Manipulative rupture
Anterior tibiofibular ligament 1. Sprain	Painful varus strain	Massage
2. Unstable mortice joint	History, foot turns over easily. Click and excessive range on varus strain	Sclerosis *or* operation
Deltoid ligament	Painful passive eversion during plantiflexion	Support and injection 2ml steroid suspension
Anterior tibiotalar ligament	Painful passive plantiflexion	Massage
Loose body	Erratic twinges on pantiflexion	Manipulative reduction
TALOCALCANEAN JOINT		
Pain on passive movement *1. Capsular conditions* Osteoarthrosis	Capsular pattern	Operation if warranted
Rheumatoid or sub-acute traumatic arthritis	Capsular pattern	Injection 2ml steroid suspension
Sudeck's atrophy	Visible radiographically	No treatment avails
2. Non-capsular conditions		
Dancer's heel	Painful passive plantiflexion at full range	Injection 2ml steroid suspension
Immobilisation limitation	Fixation in mid-position following immobilisation	Mobilisation
Subcutaneous nodules	Nodules palpable in subcutaneous fascia	Tenotomy *or* adapted footwear
Plantar fasciitis	Examination negative apart from tender spot. History of pain on first few steps of walking	Support *or* injection 2ml steroid suspension

MID-TARSAL JOINT

Pain on passive movement *1. Capsular conditions*		
Osteoarthrosis	Normally symptomless of itself	No treatment warranted
Mon-articular rheumatoid arthritis	Capsular pattern	Immobilisation
Subacute arthritis in middle age	Any movement towards inversion restricted by muscle spasm	Injection 2ml steroid suspension *or* support
Subacute arthritis in adolescence	Valgus of the heel and abduction of the forefoot maintained by muscle spasm	Support and strapping
2. Non-capsular conditions Mid-tarsal ligaments		
1. Strain	Pain at extremes of passive range	Support, exercises *and* mobilisation. Injection steroid suspension if necessary
2. Contracture	History and limitation at mid-tarsal joint; no muscle spasm	Injection 2–5ml steroid suspension

CUNEO-FIRST-METATARSAL JOINT

Osteoarthrosis	History of adolescent osteochondrosis	Adapted footwear *or* operation

METATARSAL SHAFTS

Marching fracture	Pain on walking, localised warmth, oedema and tenderness	Spontaneous recovery six weeks from onset

FIRST METATARSOPHALANGEAL JOINT

Capsular conditions		
Arthritis in adolescence	Capsular pattern	Adapted footwear
Rheumatoid arthritis	Capsular pattern	Injection 1ml steroid suspension
Osteoarthrosis	Capsular pattern	Injection 1ml steroid suspension
Gout	Capsular pattern	Phenylbutazone, indomethacin

SESAMO-FIRST-METATARSAL JOINT

Traumatic arthritis	Pain on resisted flexion of the hallux	Injection 1ml steroid suspension

OTHER METATARSOPHALANGEAL JOINTS

1. Capsular conditions Rheumatoid or traumatic arthritis	Capsular pattern	Injection 1ml steroid suspension
2. Non-capsular conditions Acute metatarsalgia	Pain on walking, at outer border of forefoot. Characteristic history (attacks); examination negative	Support *or* operation
Chronic metatarsalgia	Pain on walking at plantar aspect of forefoot (middle three toes)	Support *and* exercises

The cervical spine

Summary
Nearly all pain of cervical origin is caused by a disc lesion compressing the dura mater or nerve roots. The symptoms and signs are usually unilateral scapular pain and limitation in the non-capsular pattern. Because compression of the parenchyma will produce weakness in the upper limb, after the cervical movements the arm is examined against resistance. A root palsy of the seventh cervical root is much the commonest.

Nearly all cervical disc lesions respond to manipulation but the most careful differential diagnosis is required to sift out those rare cases where manipulation could prove dangerous.

Capsular pattern
Approximately equal limitation of all six movements except flexion

Non-capsular pattern characteristic of internal derangement
Pain/limitation on two, three or four movements.

End-feel
A hard end-feel accompanies the capsular pattern except in rheumatoid arthritis.

Differential diagnosis
Pancoast's tumour
Neurofibroma
Basilar ischaemia
Drop attacks
Osteophytic root palsy
Neuralgic amyotrophy
Acroparaesthesia
Thoracic outlet syndrome
Carpal tunnel syndrome
Soft-tissue lesion at shoulder

Fig IV.11 *The area within which pain may be referred by a cervical disc lesion compressing the dura mater.*

Examination

Six active cervical movements (extension, both side-flexions, both rotations, flexion): pain of cervical origin.
Five passive cervical movements (as above excluding flexion): painful/limited in non-capsular pattern characteristic of internal derangement.
Six resisted cervical movements (as above): painless if displacement present.
Active shoulder girdle elevation: scapular mobility.
Resisted shoulder girdle elevation: C2, C3 or C4 root palsy if weak.
Scapular approximation: dural mobility.
Shoulder girdle forwards: dural mobility.
Active arm elevation: lesion at shoulder.
Resisted abduction: C5 root palsy if weak (or supraspinatus if painful).
Resisted adduction: C7 root palsy.
Resisted medial rotation: rupture of subscapular tendon (rare).
Resisted lateral rotation: C5 root palsy, neuritis (or infraspinatus if painful).
Resisted elbow flexion: C5 or C6 root palsy (or biceps if painful).
Resisted elbow extension: C7 root palsy.

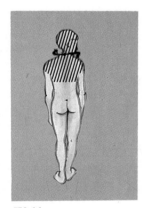

IV.11

Resisted wrist extension: C6 root palsy (or extensores carpi radialis if painful).
Resisted wrist flexion: C7 root palsy (or common flexor tendon if painful).
Resisted ulnar deviation: C8 root palsy.
Resisted thumb adduction: C8 root palsy.
Resisted thumb extension: C8 root palsy.
Resisted thumb abduction: Cervical rib.
Resisted finger adduction: TI root palsy.
Brachoradialis jerk: C5 root palsy.
Biceps jerk: C5 or C6 root palsy.
Triceps jerk: C7 root palsy.
Plantar response: Cord sign.

TREATMENT OF A CERVICAL DISPLACEMENT

Manipulation

The treatment of choice for a cartilaginous displacement is manipulation. Nearly all cervical displacements are cartilaginous. After each manoeuvre the patient is re-examined to assess progress.

Technique
The object is to reduce the displacement. One assistant is required to supply traction; a high couch is used.

    Rotation during traction 1
    Rotation during traction 2
    Side-flexion during traction
    Antero-posterior gliding – if extension remains painful.
    Lateral gliding – if residual ache.
    Traction with leverage – postero-central displacement.
    Bateman's – acute torticollis, nuclear displacement.

Contraindications to manipulation – dangerous
Cord signs
Basilar ischaemia
Drop attacks
Rheumatoid arthritis
Gross cervical deformity   } special
Postero-central protrusion } technique
                             practicable
Patient on anti-coagulants

Contraindications – ineffective
1. Root palsy
2. Brachial pain after first two months
3. Cervical movements cause pain down arm
4. Primary postero-lateral displacement

The thoracic spine

Summary
Some thoracic pain is caused by disc lesions compressing the dura mater or nerve roots. The ache may be anterior only. There are no root signs and consequently examination is confined to the trunk with resisted movements playing their part to detect muscular lesions.

It is not always easy to differentiate visceral disorder from a disc lesion and history must be given its full weight. With a displacement the passive rotations are the movements most likely to hurt; disc lesions are particularly responsive to manipulative reduction, repeated as necessary on relapse.

Capsular pattern
Equal and severe limitation of movement in every direction.

Non-capsular pattern characteristic of internal derangement
Pain and/or limitation on some but not all movements.

Differential diagnosis
Visceral disorder
Neuroma
Adolescent osteochondrosis
Adult osteochondrosis
Senile osteoporosis
Ankylosing spondylitis
Osteitis deformans
Fractured rib
Neuritis
Neuralgic amyotrophy
Diaphragmatic or cardiac pain
Thrombosis of the lower aorta
Cervical disc lesion

Examination

Neck flexion: dural mobility.
Scapular approximation: dural mobility.
T1 stretch: T1 nerve root.
Six active thoracic movements (extension, both side-flexions, both rotations, flexion): painful/limited in non-capsular pattern characteristic of internal derangement.
Passive rotations: extreme of range often painful if displacement present.
Six resisted thoracic movements (as above): contractile structures.
Plantar response: cord signs

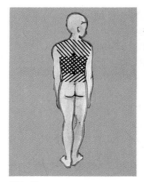

Fig IV.12 *The area within which pain may be referred by a thoracic disc lesion compressing the dura mater.*

IV.12

TREATMENT OF A THORACIC DISPLACEMENT

Manipulation

The treatment of choice for a cartilaginous displacement is manipulation. Nearly all thoracic displacements are cartilaginous. After each manoeuvre the patient is re-examined to assess progress. Relapse frequently occurs and may be countered either by manipulative reduction or sclerosants.

Contraindications – danger
Cord signs
Patient on anti-coagulants

Contraindications – ineffective
None

Technique
The object is to reduce the displacement. Two assistants are required to supply traction; a low couch is used.

Extension during traction 1
Extension during traction 2
Rotation during traction 1 ⎱ Rotary
Rotation during traction 2 ⎰ manipulations
Rotation during traction 3 ⎱ of increasing
Rotation during traction 4 ⎰ strength
Upper thoracic rotation – for upper thoracic disc lesions (rare)

Prophylaxis

Sclerosants: The object is to shorten the posterior ligaments, thus forestalling relapse. The displacement must first be reduced.
Technique: Injection 1ml P2G solution into each ligamento-periosteal junction at both ends of the supraspinous ligaments and into the outlying facet joints. The injections at each site are given a total of three times at weekly intervals.

The lumbar spine

Summary
Much pain of lumbar origin is caused by minor and remediable displacements of disc material compressing the dura mater or nerve roots. Disc lesions are particularly common at the L4 and L5 levels. Compression of the parenchyma produces weakness in the lower limb; this is examined by resisted movements after the lumbar movements have been tested. Root signs may be polyradicular.

Most displacements are cartilaginous and respond to manipulation. Some displacements are of nuclear material and require sustained traction. The pain from an otherwise irreducible (i.e. large) displacement can be abolished or permanently diminished by an injection of epidural local anaesthetic. Operation is hardly ever called for. History is particularly important.

Capsular pattern
Approximately equal limitation of both side-flexions; extension and flexion also limited.

Non-capsular pattern characteristic of internal derangement
Pain and/or limitation on some but not all movements or asymmetric limitation in all directions (e.g. lumbago).

Examination

Fig IV.13 *The area within which pain may be referred by a lumbar disc lesion compressing the dura mater.*

Inspection, palpation: bony signs.
Four active lumbar movements (extension, both side-flexions, flexion): capsular pattern, or non-capsular pattern characteristic of internal derangement.
Standing on tiptoe: S1 or S2 root palsy.
Straight-leg raise: dural mobility (bilateral limitation); nerve root mobility at L4, L5, S1 and S2 (unilateral limitation).
SIJ strain (supine): anterior sacroiliac ligaments.
Resisted hip flexion: L2 or L3 root palsy.
Resisted ankle dorsiflexion: L4 root palsy.
Resisted toe extension: L4 or L5 root palsy.
Resisted eversion: L5 or S1 root palsy.
Knee jerk: L3 root palsy.
Ankle jerk: S1, S2 or L5 (rare) root palsy.
Passive knee flexion: nerve root mobility at L3.

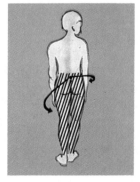

IV.13

Resisted knee extension: L3 root palsy.
Resisted knee flexion: S1 or S2 root palsy.
Wasting of glutei: S2 root palsy.
Plantar response: cord signs.
Cutaneous analgesia: sensory defect.

TREATMENT OF A LUMBAR DISPLACEMENT		
Manipulation The treatment of choice for a small cartilaginous displacement is manipulation. Most lumbar displacements are cartilaginous. After each manoeuvre the patient is re-examined to assess progress.	**Traction** The treatment of choice for a small nuclear displacement is traction. This reduces intervertebral pressure, creating negative pressure within the joint and sucking the semi-liquid protrusion back.	**Epidural local anaesthesia** The treatment of choice for a large lumbar displacement is epidural local anaesthesia. This desensitises the dura mater and nerve roots.
Technique The object is to reduce the displacement. No assistants are required; a low couch is used. Rotation Strain 1 ⎤ rotary Rotation Strain 2 ⎟ manipulations Rotation Strain 3 ⎬ of Rotation Strain 4 ⎟ increasing Rotation Strain 5 ⎦ strength Forced extension 1 ⎤ extension Forced extension 2 ⎟ manipulations Forced extension 3 ⎬ normally Forced extension 4 ⎟ reserved for Forced extension 5 ⎦ the elderly Correction of lateral deviation 1 Correction of lateral deviation 2	*Technique* The distracting force is the maximum the patient can stand without discomfort (min. 30 kg, max 80 kg). Treatment is sustained for half an hour daily for a minimum of two weeks. The patient is re-examined before each treatment.	*Technique* Inject via the sacral hiatus, using 50ml 1:200 procaine. General anaesthesia is not required and the injection proceeds over several minutes. Strict asepsis must be observed. The patient is re-examined after a week and the injection is repeated as necessary up to, say, three times.
Contraindications – danger Cord signs S4 signs Bilateral sciatica Spinal claudication Hyper-acute lumbago	*Contraindications – danger* Acute lumbago Sciatica with gross lumbar deformity Respiratory embarassment S4 signs	*Contraindications – danger* Sensitivity to local anaesthetic. Follow procedure and observe strict asepsis.
Contraindications – ineffective 1. Root signs (i.e. weakness) 2. Root pain for 6 months plus (if patient under 60) 3. Sciatica with patient fixed in lateral deviation or flexion 4. Trunk movements suggest a nuclear protrusion 5. Post laminectomy	*Contraindications – ineffective* 1. Root signs (i.e. weakness) 2. Root pain for 6 months plus	*Contraindications – ineffective* 1. Indications that manipulation or traction will succeed 2. Pre-1950 laminectomy
Prophylaxis 1. Posture – maintain lumbar lordosis. 2. Corset to maintain (not achieve) reduction, *cf* a plaster cast. 3. *Sclerosants* The object is to shorten the posterior ligaments thus forestalling relapse. The displacement must first be reduced.	*Technique* Injection 1ml P2G solution into each end of: Week 1 – supraspinous and interspinous ligaments. Week 2 – facet ligaments. Week 3 – deep lumbar fascia.	

V TEACHING FACILITIES

To date, teaching of orthopaedic medicine has been conducted on an *ad hoc* basis. Excellent individual practitioners exist; some hospital departments are well-versed and provide sound grounding. Others aspire to no such service; some claim to with no great justification. On this basis it has hitherto been impossible to give any rule-of-thumb guidance; only through a flurry of belated activity over the past few years has concrete progress been achieved.

As in the past, I myself continue to hold five-day courses open to both doctors and physiotherapists. A formal examination system has now been instituted; participants are offered the opportunity to take an oral, written and practical exam leading to certification for successful candidates. There are two grades, 'practitioner' and 'teacher'. This book amply covers the full syllabus to the former level; ideally, participants attend a total of three courses over a period of one year to eighteen months. The course administration is now run under the aegis of the Cyriax Foundation, recently registered as a charity with the principal aim to provide a clinical and teaching centre. Courses can cope with anywhere up to a hundred participants and the lecturing service operates internationally, whether for full scale courses or individual lectures, by arrangement with the Foundation's Course Organiser.

The other prime teaching organisation, working energetically along similar lines, is the Belgian Scientific Society of Orthopaedic Medicine (Cyriax). Their preferred approach is an 18 day course spread over a period of two years; at time of writing they have six teachers personally examined and certified by me. Their demonstrators are fluent in three languages (English, French, Flemish) and again their team lectures internationally. Examination standards dovetail with the UK system.

Four of the Belgian Society's teachers are on the staff of the Eindhoven School whose syllabus—originally a fairly ecclectic affair—leans progressively towards orthodox tuition in orthopaedic medicine; I understand the full transition, bringing tuition on the spine into line with modern thinking, is to be completed in the course of 1983. Germany is well represented by Dr P. Hirschfeld's organisation based in Bremen. Participants attend five to six weekend courses spread over two years; two groups, each eighty strong, are currently under tuition with the option of a concluding exam.

In the United States, two five-day courses are organised for me each year at the Strong Memorial Hospital, Rochester, NY. They are held in spring and autumn, and similar courses are given in Canada or the USA, just before and just after, when universities request it. Information is available from the Foundation's Course Organiser in London. In Spain, Salvador Cornesa MD gives a six-day course in Murcia for doctors once every two years.

It is clearly a matter of priority that standard medical training be extended to incorporate rational diagnosis and treatment of soft-tissue lesions. The immediate need is for recognised teachers able to train up other practitioners and start local groups. In this connection the reader may care to note that the teaching facilities outlined above can be supplemented by further educational aids obtainable through OM Publications in the form of audio and audio-visual material, including a complete video series.

An English society of orthopaedic medicine was founded in 1978 but, following my resignation from its Presidency, withdrew from the educational arena. In Holland an academy of orthopaedic medicine runs courses led by two physiotherapists certified by me as teachers; otherwise I have no connection with their organisation.

Overall, the reader will appreciate use of the term 'orthopaedic medicine' or unauthorised use of the name Cyriax does not convey any seal of approval and the reader must make up his own mind about the intentions and bona fides of any group.

The Cyriax Foundation will be pleased to hear from any individuals or institutions providing education in orthopaedic medicine, for listing in subsequent editions. Information supplied should be as comprehensive as possible; the author apologises in advance for any omissions from this the first edition. Reciprocally the Foundation is anxious to help by handling enquiries to put individual practitioners in contact.

The Cyriax Foundation
206 Albany Street
London NW1
United Kingdom

Belgian Scientific Society of Orthopaedic Medicine (Cyriax)
Peter Benoitlaan 27
8420 de Haan
Belgium

Foundation of Manual Medicine
Stratumsedigk 26
Eindhoven
Holland

Strong Memorial Hospital
Orthopaedic Department
601 Elmwood Avenue
Rochester NY 14642
United States of America

Hospital Arrixaca
S. Cornesa, MD
Orthopaedic Medicine Department
Murcia
Spain

Dutch Academy of Orthopaedic Medicine
Brahms Avenue 4
2625 BW Delft
Holland

Arbeitsgemeinschaft Orthopaedische Medicin nach Cyriax
Zentralkrankenhaus
St.–Jürgen–Strasse
2800 Bremen 1
Germany

INDEX